Compilation Techniques for Reconfigurable Architectures

João M. P. Cardoso · Pedro C. Diniz

Compilation Techniques for Reconfigurable Architectures

Springer

João M. P. Cardoso
Technical University of Lisbon/IST
INESC-ID, Rua Alves Redol n.9
1000-029 Lisboa, Portugal
jmpc@acm.org

Pedro C. Diniz
Technical University of Lisbon/IST
INESC-ID, Rua Alves Redol n.9
1000-029 Lisboa, Portugal
pedro@isi.edu

ISBN: 978-0-387-09670-4 e-ISBN: 978-0-387-09671-1
DOI: 10.1007/978-0-387-09671-1

Library of Congress Control Number: 2008929498

Printed on acid-free paper

springer.com

To Teresa, Rodrigo, and Frederico
(João M. P. Cardoso)

To Mariana de Sena and Rafael Nuno
(Pedro C. Diniz)

Preface

The extreme flexibility of reconfigurable architectures and their performance potential have made them a vehicle of choice in a wide range of computing domains, from rapid circuit prototyping to high-performance computing. The increasing availability of transistors on a die has allowed the emergence of reconfigurable architectures with a large number of computing resources and interconnection topologies. To exploit the potential of these reconfigurable architectures, programmers are forced to map their applications, typically written in high-level imperative programming languages, such as C or MATLAB, to hardware-oriented languages such as VHDL or Verilog. In this process, they must assume the role of hardware designers and software programmers and navigate a maze of program transformations, mapping, and synthesis steps to produce efficient reconfigurable computing implementations. The richness and sophistication of any of these application mapping steps make the mapping of computations to these architectures an increasingly daunting process. It is thus widely believed that automatic compilation from high-level programming languages is the key to the success of reconfigurable computing.

This book describes a wide range of code transformations and mapping techniques for programs described in high-level programming languages, most notably imperative languages, to reconfigurable architectures. While many of these transformations and mapping techniques have been developed in the context of compilation for traditional architectures and high-level synthesis, their application to reconfigurable architectures poses a whole new set of challenges, in particular when targeting fine-grained reconfigurable architectures such as contemporary Field-Programmable Gate-Arrays (FPGAs). Their ability to emulate virtually any execution paradigm and to configure their logic blocks as either storage or computing resources forces compilers to evaluate a huge number of possible mapping alternatives in search for effective hardware implementations on these reconfigurable architectures.

This book is primarily intended for researchers and graduate students in the areas of study of hardware compilation and advanced computing architectures in the fields of Electrical and Computer Engineering and Computer Science. As it focuses on the specific topic of compilation from high-level program descriptions to reconfigurable architectures, this book can easily support advanced compiler and computer architecture courses related to reconfigurable computing. Through this book, we hope to motivate further discussions on the challenging topic of compilation for reconfigurable architectures, and also hope this book can be a reference for researchers, educators, and students to learn more about the most prominent efforts on this subject in recent years.

This book was only made possible with the unabated comprehension, relentless, and unconditional support of our families who allowed us to devote to it countless many hours, some of them late at night. It is to them we dedicate this book, in particular to Teresa, Rodrigo, Frederico, Mariana, and Rafael. We are also truly indebted to our parents, Cristina and Luís and Mariana and Mário, for their lifelong support and encouragement. Lastly, we would also like to thank our friends for their support and friendship.

We would like to take this opportunity to acknowledge the support of the Springer staff, Amy Brais (Springer Publishing Editor) for the opportunity to publish this book, and Deborah Doherty (Springer Author Support) for her prompt help and guidance throughout the editing and publishing process.

We would also like to acknowledge the financial support of the Portuguese Foundation for Science and Technology ("Fundação para a Ciência e Tecnologia, FCT") under the research grants PTDC/EEA-ELC/71556/2006, PTDC/EEA-ELC/70272/2006, and PTDC/EIA/70271/2006.

We would like to acknowledge and thank the many contributions to a survey about compilation techniques for reconfigurable computing platforms that inspired this book by Markus Weinhardt (PACT XPP Technologies, AG., Germany). We are also grateful to a number of colleagues who have carefully reviewed early drafts of the chapters in this book, in particular, Leonel Sousa (INESC-ID/IST/UTL, Lisbon, Portugal), José Alves (FEUP, Porto, Portugal), Koen Bertels (TU Delft, Delft, The Netherlands), Horácio Neto (INESC-ID/IST/UTL, Lisbon, Portugal), Mihai Budiu (Microsoft Research SVC, Montain View, CA, USA), Timothy Callahan (CMU, PA, USA), Michael Hübner (Univ. of Karlsruhe, Karlsruhe, Germany), Benjamin Gerdemann (INESC-ID/IST/UTL, Lisbon, Portugal), Ricardo Ferreira (Federal Univ. of Viçosa, Brazil) and Jecel Assumpção, Jr. (Univ. of São Paulo, São Carlos, Brazil). Lastly, a very special thanks to Eduardo Marques (Univ. of São Paulo, São Carlos, Brazil) for all his support while completing the final stages of this book during our visit to the University of São Paulo in São Carlos, Brazil. Lastly, we are grateful to Markus Weinhardt for his contributions to a survey about compilation techniques for reconfigurable computing platforms that inspired this book.

Lisbon, Portugal,
April 2008

João M. P. Cardoso
Pedro C. Diniz

Contents

1 **Introduction** ... 1
1.1 The Promise of Reconfigurable Architectures and Systems ... 1
1.2 The Challenge: How to Program and Compile for Reconfigurable Systems? ... 3
1.3 This Book: Key Techniques when Compiling to Reconfigurable Architecture ... 4
1.4 Organization of this Book ... 5

2 **Overview of Reconfigurable Architectures** ... 7
2.1 Evolution of Reconfigurable Architectures ... 7
2.2 Reconfigurable Architectures: Key Characteristics ... 8
2.3 Granularity ... 10
2.3.1 Fine-Grained Reconfigurable Architectures ... 12
2.3.2 Coarse-Grained Reconfigurable Architectures ... 14
2.3.3 Hybrid Reconfigurable Architectures ... 16
2.3.4 Granularity and Mapping ... 19
2.4 Interconnection Topologies ... 20
2.5 System-Level Integration ... 21
2.6 Dynamic Reconfiguration ... 24
2.7 Computational and Execution Models ... 29
2.8 Streaming Data Input and Output ... 31
2.9 Summary ... 31

3 **Compilation and Synthesis Flows** ... 33
3.1 Overview ... 33
3.1.1 Front-End ... 34
3.1.2 Middle-End ... 35
3.1.3 Back-End ... 37
3.2 Hardware Compilation and High-Level Synthesis ... 39
3.2.1 Generic High-Level Synthesis ... 40
3.2.2 Customized High-Level Synthesis for Fine-Grained Reconfigurable Architectures ... 41

3.2.3 Register-Transfer-Level/Logic Synthesis ... 45
3.2.4 High-Level Compilation for Coarse-Grained Reconfigurable Architectures ... 48
3.2.5 Placement and Routing ... 49
3.3 Illustrative Example ... 51
3.3.1 High-Level Source Code Example ... 51
3.3.2 Data-Flow Representation ... 52
3.3.3 Computation-Oriented Mapping and Scheduling ... 53
3.3.4 Data-Oriented Mapping and Transformations ... 55
3.3.5 Translation to Hardware ... 58
3.4 Reconfigurable Computing Issues and Their Impact on Compilation ... 59
3.4.1 Programming Languages and Execution Models ... 61
3.4.2 Intermediate Representations ... 62
3.4.3 Target Reconfigurable Architecture Features ... 64
3.5 Summary ... 65

4 Code Transformations ... 67
4.1 Bit-Level Transformations ... 67
4.1.1 Bit-Width Narrowing ... 68
4.1.2 Bit-Level Optimizations ... 72
4.1.3 Conversion from Floating- to Fixed-Point Representations ... 75
4.1.4 Nonstandard Floating-Point Formats ... 77
4.2 Instruction-Level Transformations ... 77
4.2.1 Operator Strength Reduction ... 78
4.2.2 Height Reduction ... 80
4.2.3 Code Motion ... 84
4.3 Loop-Level Transformations ... 87
4.3.1 Loop Unrolling ... 87
4.3.2 Loop Tiling and Loop Strip-Mining ... 90
4.3.3 Loop Merging and Loop Distribution ... 94
4.4 Data-Oriented Transformations ... 95
4.4.1 Data Distribution ... 95
4.4.2 Data Replication ... 96
4.4.3 Data Reuse and Scalar Replacement in Registers and Internal RAMs ... 96
4.4.4 Other Data-Oriented Transformations ... 99
4.5 Function-Oriented Transformations ... 101
4.5.1 Function Inlining and Outlining ... 101
4.5.2 Recursive Functions ... 104
4.6 Which Code Transformations to Choose? ... 105
4.7 Summary ... 107

5 **Mapping and Execution Optimizations** 109
5.1 Hardware Execution Techniques 109
5.1.1 Instruction-Level Parallelism 110
5.1.2 Speculative Execution 112
5.1.3 Predication and if-conversion 114
5.1.4 Multi Tasking 116
5.2 Partitioning 118
5.2.1 Temporal Partitioning 119
5.2.2 Spatial Partitioning 124
5.2.3 Illustrative Example 125
5.3 Mapping Program Constructs to Resources 127
5.3.1 Mapping Scalar Variables to Registers 127
5.3.2 Mapping of Operations to FUs 129
5.3.3 Mapping of Selection Structures 130
5.3.4 Sharing Functional Units FUs 131
5.3.5 Combining Instructions for RFUs 132
5.4 Pipelining 134
5.4.1 Pipelined Functional and Execution Units 135
5.4.2 Pipelining Memory Accesses 138
5.4.3 Loop Pipelining 139
5.4.4 Coarse-Grained Pipelining 144
5.4.5 Pipelining Configuration–Computation Sequences 145
5.5 Memory Accesses 146
5.5.1 Partitioning and Mapping of Arrays to Memory Resources 146
5.5.2 Improving Memory Accesses 148
5.6 Back-End Support 150
5.6.1 Allocation, Scheduling, and Binding 150
5.6.2 Module Generation 151
5.6.3 Mapping, Placement, and Routing 153
5.7 Summary 153

6 **Compilers for Reconfigurable Architectures** 155
6.1 Early Compilation Efforts 155
6.2 Compilers for FPGA-Based Systems 157
6.2.1 The SPC Compiler 157
6.2.2 A C to Fine-Grained Pipelining Compiler 158
6.2.3 The DeepC Silicon Compiler 158
6.2.4 The COBRA-ABS Tool 158
6.2.5 The DEFACTO Compiler 159
6.2.6 The Streams-C Compiler 159
6.2.7 The Cameron Compiler 160
6.2.8 The MATCH Compiler 160
6.2.9 The Galadriel and Nenya Compilers 161
6.2.10 The Sea Cucumber Compiler 161

6.2.11 The Abstract-Machines Compiler ... 161
6.2.12 The CHAMPION Software Design Environment ... 162
6.2.13 The SPARCS Tool ... 163
6.2.14 The ROCCC Compiler ... 163
6.2.15 The DWARV Compiler ... 163
6.3 Compilers for Coarse-Grained Reconfigurable Architectures ... 164
6.3.1 The DIL Compiler ... 164
6.3.2 The RaPiD-C Compiler ... 165
6.3.3 The CoDe-X Compiler ... 165
6.3.4 The XPP-VC Compiler ... 166
6.3.5 The DRESC Compiler ... 166
6.4 Compilers for Hybrid Reconfigurable Architectures ... 167
6.4.1 The Chimaera-C Compiler ... 167
6.4.2 The Garp and the Nimble C Compilers ... 168
6.4.3 The NAPA-C Compiler ... 168
6.5 Compilation Efforts Summary ... 169

7 Perspectives on Programming Reconfigurable Computing Platforms ... 177
7.1 How to Make Reconfigurable Computing a Reality? ... 177
7.1.1 Easy of Programming ... 178
7.1.2 Program Portability and Legacy Code Migration ... 179
7.1.3 Performance Portability ... 180
7.2 Research Directions in Compilation for Reconfigurable Architectures ... 181
7.2.1 Programming Language Design ... 181
7.2.2 Intermediate Representation ... 181
7.2.3 Mapping to Multiple Computing Engines ... 182
7.2.4 Code Transformations ... 182
7.2.5 Design-Space Exploration and Compilation Time ... 183
7.2.6 Pipelined Execution ... 184
7.2.7 Memory Mapping Optimizations ... 185
7.2.8 Application-Specific Compilers and Cores ... 185
7.2.9 Resource Virtualization ... 186
7.2.10 Dynamic and Incremental Compilation ... 186
7.3 Tackling the Compilation Challenge for Reconfigurable Architectures ... 187
7.4 Reconfigurable Architectures and Nanotechnology ... 189
7.5 Summary ... 189

8 Final Remarks ... 191

References ... 193

List of Acronyms ... 213

Index ... 217

Chapter 1
Introduction

The increasing number of transistors on a chip [221,278] has enabled the emergence of reconfigurable architectures and systems with a wide range of implementation flavors [145, 308]. While they were once confined to glue-logic applications, given their very limited device capacities, reconfigurable architectures now cover a wide range of application domains, including high-performance computing where they deliver complete multicore solutions on a single chip [228, 270, 303]. The diversity of reconfigurable architectures is astounding. At one end of the spectrum, reconfigurable architectures are composed of a very large number of fine-grained configurable elements as is the case in Field-Programmable-Gate-Arrays (FPGAs) [5, 14, 54, 111]. In this case, one can build very specialized storage and custom computing elements in response to specific domain requirements such as input data rates or stringent real-time requirements. At the other end of the spectrum, many computing cores such as general-purpose processors (GPPs) can be interconnected with other processors or memory via a customized reconfiguration network [37, 211, 303]. In between these two extremes lies a range of architectural options where multiple, and possibly heterogeneous, custom processing elements and storage structures can be interconnected in an almost infinite set of possibilities [145].

1.1 The Promise of Reconfigurable Architectures and Systems

Not surprisingly, the last decade has witnessed a growing interest in computing architectures and systems with hardware elements that can be reconfigurable, possibly even dynamically, on-the-fly and on demand. The configurability of the individual computing and storage elements and their interconnectivity allows these architectures to emulate a wide range of computing paradigms. For example, reconfigurable architectures can be organized as a collection of independently executing processing elements, thus as a parallel computer, or as a collection of cooperating and tightly synchronized functional units (FUs) as in a pipelined architecture.

J.M.P. Cardoso, P.C. Diniz, *Compilation Techniques for Reconfigurable Architectures*,
DOI 10.1007/978-0-387-09671-1_1,

The extreme flexibility of reconfigurable architectures and their potential performance, measured in a wide range of performance metrics, such as energy consumption and execution time, have allowed them to become the vehicle of choice in several computing domains, namely:

- **Custom Computing Machines:** The ability to be reconfigured as specific hardware structures, such as highly parallel data-paths or supporting custom arithmetic formats, makes reconfigurable architectures a prime vehicle for custom computing machines. For example, a signal processing application might require only 12-bit fixed-point precision arithmetic and use custom rounding modes [279] or make intensive use of a 14-bit butterfly routing network used for parallel computation of a fast Fourier transform (FFT). In other domains, such as robotics, cost, flexibility, and real-time capabilities might be critical requirements traditional architectures cannot meet. In many such domains and application settings, reconfigurable architectures exhibit computing densities superior to traditional computing architectures [88].
- **Fast Prototyping and Emulation Systems:** In addition, to their potential as custom machines, their reconfigurability also makes them an ideal vehicle for deployment scenarios where the computational needs cannot or are not fully defined at design time. This is the case in early system prototyping where not all the engineering requirements might be defined. Fabricating an Application-Specific Integrated Circuit (ASIC) to detect a posteriori a manufacturing error or simply an engineering miscalculation might prove to be a costly design solution. The field-programmability of reconfigurable architectures allows them to mitigate these issues as the recent increase in device capacity has enabled them to emulate a wide range of ever increasing system functionalities. In other settings, like communication protocols, where the parameters of operation might not be well defined at deployment time, reconfigurable architectures may facilitate future design upgrades that would have to be relegated to software-only solutions in traditional systems [33].
- **High-Performance Computing:** Enabled by the large increase in fabrication device capacity, high-end reconfigurable architectures can also deliver impressive performance by virtue of exploiting massive amounts of concurrency, as these architectures can leverage parallelism at several levels (operation, basic block, loop, function, etc.), and support multiple flows of control. In addition, high-end reconfigurable architectures include multiple internal traditional cores (see, e.g., the Virtex-II Pro [340] and Virtex-5 [342] FPGAs with PowerPC [280] cores) and large, customizable, internal storage components. Several applications areas such as security (encryption) and image/signal processing have highlighted the true potential of configurable architectures in the high-performance arena [83].
- **Submicron and Nanoscale Computing Systems:** An undesired effect of the diminishing VLSI feature size in submicron fabrication processes is the increase in transient and permanent hardware failures [277]. In some contexts, the use of traditional fault-tolerant approaches might not be satisfactory and thus design mapping and run-time techniques might be needed. In promising new computing technologies, such as nanoscale computing systems [89, 286], where

failure/defect rates are non-negligible, reconfiguration is seen as a key technique for dealing with defective resources [93] and transient faults [277].

This promise and potential of reconfigurable architectures was recognized very early on by Gerald Estrin [104] and more recently by the academic research community. During the past 10 years, a large number of reconfigurable computing systems have been developed by the research community, achieving high performance for a selected set of applications [145, 151]. Such systems combine, synergetically, microprocessors and reconfigurable hardware, thus exploiting the advantages of both computing paradigms (e.g., [125]). Other researchers have developed reconfigurable architectures based solely on commercially available FPGAs [96], in which the FPGAs act as processing nodes of a large multiprocessor machine possibly accommodating on-chip *softcore* or *hardcore* processors. In yet another thrust, researchers have developed dedicated reconfigurable architectures using as internal building blocks multiple FUs such as adders and multipliers interconnected via programmable routing resources (e.g., [101, 234]).

The tremendous increase of available transistors on a die coupled by the regularity of many of the VLSI designs commercial reconfigurable architectures have, as is the case of fine-grained devices, allowed these architectures to be propelled by Moore's Law [221] and poise themselves as versatile computing platforms capable of challenging traditional architectures as mainstream computing engines.

1.2 The Challenge: How to Program and Compile for Reconfigurable Systems?

Despite their enormous potential, reconfigurable architectures are extremely hard to program. Currently, programmers must assume the role of software programmers and hardware designers to effectively exploit the potential of the target reconfigurable devices. They will not only have to master two programming languages, and bridge the semantic gap between them, but will also have to deal with all the low-level details of mapping computations expressed in high-level programming languages to these architectures. The lack of programming tools and effective methodologies results in programmers engaging in long and error-prone mapping processes, with the net result of not fully exploiting the capabilities of reconfigurable architectures.

It is thus widely believed that automatic compilation from established high-level imperative programming languages, such as C or MATLAB, is a key approach to the success of reconfigurable computing, as the design expertise required for developing applications to reconfigurable computing platforms is excessively complex for the typical user (e.g., embedded systems programmer) to handle. For reconfigurable computing to become widely accepted, we believe that compilation times for reconfigurable architectures should be comparable to those of current software compilation, and, yet, generate solutions that are competitive, in terms of execution time and hardware resources used, with hand-coded hardware solutions.

A current challenge in this area is the establishment of efficient compilation approaches, which would help the programmer accomplish an efficient hardware implementation without the need to be involved in complex and low-level hardware programming. Although mature design tools exist for logic synthesis, for placement and routing, and for multiunit spatial partitioning for programmable logic devices,[1] there is a lack of robust integrated tools that take traditional sequential programs and automatically map them to reconfigurable computing architectures. In addition, High-Level Synthesis (HLS)[2] tools have been mostly developed for ASICs and neither wield the special characteristics of the reconfigurable architectures nor desired high-level abstractions. These tools are commonly based on resource sharing schemes [114] that target the layout flexibility of ASICs. They are, typically, less efficient when considering the predefined logic cell architecture and limited routing resources of fine-grained Reconfigurable Processing Units (RPUs), e.g., FPGAs, where resource sharing is often inadequate. The inherent characteristics of the target reconfigurable architectures require specialized (architecture-oriented) compilation and synthesis approaches.

1.3 This Book: Key Techniques when Compiling to Reconfigurable Architecture

This book presents a comprehensive description of the most significant work on compilation for reconfigurable computing platforms. The widespread dissemination of embedded systems and their increased integration level with reconfigurable devices exacerbate the difficulties of current programming methodologies for these systems and architectures.

A major goal of this book is to aid the reader bridge the gap between the software compilation and the hardware synthesis domains as these subjects are seldom taught jointly as part of Computer Engineering curricula in any advanced engineering degree. This book is thus intended for computer professionals, graduate students, and advanced undergraduates who need to understand the issues in both compilation and synthesis domains. This book also relates the technical aspects of the most significant commercial efforts in the area of compilation for reconfigurable computing with the techniques described here. This effort will, we hope, increase the understanding of these efforts and their techniques, ultimately increasing the acceptance of reconfigurable architectures and more broadly of reconfigurable computing.

Naturally, the work presented in this book is derived from the research efforts in the areas of compilation, parallelizing compilers, and hardware synthesis. With the growing number of hardware resources in today's VLSI chips, reconfigurable architectures are effectively becoming parallel architectures with heterogeneous and configurable internal topologies. Naturally, many of the compiler analyses and

[1] In this book we make no distinction between FPGAs and PLDs.

[2] We make no distinction between the terms: high-level synthesis, architectural synthesis, and behavioral synthesis.

mapping techniques described in Chaps. 4 and 5, respectively, are derived from the parallelizing compilation research community and molded to fit the increased degrees of freedom reconfigurable architectures enable. Despite this morphosis as parallel architectures, at their core, reconfigurable architectures are still hardware-centric. The mapping of computations inevitably includes the fundamental steps of spatial partitioning of computations among various reconfigurable devices in a board, and/or its temporal partitioning when the computations require more hardware resources than the physically available, respectively. Further, data must be allocated and managed between the available memories (on- and/or off-chip memories) and between registers. Lastly, and because it is a very important execution technique, the mapping can exploit pipelining execution schemes at either a fine- or coarse-grain level. Many, if not the vast majority, of these techniques originated from the hardware synthesis community and were given a new emphasis with the increased device capacity and flexibility of these reconfigurable architectures.

The maturity of some of the compiler techniques for reconfigurable architectures and the stability in the underlying reconfigurable technology have enabled the emergence of commercial companies with their own technical compilation solutions to help port, with some degree of effort, applications written in high-level programming languages to reconfigurable devices. We include a chapter devoted to the most prominent efforts highlighting the use of the techniques described here and their technical solutions.

Complementary to this book, the reader can find survey-like literature focusing on specific features of reconfigurable computing platforms and on software tools for developing FPGA-based designs. Hartenstein [145] presents a summary of a decade of research in reconfigurable computing, whereas Compton and Hauck [81] present a survey on systems and software tools. Other authors present surveys that focus on specific application domains or reconfigurable architectures [306, 308, 350].

In addition, other books have been published on reconfigurable computing [90] or the use of reconfigurable hardware designs to solve specific problem domains [122]. This book complements these efforts in that, rather than describing specific application or domain solutions, it provides a comprehensive description of the base techniques programmers and designers expect to find in high-level compilation and synthesis tools for these reconfigurable architectures. Understanding how a compiler views its design space will ultimately allow programmers and designers to better understand and thus become more productive users of the tools.

1.4 Organization of this Book

This book is organized into eight chapters with distinct perspectives. In Chap. 2, we provide a brief description of current architectures for reconfigurable computing platforms with the goal of giving the readers a good perspective of the wide diversity of reconfigurable architectures and their preferential execution model. In Chap. 3, we present an overview of generic compilation and synthesis flows for reconfigurable architectures. In this chapter, we focus on the aspects of the compilation and synthesis process that are exacerbated by the reconfigurability of the target architectures, but also address the important and often neglected aspects of the input programming paradigm. In Chap. 4, we describe in detail a wide range of code transformations enabled or emphasized by the nature of the reconfigurable target architecture at hand. This chapter includes many illustrative examples using an imperative source programming language, so that the reader can understand the underlying transformation of the code either as the source- or intermediate-level representation. In Chap. 5, we describe mapping techniques for reconfigurable architectures with a special emphasis on temporal and spatial partitioning of the computation and the corresponding mapping of data to various storage structures. In Chap. 6, we present a selected sample of existing compilers and tools for mapping high-level languages to reconfigurable architectures. In Chap. 7, we present our overall perspective on reconfigurable computing, highlighting what we believe are key issues that need to be addressed to make this promising technology a reality. In this chapter, we also describe a set of possible research directions in this area and provide a vision for a future compilation and synthesis flow that aims at mitigating some of the hard compilation problems reconfigurable architectures raise. Finally, in Chap. 8, we conclude with our overall remarks on the state and possible evolution of compilers for reconfigurable computing systems.

Chapter 2
Overview of Reconfigurable Architectures

In this chapter, we describe the main features of reconfigurable architectures and systems, focusing on reconfigurable fabrics, the underlying vehicle for reconfigurable computing. We begin with a short historical perspective followed by a description and categorization of reconfigurable architectural features, such as their granularity, interconnection topologies, and system-level integration. We describe dynamic reconfigurable features some architectures exhibit as well as the execution models these architectures preferentially expose. Throughout this chapter we illustrate specific architectural features using representative examples of commercial and academic reconfigurable architectures, but without aiming to survey all the efforts on reconfigurable computing architectures.

As this book mainly focuses on compilation techniques for computations expressed in high-level programming languages when targeting reconfigurable architectures, we do not extensively describe system-level issues such as overall system organization or integration. Similarly, we have omitted detailed descriptions of architectural approaches that rely on the reconfigurable fabric as building blocks of complex systems. Examples of these blocks are configurable processors and synthesizable IP-cores with parameterized features, e.g., related to register windows, pipeline stages, or instruction-set customizations. We see these architectural definition efforts as the application of domain-specific mapping approaches, of limited scope, but complementary to the general techniques described in Chaps. 4 and 5.

2.1 Evolution of Reconfigurable Architectures

Reconfigurable architectures might have had their origin in the seminal work of Gerald Estrin et al. [104–106] with the development of the concept of restructurable computers. This work was the focus of attention in the 1970s by Miller and Cocker [215] and later by Reddi and Feustel [259]. Despite the interesting potential performance advantages over traditional computers, the concept of reestructurable computers was never integrated in general-purpose computing systems at

J.M.P. Cardoso, P.C. Diniz, *Compilation Techniques for Reconfigurable Architectures*,
DOI 10.1007/978-0-387-09671-1_2,

that time, due mainly to the high costs and the inexistent appropriate technology to build those machines. More constraint-driven architectures based on the von-Neumann paradigm (RISC and CISC) were the preferable engines for mainstream computing [154].

The work by Altera Corp. and Actel Corp. in programmable logic devices [14] and in reconfigurable interconnections [5] and the work in the early 1980s, by Freeman from Xilinx Inc., in the definition of the configurable logic array [111] have contributed to the birth of a new breed of reconfigurable architectures named Field-Programmable Gate-Arrays (FPGAs). Given their limited device capacity, early FPGAs were thus limited to fast-prototyping and glue-logic functions in products that did not justify ASIC solutions. Recent technological advances and the regularity of FPGAs have allowed them to evolve to very powerful reconfigurable devices [83] with the potential to implement almost any circuit from simple hardware designs to entire multicore systems [228]. FPGAs are now seen as a technology able to implement entire systems, some including hardwired traditional microprocessors (e.g., Virtex-II Pro from Xilinx [340]).

The extraordinary growth in FPGA capacity has enabled researchers in academia to experiment and validate novel computing paradigms. In the late 1980s researchers developed several prototype architectures based on FPGAs (see, e.g., [135, 331]) which, among other efforts, can be considered the main roots of reconfigurable computing. Reflecting the growing interest in reconfigurable computing in academia and industry, the 1990s saw the birth of numerous academic forums for discussion of reconfigurable computing related research. Academic forums such as the International Conference on Field-Programmable Logic and Applications (FPL), the IEEE Symposium for Field-Programmable Custom Computing Machines (FCCM), and the ACM International Symposium on Field-Programmable Gate Arrays (FPGA) are today well-established venues for the presentation and dissemination of academic and industry related findings and experiences in reconfigurable computing.

2.2 Reconfigurable Architectures: Key Characteristics

In this description we distinguish between reconfigurable architectures, as the fundamental architectural hardware elements, and reconfigurable processing units (RPUs) as reconfigurable architectures with associated execution control and operations. While reconfigurable architectures present the basic hardware elements, RPUs organize these configurable elements exposing to the software layer an abstraction level that ranges from the very low-level bit-oriented instructions to higher-level instructions. The abstraction and capabilities of RPUs critically depend on the granularity and interconnection of the underlying reconfigurable fabric resources, namely:

- Functional Units (FUs) – each one programmed to select a finite number of behaviors. The complexity of those behaviors can range from an ALU (Arithmetic Logic Unit) operation to a simple boolean function, depending on the granularity of the reconfigurable device.

- Memory Elements (MEMs) – each one with finite size capacity that can usually be customized to implement application storage requirements. For example, internal memory banks can be used for partitioning of data and registers can be organized to form tapped-delay lines.
- Interconnection Resources (IRs) – consisting of channels, programmable connection switches, and programmable routing switches or buses. These resources are programmed to connect resources in the device, for instance to define specific FU to Memory topologies, or inter-FU communication topologies (e.g., linear or two-dimensional torus).
- Control Units (CUs) – can range from custom, very specific, finite-state machines (FSMs), typically seen in fine-grained reconfigurable architectures to microprogrammed VLIW (Very Long Instruction Word) based architecture controllers commonly found in coarse-grained architectures. Depending on the architecture, these CUs may offer some degree of customization or may consist of fixed resources, e.g., controlling the execution of the FU, not exposed to the programmer.
- Input/Output Buffers (IOBs) – used to interface devices and/or units and can be configured to meet specific timing/bandwidth requirements.

Of these elements, the very fine-grained FUs present in contemporary FPGAs offer a unique aspect seldom found in other reconfigurable architectures. With its configurable logic blocks, it is possible to interchange part of the available resources between functional and storage elements. This unique capability makes these reconfigurable devices even more challenging to program as tools must gage the cost/benefits of using the configurable resources either for computation or for storage.

Another important aspect of reconfigurable architectures deals with its synchronicity. Although there have been various research efforts regarding asynchronous reconfigurable computing architectures (e.g., [304]), the vast majority of reconfigurable architectures are synchronous. Most fine-grained reconfigurable architectures, such as FPGAs, and in spite of their intrinsic maximum clock frequencies, operate at frequencies dependent on each configuration, dictated by the critical path delay of the hardware structures. The operating frequency is dictated not only by the characteristics of the design but also by the ability of the mapping tools to place and route (P&R) the designs, so that the maximum delay between sequential elements (e.g., registers and memories) is as short as possible. Conversely, coarse-grained reconfigurable architectures usually have a fixed frequency clocking scheme synchronizing the transfer of data between the elements. This strategy limits flexibility, but renders easier programmability, performance estimation models, and predictability.

In addition to the many possible configurations of the architectural elements in specific topologies, RPUs offer an almost infinite number of higher level programming abstractions and execution schemes. At one end of the spectrum of possibilities, RPUs can be organized internally as VLIW architectures [110] offering a VLIW programming ISA. In common VLIW architectures there exist a number of programmable FUs, without direct interconnections between them. The flow of data between FUs is accomplished through register files. In these VLIW architectures no

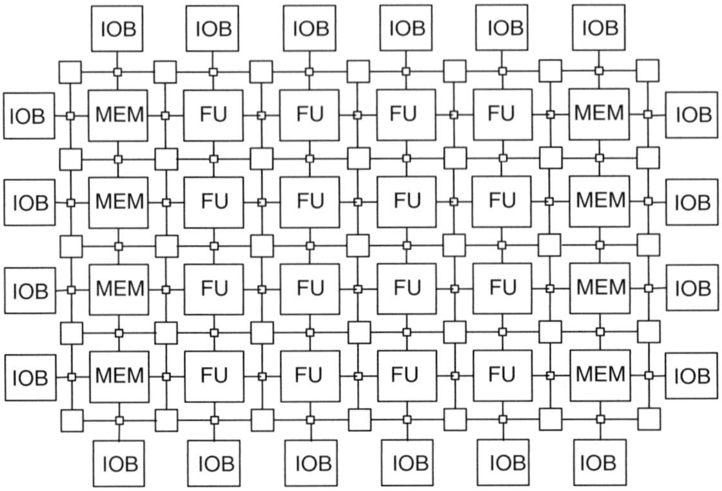

Fig. 2.1 Possible two-dimensional structure for a reconfigurable architecture

traditional placement and routing a complex step is needed. In this case, the placement can be seen as a sequential assignment of the instructions to the FUs. A routing step is not present as there is usually no need to establish the routing paths using the interconnection resources as in the case of common reconfigurable fabrics. On the opposite end of the spectrum, the various FUs can have a localized controller capable of interpreting specific instruction streams behaving as Network-on-a-Chip (NoC) architectures [37, 211], where elements communicate via data packets using dynamic or static routing schemes.

We now describe different reconfigurable computing architectures according to their granularity. We begin by describing fine-grained reconfigurable fabrics represented by FPGAs and then focus on academic research and industry efforts considering coarse-grained and hybrid reconfigurable architectures.

2.3 Granularity

Granularity is one of the key aspects that differentiate reconfigurable architectures as it indirectly dictates the level of effort required to map computations or other high-level abstractions to the underlying reconfigurable fabric. We summarize in Table 2.1 various reconfigurable architectures, their typical organization, and the atomic granularity of their hardware resources.

According to the granularity of their cells (e.g., processing elements (PEs)), we classify reconfigurable architectures in three broad categories, namely:

- Fine-Grained: The configurable cells of these RPUs, often referred to as "sea-of-gates," include logic gates thus allowing the implementation of arbitrary and specialized data-path hardware designs.

Table 2.1 Examples of architectures with different granularities (Virtex [343], Stratix [15] DPGA [87], Garp [60], PipeRench [132], rDPA [149], MATRIX [217],XPP [31], MorphoSys [282], ADRES [208], ARRIX FPOAs [203], RAW [303])

Cell granularity	Canonical Operations	Examples of devices	Shape	Cell type	Bit-width
Fine (wire)	Logic functions of 2–5 bits	FPGAs, Xilinx Virtex and Altera Stratix	2D array	CLB, LUTs, multiplexer, register MULT, DSP blocks RAM Blocks	2–5 1 18 Customizable
		DPGA	2D array	LUT	4
		Garp (reconfigurable logic array)	2D array	CLB	2
Coarse (operand)	ALU operations of 4–32 bits	PipeRench	2D array	ALU + Pass Register File	2–32 (parametrizable before fabrication)
		rDPA/KressArray (Xputer)	2D array	ALU + register	32 (parametrizable before fabrication)
		MATRIX	2D array	ALU with multiplier + memory	8
		RaPiD	1D array	ALU, multipliers, registers, RAM	16
		XPP	2D array	ALU with multiplier, RAM	4–32 (parametrizable before fabrication)
		MorphoSys	2D array	ALU + multiplier + register file	28
		ADRES	2D array	ALU + multiplier + register file	32
		ARRIX FPOAs	2D array	ALU + MAC + register file	16
Mix-coarse	Sequence of assembly instructions	RAW	2D array	RISC + memory + switch network	32

- Coarse-Grained: The configurable cells of these RPUs, often designated as Field-Programmable ALU Arrays (FPAAs), include ALUs, multiplier blocks, and distributed memories.
- Mix-Coarse-Grained: The configurable cells of these RPUs include microprocessor cores combined with very fine-grained reconfigurable logic.

There are cases of architectures that crosscut different granularity categories. For instance, the PipeRench [131, 132] (see Table 2.1) can be classified either as a fine- or as a coarse-grained architecture. In PipeRench, the parameterized bit-width of each PE can be set before fabrication ranging from a few bits to a larger number of bits [132], as is typical in coarse-grained architectures. Another example of a coarse-grained architecture with variable bit-width is the XPP [31] (see Table 2.1).

Some approaches use a layer of abstraction implemented by architectural templates as is the case of the dynamic processor cores in fine-grained RPUs, such as the DISC (Dynamic Instruction Set Computer) [327]. A differentiating aspect of the DISC approach is that it allows the dynamic reconfiguration of dedicated hardware units, when presented with a new instruction corresponding to a unit that has not yet been configured.

In the next sections, we discuss in more detail fine- and coarse-grained reconfigurable architectures.

2.3.1 Fine-Grained Reconfigurable Architectures

Fine-grained reconfigurable architectures, such as FPGAs, can be viewed as reconfigurable hardware devices consisting of fine-grained FUs interconnected by an arbitrary programmable network. These fine-grained, programmable FUs are able to implement low-level bit-oriented logic functions for a specific number of inputs and outputs. For example, a simple fine-grained reconfigurable FU can be implemented as a Look-Up Table (LUT) with two inputs and one output as depicted in Fig. 2.2. In this example, the logic function implemented by the two-input LUT is selected by the addressing value of the tuple (`x1`, `x2`) which selects one of the four table bits (`bit0` through `bit3`) as its output. The loaded configuration of the table bits thus defines the specific logic function of the two inputs `x1` and `x2`.[1] The FU illustrated allows the connection to `y1` of either a nonregistered or a registered output of the LUT by controlling the output multiplexer via the `s1` signal.

Contemporary FPGAs use FUs more complex than the one in the example given above. In Xilinx FPGAs the FUs are called Configurable Logic Blocks (CLBs) and consist of a number of Slices, typically two, where each Slice includes two LUTs. Typical input/output lines for each LUT are 4 and 1, respectively. Besides the LUTs, each CLB also includes multiplexers and flip-flops (FFs). Existing high-end FPGAs include specific FUs such as multipliers, digital signal processing (DSP) blocks, and distributed memory blocks [342]. Common CLBs can still be used to implement storage elements such as small RAMs, FIFOs, and shift registers [175].

The logic functions implemented by each CLB are programmed by modifying the table of bits for each LUT and the multiplexer's selection lines. One possible

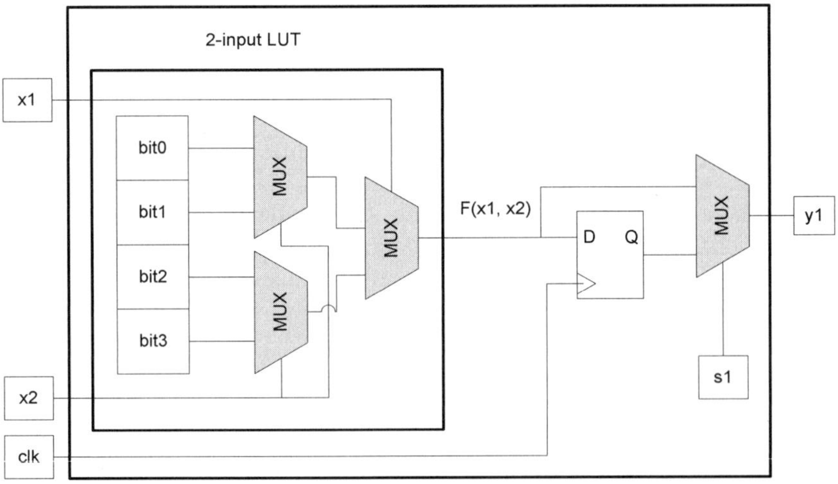

Fig. 2.2 Example of a simple FU with a 2-input LUT

[1] Using this LUT-based approach an LUT with n inputs is able to implement 2^{2^n} different logic functions.

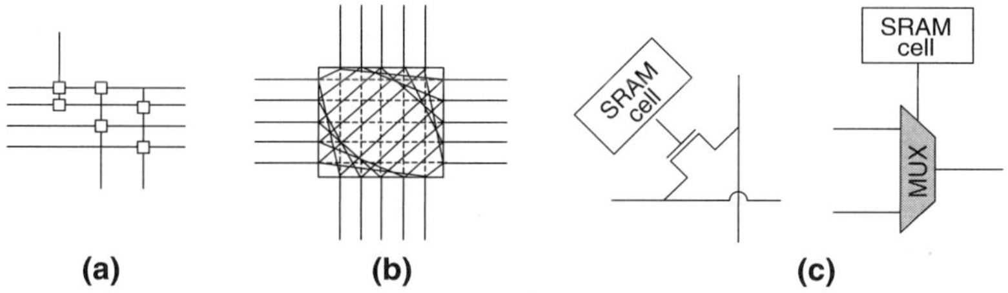

Fig. 2.3 Elements used for establishing routing channels between architectural components: (**a**) programmable connection switch; (**b**) programmable routing switch; (**c**) SRAM-based programmable connections between wires

approach for device programmability consists of using SRAM-based configuration cells [294], containing not only the contents of each LUT table, but also the configuration of the interconnections between resources. Interconnecting CLBs allows the architecture to implement arbitrary complex logic functions.

The way FUs (e.g., CLBs) are distributed and interconnected in the architecture defines the topology of the reconfigurable architecture. Common FPGAs use an island-style topology consisting of tiles where each tile includes an FPGA component (e.g., FU, memory block). Wire segments and programmable routing switches are used to establish the connections between reconfigurable components as illustrated in Fig. 2.3. These routing resources can be organized into two main schemes often present in the same architecture. A flat single level of interconnection is used to promote fast localized connectivity, whereas a hierarchical, device-wide, interconnection scheme is used for long range connectivity.[2]

Despite their extreme flexibility, fine-grained reconfigurable architectures, such as FPGAs, do exhibit some disadvantages. Their fine granularity and large number of programmable points impose large configurations (bit-streams) and thus long reconfiguration times. Large number of hardware synergies for reconfigurability purposes is also problematic in terms of power dissipation given the increasing leakage current effects of leading edge manufacturing processes.

Programming these architectures is also a challenge as they require the use of hardware-oriented programming languages, such as VHDL [162] and Verilog [163], to bridge the gap between the very low-level bit-oriented reconfigurable devices and the high-level programming structures. Despite the ability of these languages to raise the level of abstraction to structural or even behavioral constructs, the abstractions they expose to the programmer are still fairly low level. The increase in device capacity only exacerbates this issue, as programmers seek to map increasingly complex computations to even larger devices. Many research efforts in academia and industry have sought to ameliorate this issue as described in Chap. 6, by offering higher-level programming abstractions and/or offering an automatic compilation and synthesis path from popular high-level programming languages such as C or MATLAB.

---

[2] The choice of the interconnection strategy has profound implications on placement and routing approaches.

2.3.2 Coarse-Grained Reconfigurable Architectures

We now describe some of the most representative efforts in reconfigurable architectures that exhibit coarse reconfigurable granularity elements.[3]

The Xputer architecture [146, 149] was one of the first coarse-grained reconfigurable architectures. The Xputer consists of a reconfigurable Data-Path Array (rDPA) organized as a uniform two-dimensional array of ALUs (32-bit width in the KressArray-1 version). The ALUs are mesh-connected via three levels of interconnection, namely: (1) nearest neighbors; (2) row/column back-buses; and (3) one global bus. The ALUs can also be used as routing resources. An address generation unit is responsible to control the flow of data to and from the rDPA. Each Xputer is connected to the host I/O bus and to its rDPA, as depicted in Fig. 2.4. The Xputer is programmed using CoDe-X [34], a co-compiler that maps the suitable portions of a C program to the rDPAs and the remainder of the program to the host system.

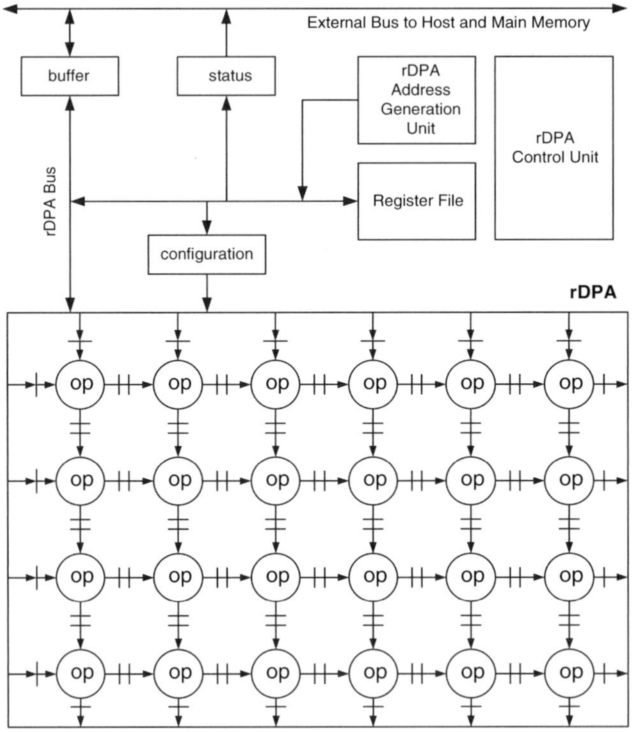

Fig. 2.4 The rDPA architecture (based on [148])

---

[3] For a more exhaustive coverage of this topic the interested reader is referred to the survey by Hartenstein [145].

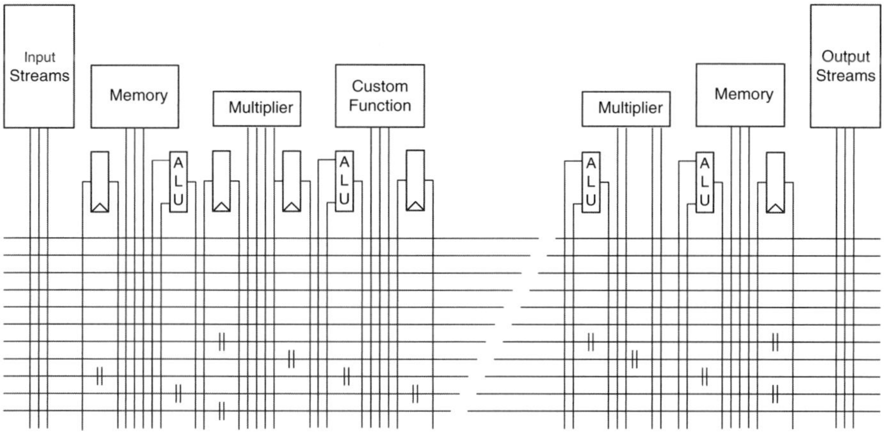

Fig. 2.5 A generic RaPiD architecture (based on [101])

The RaPiD [101], depicted in Fig. 2.5, is another coarse-grained reconfigurable architecture composed of multiple functional units such as ALUs, multipliers, registers, and RAM blocks organized linearly over a programmable segmented bus structure, and communicating through registers in a pipeline fashion. There are no cache memories as data is streamed in and out directly from external memory, or input/output devices, respectively. The architecture includes programmed controllers that generate an instruction stream, which is decoded as it flows through the datapath. Rather than having a global register file, data and intermediate results are stored locally in registers and small RAMs, close to their destination FUs. RaPiD is also a dynamically reconfigurable architecture as it allows data to be redirected or bypass selected elements in a programmable and data-dependent fashion, i.e., the routing of data can reflect the outcome of an operation. To facilitate the mapping of applications, an imperative C-like programming language was developed, which exposes to the programmer the pipelining of the architecture [84].

A radically distinct coarse- or mixed-grained reconfigurable architecture is the PipeRench [132], illustrated in Fig. 2.6. PipeRench is naturally geared for streaming and pipelining of computations with virtually unlimited number of pipeline stages implemented as *hardware stripes*. Each hardware stripe has an array of PEs exclusively connected to the previous and to the next stripes. Each PE consists of an ALU and a pass register file allowing the data to bypass the ALUs of a specific stripe. As it does not have explicit support for iterative constructs such as loops, PipeRench requires the compiler to fully unroll loops and to schedule the flow of data between stripes and memory. Programmers use the compiler to map their applications, written in DIL [55], by splitting their computations in stripes (possibly using more stripes than the physically available). The compiler generates a schedule of the virtual stripes and relies on hardware support for swapping in and out, on demand, the configuration for each stripe.

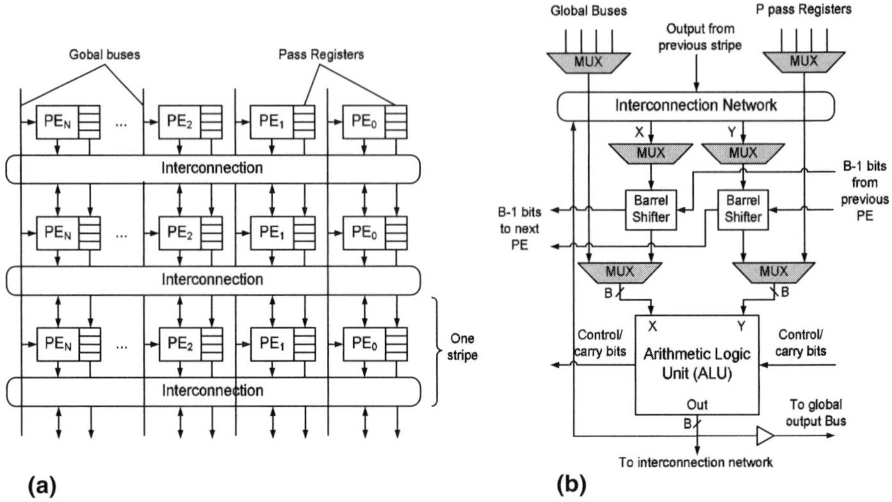

Fig. 2.6 The PipeRench architecture (based on [132]): (**a**) a stripe consists of PEs and interconnections; (**b**) PE structure

Another coarse-grained architecture is the Architecture for Dynamically Reconfigurable Embedded Systems (ADRES) [208]. ADRES is composed of two major components, a VLIW engine and a reconfigurable array, able to communicate via direct interconnection resources as depicted in Fig. 2.7. The reconfigurable array consists of a two-dimensional array of coarse-grained 32-bit PEs, each of which is composed internally of an FU and a local Register File (RF). The reconfigurable array is responsible for exploiting parallelism in highly pipelined kernels (e.g., loops) while the VLIW engine is responsible for exploiting ILP on nonkernel parts of the application. In this architecture, FUs support predicated execution and along with normal operands, the predicate signals are also routed between FUs. The authors have developed a C compiler for ADRES architecture templates [206]. The compiler maps to the two-dimensional array structures kernel computations identified through execution profiling techniques [207].

2.3.3 Hybrid Reconfigurable Architectures

We define hybrid reconfigurable architectures as architectures where the reconfigurable computing component resides with a host microprocessor on the same chip using either fine- or coarse-grained RPUs. Examples of hybrid reconfigurable architectures range from an architecture configuration arrangement where a microprocessor is connected to a fine-grained reconfigurable logic (Garp [60] and SCORE [72]) or a coarse-grained array (MorphoSys [282] and ADRES [208]) to an architecture configuration arrangement such as RAW [303] where an array of RISC-based cells

(a)

(b)

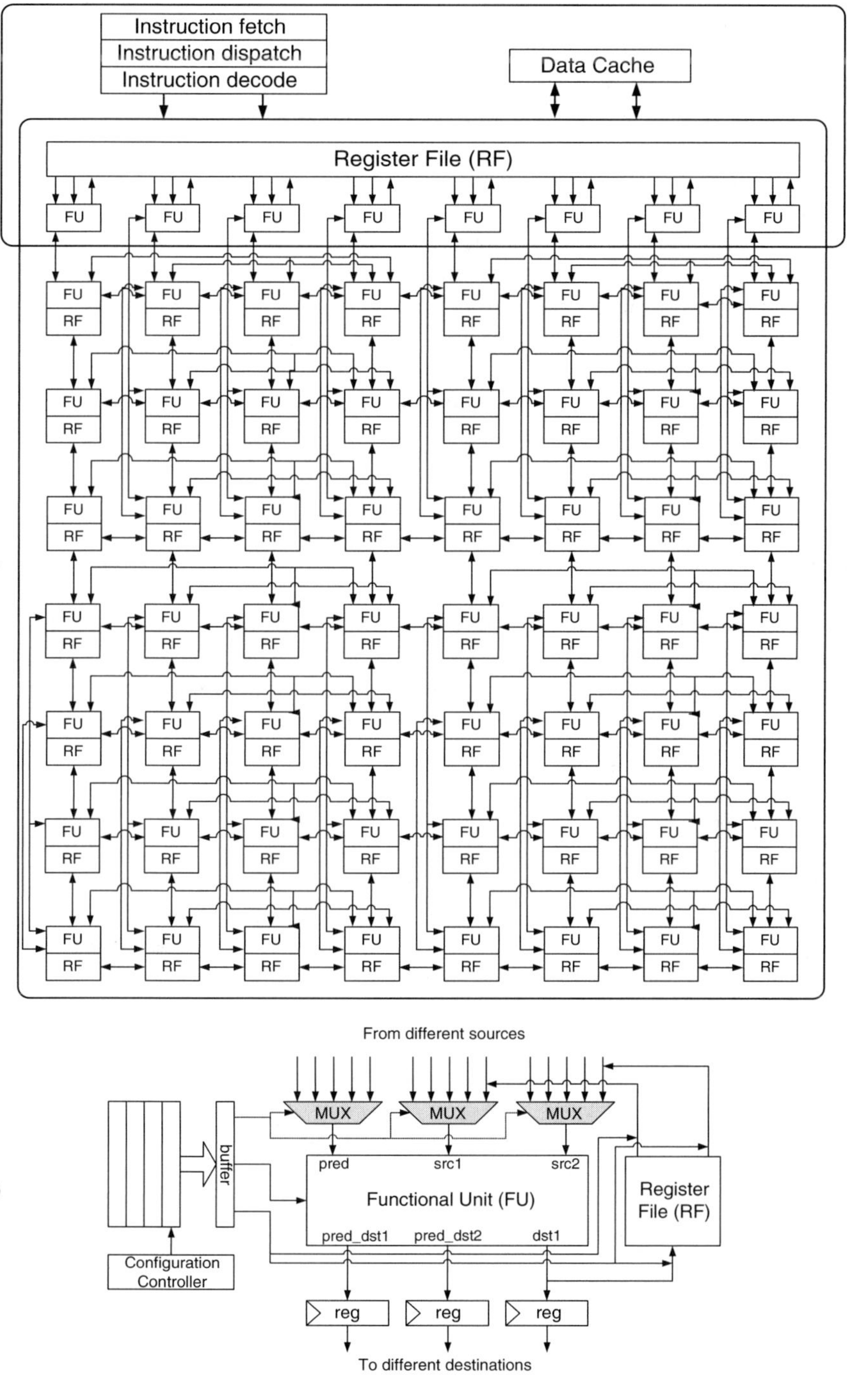

Fig. 2.7 The ADRES architecture (based on [208]): (**a**) typical architecture template; (**b**) its PE

each of which possibly containing some amount of dedicated configurable logic.[4] Companies such as Triscend [312], Chameleon [267], and Altera [13][5] have commercialized devices integrating one or more hard-wired microprocessors with reconfigurable logic. From the major FPGA vendors, only Xilinx [338] currently includes in its family of devices FPGAs [340] with one or more *hardcore* PowerPC processors [344]. We now present illustrative examples of architectures in this class.

The Garp architecture [60] integrates a MIPS core with an RPU used as a coprocessor accelerator. The RPU uses a fixed clocking scheme and consists of a fine-grained two-dimensional reconfigurable array of CLBs interconnected by programmable wiring. Each array row has a section dedicated to memory interfacing and control. The array has direct access to memory for fetching either data or configuration data, hence avoiding both data and reconfiguration bottlenecks. An ANSI C compiler has been developed for the Garp architecture [60] that uses the hyperblock [256] intermediate representation to extract loop kernels suitable to be mapped to the Garp array [61].

The MorphoSys architecture [282] also integrates an RISC processor core with an RPU and a memory interface unit. The RPU consists of an 8-by-8 reconfigurable array of coarse-grained cells, each internally composed of an ALU, using 28-bit fixed-point precision arithmetic and capable of 1 of 25 functions, a multiplier (16×12 bits), and a register file (composed of 4 16-bit registers). Before mapping a C program to Morphosys, suitable functions for the reconfigurable array are manually identified by the user. Then, those functions are mapped and programmed on the reconfigurable array using the MorphoSys assembly language [281].

The SCORE (Stream Computations Organized for Reconfigurable Execution) system [72] connects a microprocessor to distributed memory modules with attached reconfigurable logic based on four-input LUT elements. SCORE supports a stream-oriented computational model where the computation is split in compute pages managed by a run-time operating system [201]. An architecture-specific language, TDF (Task Description Format) [92], was developed, as well as a tool to translate TDF programs to RTL Verilog code, mapped to reconfigurable resources using specific back-end tools.

Lastly, the RAW Machine [303] is a coarse-grained two-dimensional tiled architecture. Each tile consists of an 8-stage pipelined 32-bit RISC processor with a pipelined floating-point unit, 32KB of instruction cache and 32KB of data cache memory, as well as programmable communication channels and routers for a static and a dynamic network. The authors use a parallelizing C compiler that partitions the computation and data among the tiles and programs the communication channels to best suit the communication patterns for each application [189].

[4] Early versions of RAW considered a reconfigurable logic unit connected to each RISC processor.

[5] Altera has discontinued the Excalibur FPGA devices, which integrated an on-chip *hardcore* ARM processor.

2.3.4 Granularity and Mapping

In commercially available fine-grained FPGAs, as is the case of the Xilinx family of Virtex devices (e.g., [343]), reconfigurable elements or CLBs consist of flip-flops and function generators that implement boolean functions of up to a specific number of variables. By interconnecting many CLBs, a designer can implement virtually any digital circuit with combinatorial and sequential behavior. Given their fine-granularity, the burden of compilation is placed on the synthesis, mapping, and placement and routing (P&R) aspects of the design. The P&R steps are notoriously difficult to predict or estimate, making the interaction between these steps and high-level compilation problematic. Their extreme flexibility, however, coupled with the tremendous increase of device capacity, has made FPGAs a very popular reconfigurable fabric in various domains, turning them into a commercial success.[6]

Coarse-grained reconfigurable architectures use ALUs as the basic reconfigurable hardware blocks [146]. This approach may provide more efficient silicon solutions, but limits the flexibility. Each reconfigurable block, an ALU, has a more compact silicon implementation than the equivalent ALU in a fine-grained reconfigurable architecture. However, it has a more rigid structure with respect to its control and possible interconnection network. The placement and routing efforts are alleviated, as the burden of translation is placed on the mapping of high-level instructions to the individual ALU instructions and the data routing between the various units.

To attempt to bridge the gap between fine-grained and coarse-grained architectures, and taking advantage of their tremendous increase in capacity, some of the newer FPGA architectures (e.g., Virtex-II [343] and Stratix [15]) include distributed multiplier and memory blocks. These architectures thus retain the fine-grained flavor of their fabric while supporting other, coarser-grained, classes of architectures commonly used for data-intensive computations.

An alternative approach to offer a coarse-grained abstract architecture, given the underlying fine-grained fabric, is to provide a mapping tool or to rely on the design of an operand-level library of macros, also known as soft-macros. These macros, possibly preplaced and/or relatively placed (e.g., as with Xilinx's Relatively Placed Macros or RPMs), provide a mapping of higher-level operators such as adders of parameterized bit-widths, to each target FPGA's specific configurable logic blocks. Libraries of such macros include multiple implementations considering different design trade-off points (e.g., area, latency, and configuration time). This soft-macro practice improves the compilation time and leads to more accurate time and area estimates.

Yet another alternative for the development of an abstraction layer in reconfigurable architectures is the use of hardware templates with specific architectures, possibly with parameterized and/or programmable features. An extreme application

[6] Despite their widespread use and commercial success, FPGAs have shown inefficiency in time and area for certain classes of problems [144, 145].

of this concept are the configurable and the *softcore* processors implemented as soft-macros on FPGAs. Given the capacity of contemporary FPGA devices, it is possible to replicate multiple cores, with distinct combinations of configuration parameters, with reconfigurable interconnections on the very same FPGA hardware configuration [333].

2.4 Interconnection Topologies

As silicon-based fabrication processes are natural planar, arrangements of devices, one-dimensional and two-dimensional array topologies for interconnecting FUs, on-chip memories, and I/O buffers, are the dominant organization in reconfigurable architectures.

In one-dimensional array architectures, a possible interconnection topology is a simple ring with wrap-around connections. While this linear topology follows the natural arrangement of the array, it exhibits a long worst-case delay/latency between end points of the array. A variant of this approach includes a secondary ring dedicated to communication in opposite directions. An alternative interconnection topology is a shared bus which avoids the potential issue of half-way latency at the expense of possible contention. An arrangement that potentially solves the issues of latency and contention is the all-to-all crossbar interconnection topology. Not surprisingly, the crossbar is only feasible for a small number of array elements. For larger number of elements, sparse topologies are often used (e.g., as in RaPiD [101]).

Regarding two-dimensional arrays, island-style architectures are the most common organizations as they allow routing and computing resources to intermingle without exacerbating possible bisection bandwidth issues. Usually, each basic tile consists of an FU and/or memory block connected to vertical and horizontal wire segments. This is the basis for the most common FPGA topologies which can be augmented by interconnection resources based on different length segments, in order to more efficiently connect non-neighboring tiles. Other two-dimensional array architectures using easily scalable topologies consist of mesh, octal, and hexagonal arrays. In these topologies, FUs have local and direct connections to their neighbors as depicted in Fig. 2.8a. To augment the routing possibilities of these topologies, some architectures use dedicated connections from each FU to other nonlocal FUs, or buses as depicted in Fig. 2.8c. To directly connect FUs or other components located at the boundaries of the two-dimensional arrays, torus-based topologies are used (see, e.g., [147]), as illustrated in Fig. 2.8d.

Other topologies used in the context of multiprocessors such as hypergraphs, trees, and hierarchical combinations of these are seldom applied in reconfigurable architectures [157].

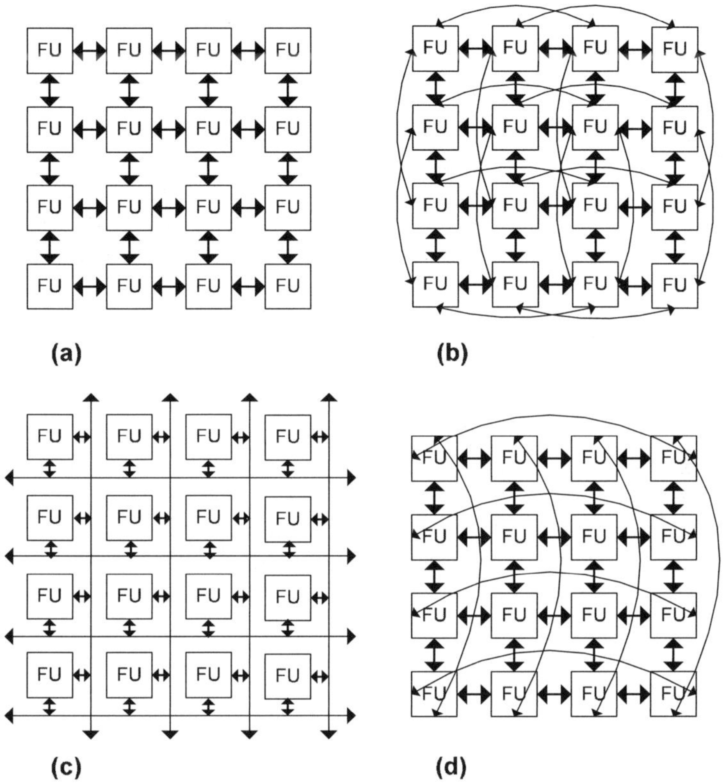

Fig. 2.8 Different interconnection topologies: (**a**) mesh; (**b**) mesh with 1-hop connections; (**c**) mesh with buses; (**d**) torus

2.5 System-Level Integration

Reconfigurable computing systems are typically organized as RPUs coupled to a host system consisting of a general-purpose processor (GPP), as illustrated in Fig. 2.9. The type of interconnection between the RPUs and the host system as well as the specific characteristics of the RPUs lead to a wide variety of possible reconfigurable architectures. While some architectures naturally facilitate some aspects of mapping of computations, no single dominant design solution has emerged for all application domains.

The type of coupling between the RPUs and the host system has a significant impact on the communication cost between the RPU and its external system. We classify this coupling into three main types, as listed below in order of decreasing communication costs:

- RPUs coupled to the host bus: The connection is accomplished via a system bus of the host subsystem. Many commercially available system boards have opted for this arrangement as it implies minimal modification of the

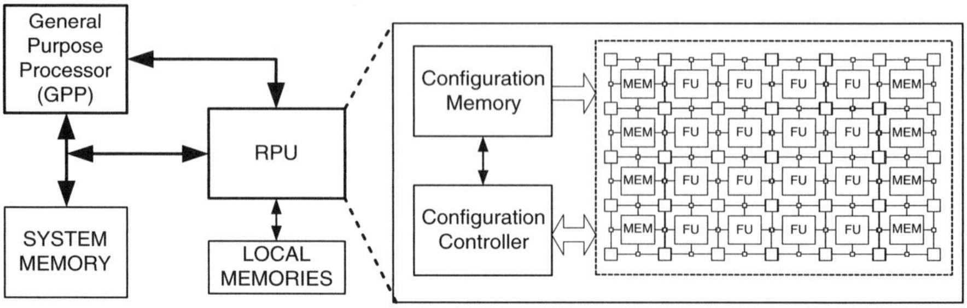

Fig. 2.9 Typical reconfigurable computing system

devices and the overall system organization such as virtual memory and system software. Boards with RPUs vary in complexity, size, and cost, the most sophisticated being composed of multiple RPUs, RAMs, and/or microprocessors. Some of these boards with RPUs connect to a PCI (Peripheral Controller Interface) bus of a PC or workstation. Examples of reconfigurable computing platforms connecting to the host via a bus include HOT-I, II [226], Xputer [146], Splash [123], ArMem [250], Teramac [17], DECPerLe-1 [220], Transmogrifier [191], RAW [319], and Spyder [164].

- RPUs coupled as coprocessors: In this case the RPU can be tightly coupled to the GPP but has autonomous execution and access to the system memory. In most architectures, when the RPU executes, the GPP is stalled. Examples of such platforms include the NAPA [264], REMARC [218], Garp [153], PipeRench [131], RaPiD [101], MorphoSys [282], and the Molen paradigm [317].
- RPUs acting like an extended data-path of the processor and without autonomous execution: The execution of the RPU is controlled by special opcodes of the GPP's instruction set. These data-path extensions are named as reconfigurable functional units (RFUs). Examples of such platforms include the Chimaera [348], PRISC [257, 258], OneChip [329], and ConCISe [168].

There is also a trend to use the fine-grained structures of high-end FPGAs to define System-on-a-Chip (SoC) solutions [35]. In these scenarios, FPGAs integrate microprocessor cores such as the PowerPC microprocessor in the Xilinx Virtex-II Pro devices [340], as hard VLSI macros. Another possibility consists of the use of *softcores*. *Softcores* based on von-Neumann architectures have been widely used. The most known examples of such microprocessor *softcores* are the Nios (I and II) [16] from Altera and the MicroBlaze [345] from Xilinx. This approach provides a simple migration path for legacy code and a clear programmer portability benefit also leveraging mature software compilation tools. *Softcores* also allow the use of highly customized interfaces between the components of the SoC. This approach of *softcores* has the attraction of allowing for domain-specific *softcores*, e.g., architecture templates based on coarse-grained arrays.

There are also examples of companies delivering their own microprocessor configurable *softcores*, usually targeting domain-specific applications. One such example is the *softcore* approach addressed by Stretch [297] which is based on the

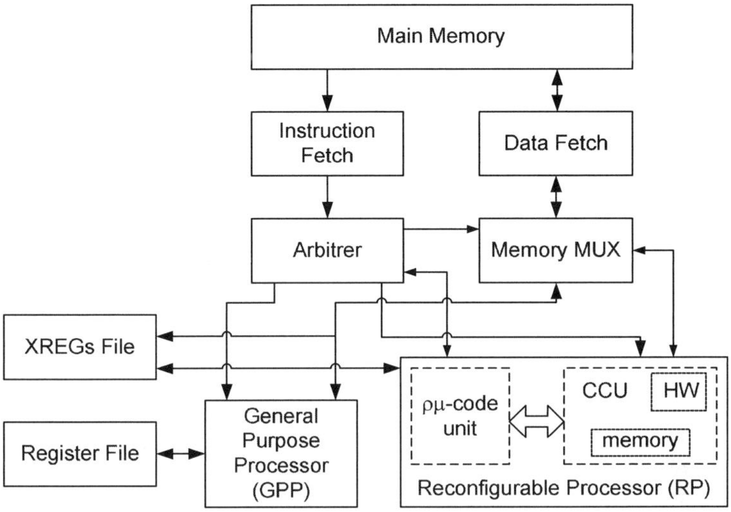

Fig. 2.10 The Molen polymorphic processor system organization

Tensilica Xtensa (a configurable RISC microprocessor) [134,305] and an extensible instruction set fabric. This approach is very valuable for fine-grained configurable architectures as it combines the benefits of a known programming environment with the performance benefits of customization.

A concrete example of a reconfigurable system integrated with a microprocessor is the Molen polymorphic processor [317] depicted in Fig. 2.10. The main PE is the GPP and the reconfigurable processor (RP), seen as the RPU of the system and typically used to accelerate key kernel operations. The communication between the GPP and the RP is performed via a special set of registers, called transfer registers or XRs resembling a software remote-procedure-call (RPC). To invoke an operation on the RP, the GPP first activates the configuration of the RP for the specific hardware operation, and in a second step prepares and sends the operation parameters by transferring data to the XRs. In the next phase, the operation is executed and the results made available to the GPP in the XR registers. The Molen concept has been evaluated using FPGAs, with the GPP as a *hardcore* or a *softcore* processor.

A key distinction between the Molen processor organization and previous reconfigurable systems, with similar organization, is the ability of the Molen machine to execute microcode for the emulation of complex operations which are executed on the RP (denoted as $\rho\mu$-code). Generic *set/execute* instructions can be used for the configuration/execution of any arbitrary operation, as long as they refer to the appropriate $\rho\mu$-code. An arbitrary number of hardware functions can be provided by architectural extension of *set/execute* instructions. Additionally, the parameters of these hardware operations are not included in the *set/execute* instructions, as they can be directly encoded in the associated $\rho\mu$-code. The flexibility of the Molen machine organization mitigates some issues with other system integration approaches as Molen does not require a new instruction for each hardware function. Furthermore, it imposes no limitation on the number of input/output parameters. The level of integration and cross-compilation transparency supported by the Molen machine organization effectively lowers the barrier for the use of reconfigurable computing machines consisting of a microprocessor coupled to an RPU.

2.6 Dynamic Reconfiguration

A unique feature of reconfigurable architectures is their capability to dynamically reconfigure the hardware resources at run-time and possibly on demand. This reconfiguration, or programming of the architecture, is typically achieved by loading the configuration data values to program reconfigurable resources. Reconfiguration can be a complete (or full) configuration (i.e., programming all the reconfigurable resources) or a localized (or partial) configuration operation (i.e., programming a set of reconfigurable resources).

This reconfiguration process can be accomplished by the use of a variety of architectural support mechanisms to store and apply configurations, namely:

- Architectures with on-chip memory, able to store a set of configurations
- Multiple on-chip configuration planes, also called contexts (see, e.g., [309]), able to switch very quickly between configurations
- On-chip configuration controllers, able to be programmed in order to orchestrate the configuration of hardware resources based on a flow of configurations

Given the nontrivial costs of reconfiguration, either to load the configuration data from an external device or simply because of the actual reconfiguration process, it is common for systems to support a pipelined operation between the programming of a given configuration and the execution with an active/existing configuration. This overlapping of reconfiguration with computation mitigates, or even eliminates, the reconfiguration time overhead. Figure 2.11 depicts an example of pipelining reconfiguration and computation for an illustrative architecture that supports partial reconfiguration. In this example, configuration 1 is being executed while portion `b` of configuration 2 is being loaded and programmed onto the reconfigurable fabric.

Partial reconfiguration can be fine- or coarse-grained. In a fine-grained partial reconfiguration, the architecture is able to individually change the logic function, ALU operation of a specific FU, a connection, or the logic values of a set of bits (e.g., to specify a new constant value). In a coarse-grained partial reconfiguration, it is possible to change sets of FUs and interconnection resources based on columns, rows, or selected regions. With RPUs that allow partial reconfiguration, it is possible to reconfigure regions of the RPU while others are executing. For architectures supporting partial reconfiguration, and depending on the amount of the resources to be reconfigured, the reconfiguration time might be substantially shorter than the one required when only full reconfiguration is supported. Reconfiguration based on

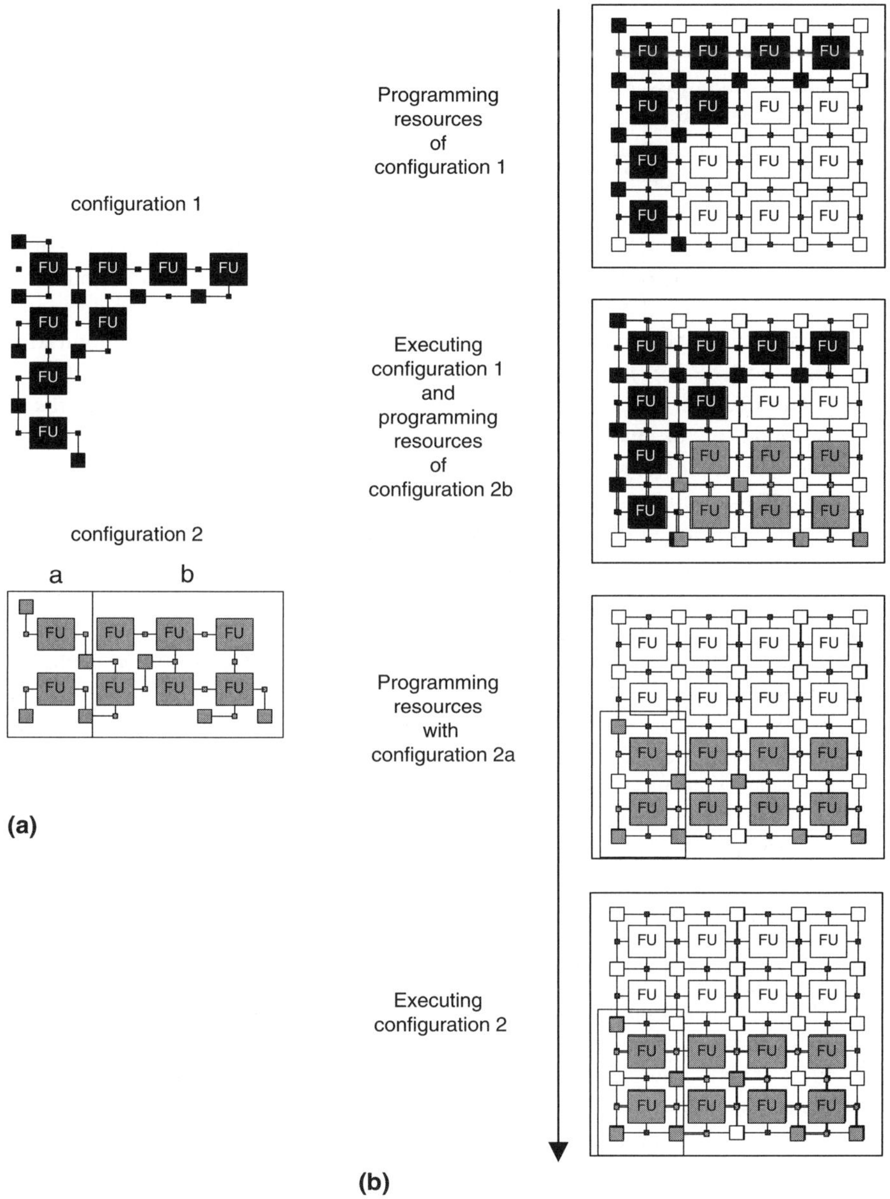

Fig. 2.11 Example of partial reconfiguration and pipelined operation: (**a**) two configurations; (**b**) execution flow

layers of on-chip configuration planes, selected by context switching, has been addressed by Ling and Amano [194, 195], DeHon [87], and Fujii et al. [113]. This technique allows an efficient time-sharing of RPUs by more than one task, or by a large task that can be partitioned in time to fit in the available reconfigurable area.

Despite its flexibility, partial reconfiguration is not widely available in today's reconfigurable devices. The lack of such support is prevalent in fine-grained reconfigurable architectures. Partial reconfiguration in fine-grained RPUs raises the issue of interference between two or more configurations, as they may dispute hardware resources (e.g., interconnection resources or configurable blocks). Usually, to avoid these interferences, designers direct tools to perform placement and routing of the designs on disjoint areas of the RPU, which can be unfeasible when both designs have to use the same resources, e.g., I/O ports. In addition, there is also the issue of data saving and data communication between configurations. For coarse-grained architectures, however, these issues are less problematic and most of them do support partial dynamic reconfiguration and data communication between configurations (see, e.g., the XPP [68]).

The architectural support for dynamic reconfiguration can also influence the execution model of the underlying architecture. In Fig. 2.12, we depict four generic illustrative examples for reconfigurable architectures using a configuration cache (Fig. 2.12a) or on-chip multicontext planes (Fig. 2.12b). In this illustration, *fetch* (F) refers to the movement of configuration data between the off-chip memory and the configuration cache or the multicontext planes, *configure* (CONF) or *context-switch* (CS) refers to the actual configuration of resources in the architecture (from the configuration data in the configuration cache or directly by context switching of the multiple contexts, respectively), and *compute* (COMP) refers to the execution of computations in the architecture with previously configured resources.

We now illustrate two scenarios with partial reconfiguration using the three stages previously described (fetch, configure, and compute). In the first scenario (see Fig. 2.12d), configurations are locally applied to different areas of the architecture. When the computation completes with the first configuration, the execution is ready to start the computation with the second configuration. In the second scenario (Fig. 2.12e), both configurations share areas of the architecture and the programming of the second configuration can only be completely carried out after the computation using the first configuration terminates. Note, however, that hiding the programming or loading of a second configuration, as presented in Fig. 2.12d, is also dependent on the computation and programming time of the two phases of reconfiguration being overlapped. Finally, we illustrate in Fig. 2.12f the concept of context switching, where configurations already stored in the hardware context planes can be activated in short time.

Dynamic reconfiguration raises the issue of the control flow of configurations. To support control flow, the reconfigurable architecture may use a scheme to communicate events to the configuration controller by means of special connections or special registers. A simple approach uses connections from the array (e.g., FU outputs) to the configuration controller to identify the next configuration or to signal the end of the computation with the current configuration. An example of an architecture supporting this is the XPP [31]. In the XPP, events generated in the array can be connected to special configuration controller ports, which can be used to trigger the next configuration.

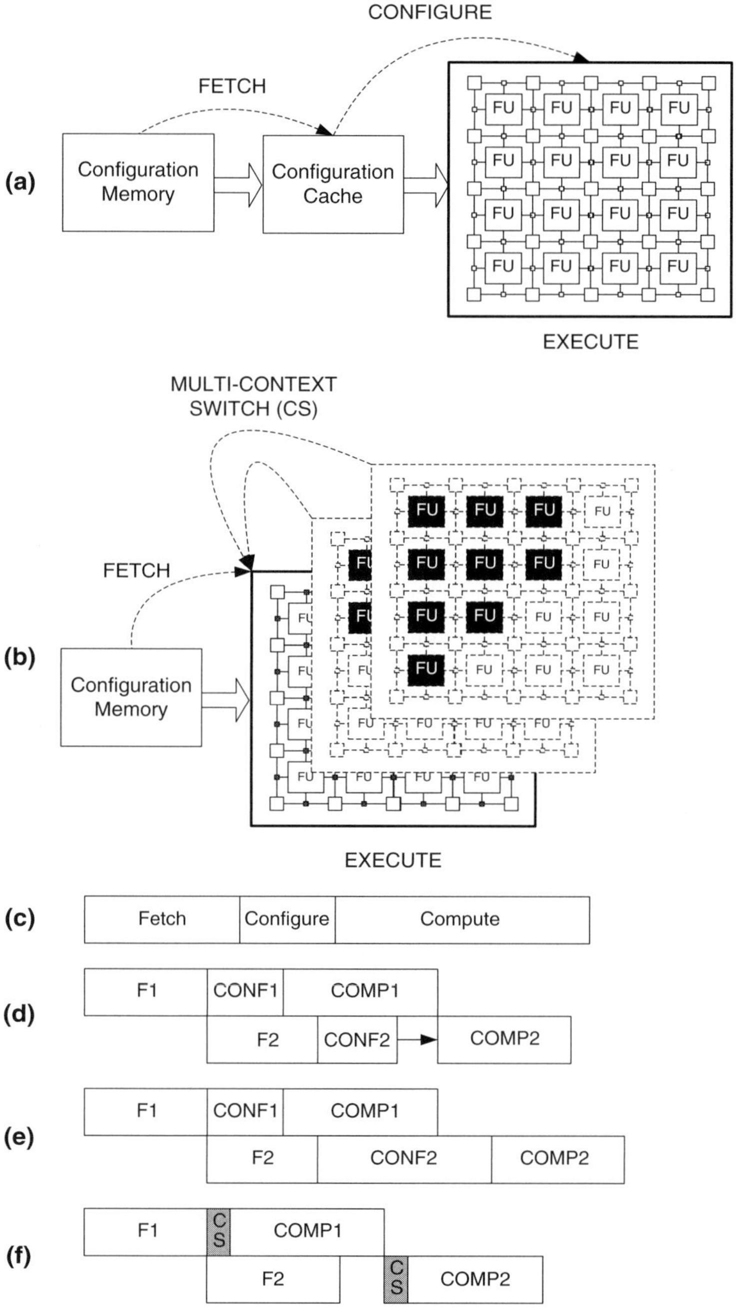

Fig. 2.12 Possible execution phases in reconfigurable architectures: (**a**) architecture with configuration cache; (**b**) architecture with on-chip memory for fast context switching; (**c**) execution stages for architecture (**a**); (**d–f**) execution examples

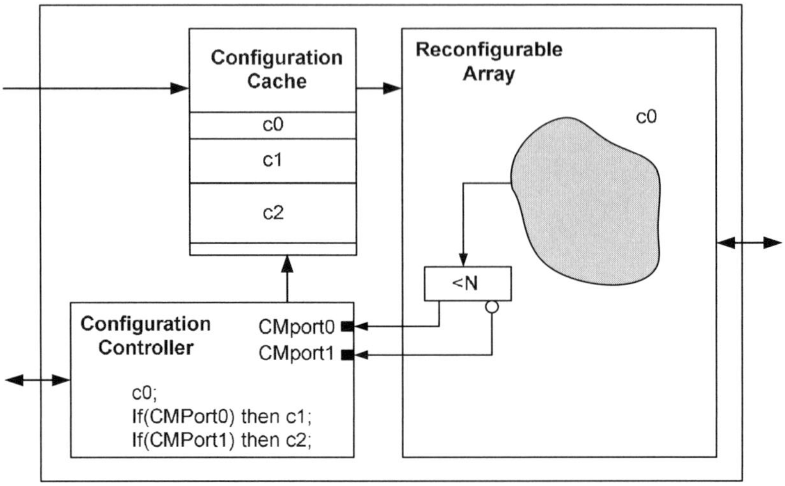

Fig. 2.13 Conditional request of configurations c1 and c2 by configuration c0

Figure 2.13 depicts a simple example where one of two configurations (c1 or c2) is configured and executed after the completion of configuration c0. Based on the comparison result, one of these two configurations c1 or c2 is requested. The configuration controller accommodates the microcode[7] to execute the flow of configurations related to the application under execution. It checks the configuration controller ports and based on the value of the event starts the next configuration step.

In this kind of architecture, prefetching is used to amortize the time required for loading the configuration data onto the internal configuration cache. However, whenever a configuration is not in cache, the configuration controller has to fetch it from the external memory. In the case of the XPP, the configuration controller initiates the programming of a subsequent configuration as soon as it is determined and the execution of the current configuration has terminated. Another, more advanced, possible reconfiguration process is to use partial reconfiguration as soon as the controller determines the subsequent configurations. As each PE has a state flag that identifies if it is being used or not, the configuration controller can use this information to overlap the execution of the current configuration with the configuration of subsequent ones. When configuring the hardware resources for a subsequent configuration, the configuration controller is able to configure first the resources not in use by the current configuration. The completion of the loading and programming of the subsequent configuration depends on the conflicting use of hardware resources between the two configurations, on the execution time of the current configuration, and on the total configuration latency of the subsequent configuration.

[7] The configuration controller can be viewed as a microcontroller, a microprocessor, or a programmable FSM.

2.7 Computational and Execution Models

Fine-grained reconfigurable architectures have the potential to emulate many (if not all) distinct computational models because of the fine granularity of their configurable elements and their extreme interconnection abilities. Using fine-grained architectures, designers can use arbitrary computational functions and storage and, more importantly, arbitrary control structures. The huge configurability space has prevented the emergence of a high-level programming and coarse-grained execution model, as designers and engineers in general wish to retain the freedom of designing their custom architectures and execution models using low-level programming languages and hardware abstractions.

Coarse-grained reconfigurable architectures have offered several distinct, yet restricted, execution models specific to certain domains of application. Typically, the functional and storage elements exhibit some configurability, but the control schemes tend to be more limited. For these architectures, a handful of execution models have naturally emerged dealing with data streaming and pipelining. Examples of those execution models have been considered in architectures such as RaPiD [101], PipeRench [132], and SCORE [72, 92].

In general, there have been different approaches to define a control scheme and the corresponding execution model for the computations to be executed in reconfigurable architectures:

- Embedded control units such as specific FSMs, implemented with the resources of reconfigurable architectures (used in FPGA designs), or control schemes based on the static dataflow model (used in the XPP architecture), where a ready/acknowledge protocol is used on each FU and specific control events may flow through the FUs.
- VLIW type of instructions with the control flow being managed by a configuration controller used in linearly oriented architectures such as RaPiD.
- A combination of the above two possibilities, where each VLIW type instruction defines a configuration consisting of control and data-path units. This approach can be used in FPGAs when the application is executed with more than one configuration or in architectures such as the XPP.

In Fig. 2.14 we illustrate the main difference between VLIW processor execution style and a coarse-grained reconfigurable architecture, in this case a one-dimensional array (Fig. 2.14c). Using VLIW control (Fig. 2.14b), the movement of data between operands is done using the register file (Fig. 2.14d). In some instances the access to the data in the register file is constrained in time, as not all FUs might have simultaneous access to all the registers (or to the same register file when in the presence of cluster-based VLIW architectures). Thus, the assignment of an operation to an FU is driven not only by the capability of that FU to execute the operation but also by the scheduling of the accesses to the registers. By exposing operation-level parallelism, the compiler can schedule groups of operations to be part of each VLIW instruction, as depicted in Fig. 2.14d.

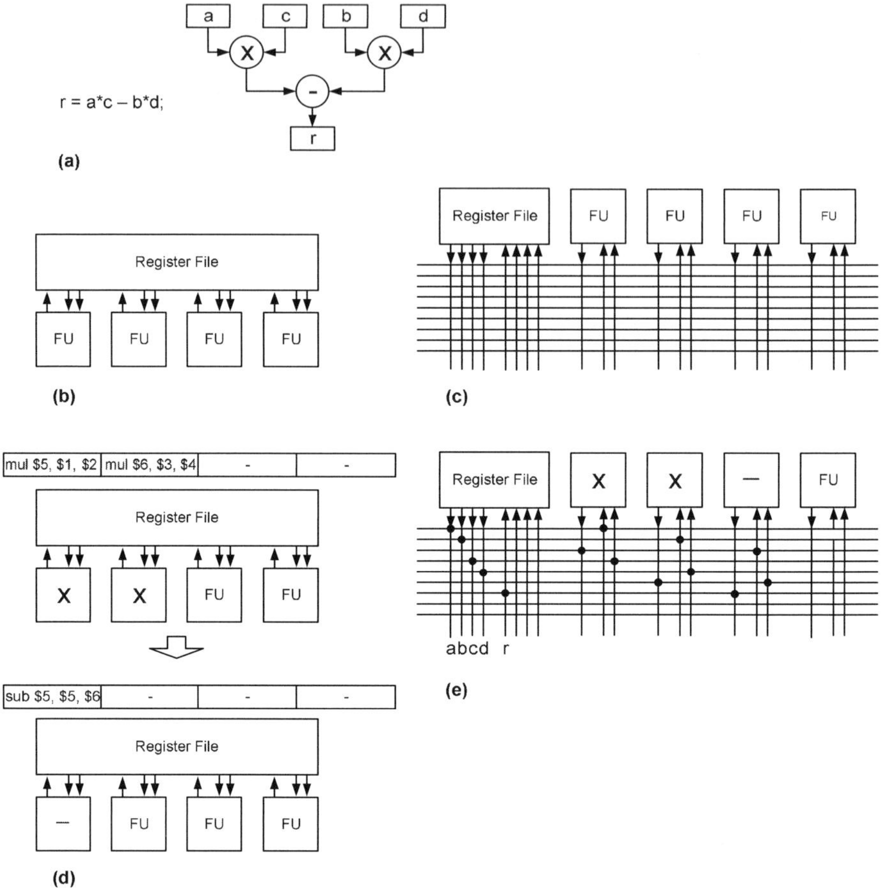

Fig. 2.14 Example comparing VLIW-style architectures to reconfigurable architectures: (**a**) input example; (**b**) VLIW architecture with a centralized register file; (**c**) reconfigurable linear array (1-dimensional); (**d**) possible execution of the example in the VLIW; (**e**) possible execution of the example in the reconfigurable linear array

Reconfigurable architectures can be viewed as a set of FUs, as in VLIW-style architectures, and programmable interconnection resources. In this case and as opposed to usual VLIW-style architectures, it is possible to directly interconnect FUs (by chaining them as depicted in Fig. 2.14c), thus allowing operands and results to be transferred directly between them. This transfer, without the use of interim storage elements (e.g., the register file), allows the implementation, in a single instruction (or configuration), of several levels of operations (Fig. 2.14e). As invariably the interconnection resources are limited, the assignment of operations to the FUs (known as placement) can be an important factor for the routability between the FUs as is usually the case in two-dimensional reconfigurable architectures. Sophisticated interconnections, however, require advanced routing algorithms leading to long placement and routing steps.

Finally, an aspect of VLIW-oriented execution model, also used by reconfigurable architectures, is the use of *if-conversion* [11] and predicated execution techniques to handle control structures (e.g., *if-then-else*). Examples of reconfigurable architectures using predicated execution include the ADRES [208] and the XPP [31] architectures.

2.8 Streaming Data Input and Output

Another key aspect of reconfigurable architectures is their unique ability to provide very high input and output data bandwidth. This is particularly significant in real-time applications or when data (possibly from various sensors) needs to be organized, processed, or classified in a short period of time. In this context, reconfigurable architectures can directly provide hardware support for data access modes (including streaming) in combination with pipelined execution techniques. This support is accomplished by several hardware mechanisms, namely:

- Specific address generation units coupled to the reconfigurable array allow it to store and load data to/from the memories to the FUs. This is the solution used by the Xputer [149] and RaPiD [101] architectures.
- Specific load/store operations in some of the cells of the architecture allow one or more FUs to perform load and store operations over shared memory. This is the solution used in the ADRES architecture [208].
- Configuration of architecture resources to create specific and distributed load/store units to access internal or external memories of the array. In this case, the memories are seen as additional array components and interconnection resources and FUs are allocated to create the needed address generation units and to route data from/to the memories to/from FUs. This is the solution used in FPGAs and in the XPP [31].

In an effort to address the important stream-oriented data paradigm, researchers have developed programming languages constructs with streaming semantics [127]. Typically, the high-level language streaming constructs are translated to FIFO buffer hardware structures with dedicated hardware controllers to orchestrate the movement of data between streams.

2.9 Summary

In this chapter we have summarized the fundamental aspects related to reconfigurable computing architectures. We have described relevant fine-grained to coarse-grained reconfigurable architectures. Although the arena of reconfigurable architectures is dominated by companies (Xilinx and Altera) providing fine-grained architectures, there have been several research efforts on coarse-grained reconfigurable computing architectures both by academia and industry. Due to the high flexibility of reconfigurable computing, supporting architectures are not tied to any specific computational model and thus different models have been proposed. This flexibility has also been the source of different compilation strategies as emphasized in the following chapters.

Chapter 3
Compilation and Synthesis Flows

When mapping applications to reconfigurable computing platforms composed of general-purpose processors (GPP) and reconfigurable architectures, compilers must assume the dual role of compiling for a known instruction-set architecture (ISA) and synthesizing an application-specific architecture to be implemented with the hardware resources of the underlying reconfigurable architecture. The compiler is thus responsible for the definition of the specific organization of the computing engine implemented in the reconfigurable processing units (RPUs). As reconfigurable systems offer the possibility of multiple processing elements (PEs), compilers must deal with the many aspects of parallel computing and all its associated compilation techniques, namely, processor synchronization, data partitioning, and code generation. It is thus not surprising that compilation for reconfigurable systems is notoriously hard as compilers must weave, in a coherent and effective way, techniques from parallel computing with techniques from traditional hardware synthesis.

In this chapter, we outline and describe the main phases of a generic compilation and synthesis flow for reconfigurable systems. We begin by highlighting the specific responsibility of each compilation phase and their interplay. Given their significance in terms of definition of the overall computing architecture, we describe in detail the internal structure of common high-level synthesis and compilation for fine-grained and coarse-grained reconfigurable architectures, respectively. We then illustrate the application of the various compilation and synthesis concepts with examples of the mapping of computations expressed in the C programming language to fine-grained and coarse-grained reconfigurable architectures. We conclude this chapter highlighting a series of issues that directly impact the complexity and the effectiveness of compilation and synthesis for these architectures.

3.1 Overview

Figure 3.1 depicts a generic compilation and synthesis flow for reconfigurable computing platforms. In this description, we focus on aspects that deal with the interaction between the high-level compilation and synthesis for RPUs, and give less emphasis to system-level organization issues.

J.M.P. Cardoso, P.C. Diniz, *Compilation Techniques for Reconfigurable Architectures*,
DOI 10.1007/978-0-387-09671-1_3,

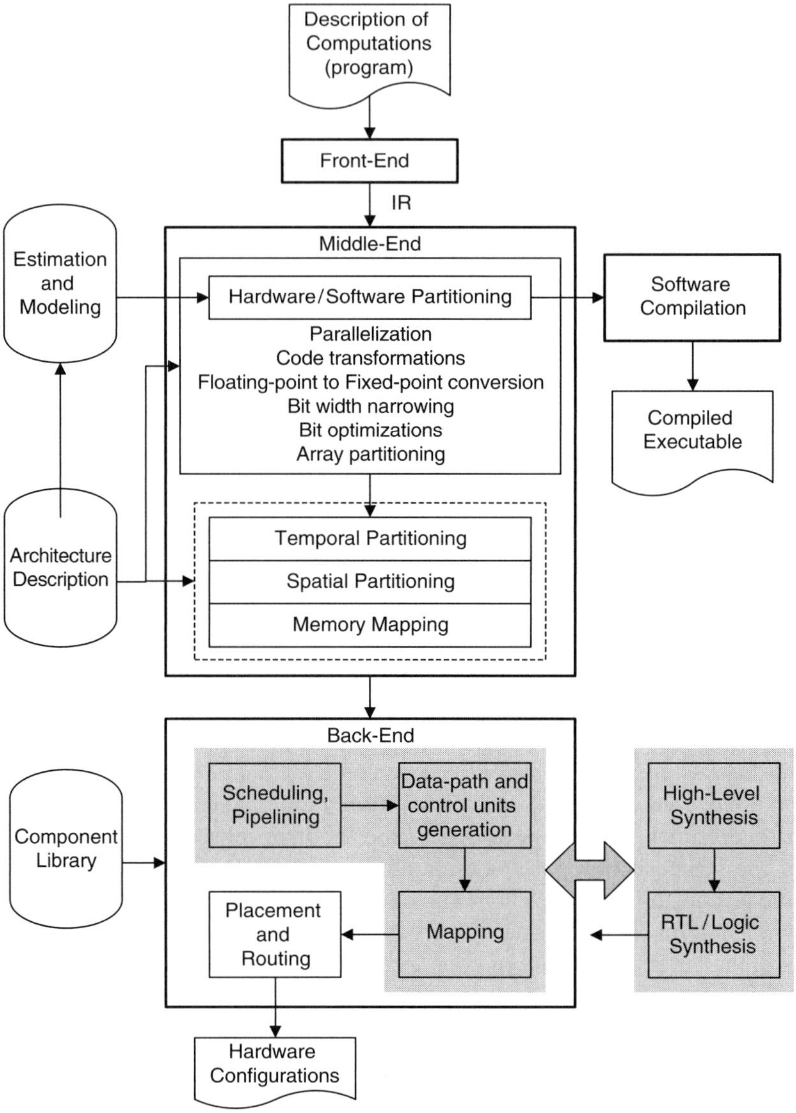

Fig. 3.1 Generic compilation/synthesis flow for reconfigurable computing systems

3.1.1 Front-End

As with traditional compilation flows, the typical compilation and synthesis flow for reconfigurable architectures is structured as a sequence of phases. First, a *front-end* phase interfaces the input program or computation specification decoupling the specific aspects of the input programming language (e.g., its syntax) from an intermediate representation. This front-end is similar to any compiler front-end for traditional programming languages in that it validates the syntax of the input program and possibly applies syntactic-level transformations such as macroexpansion or function inlining. Depending on the input language, the front-end may map constructs in the input code to sequences of intermediate representation instructions exposing their underlying sequential and concurrent nature while preserving the semantics of the input language. For instance, for languages with nondeterminist evaluation order, the front-end can impose a specific order or generate a concurrent evaluation representation. It is uncommon for front-ends to apply source-to-source transformations that are specific to the underlying reconfigurable architecture, but rather relegate these transformations to the middle-end.

3.1.2 Middle-End

Next, the flow is composed of a middle-end where it applies a diversity of architecture-independent transformations (e.g., elimination of redundant memory accesses) and architecture-dependent transformations (e.g., array data partitioning) without engaging in specific code generation or synthesis for the target reconfigurable devices.

As many of the reconfigurable computing platforms include a traditional GPP, the partitioning of the overall computation and data between the GPPs, called the software components, and the RPUs, called the reconfigurable hardware component, is a key aspect in this phase. This hardware/software partitioning [192] is typically guided by estimates of specific performance metrics such as execution time, hardware resources needed, power dissipation, and/or consumed energy.

Given the high costs of reconfiguration in current architectures, this partitioning can also be instrumental in hiding the latency of the reconfiguration processes. By scheduling the reconfigurations at appropriate points in the execution of the program, the overlapping between reconfiguration and execution can be maximized hence hiding, in some cases even completely, the execution time cost of reconfiguration [237].

After hardware/software partitioning, the software component is compiled onto a target GPP using a native compiler for that specific processor. The components of the solution mapped to the RPU are subject to different compilation approaches according to the RPU type. Two main approaches are common for this compilation. For fine-grained reconfigurable architectures (e.g., FPGAs) the middle-end (in co-operation with the back-end) will be responsible by the complete definition of the RPU component of the system and the communication scheme between the RPU and the GPP or in the case of a system with multiple RPUs, the communication between them. For these fine-grained architectures this definition is accomplished using a hardware-oriented synthesis tool. For coarse-grained reconfigurable architectures, where some of these communication aspects may already be directly supported by the underlying architecture, the definition of the communication schemes is performed by synthesis-related steps of the flow that establish the routing of the data through the various RPUs and the GPP.

Irrespective of the granularity of the target architecture, the middle-end still needs to partition that data and the computation, and orchestrate the execution of the computation among the many units by the insertion of communication primitives or instructions to ensure the communication of data in a timely fashion. The partitioning process may be even more complex when the target architecture has multiple PEs and/or when the communication schemes between them have been defined at design time, as is common for embedded systems [212].

The existence of a truly multiprocessing execution environment also requires the compiler to make decisions about the execution models to use, such as pipelining, either fine- or coarse-grained, or whether to take advantage of multithreading execution techniques to exploit as much concurrency as possible. While some code transformations used by the middle-end exploit high-level architectural aspects, such as the existence of multiple RAM modules to increase the availability of data, other transformations exploit the ability to customize specific functional units (FUs) to directly implement high-level instructions in hardware.

We can thus classify the transformations the middle-end applies in three broad categories, namely:

- **Spatial-Oriented:** Given the spatial nature of reconfigurable architectures and their inherent limited resources, the compiler must perform spatial partitioning of the data and computations. These transformations include the partitioning, allocation, and management of data between internal storage resources so that data and computation are collocated.
- **Temporal-Oriented:** In this class of transformations, we include all execution-related transformations that schedule, either using fine- or coarse-grained techniques, the computation onto the available RPUs. These include pipelining execution, assigning to each RPU a specific function, or partitioning, in a time-shared fashion, the computations among the available resources.
- **Custom-Oriented:** The transformations in this class exploit application-specific arithmetic formats and operations. These include arithmetic conversions between operations in floating-point formats to use fixed-point or nonstandard bit-width formats, representations, or rounding modes.

As highlighted in Fig. 3.1, memory mapping of the data, in space and time, is a key aspect in a reconfigurable system. At a high-level system organization, there is rarely the abstraction of a single address space. Common reconfigurable architectures have local RAMs and/or memory modules that can be programmed to be organized in a variety of bit-width memory sizes and depths. Each memory has its own addressing space and corresponding addressing hardware structures. As a result, it is uncommon to have hardware translation mechanisms that enforce any sort of data consistency between memories. The reconfigurable features, both on routing data and customizing storage units, place a burden on the compiler to orchestrate the flow of data between the various memories to match in space and in time with the execution of the computations in the various RPUs.

A typical middle-end thus largely supports the bulk of the efforts in the compilation flow and commonly makes use of supporting mechanisms and techniques, namely:

- **Architecture Description:** This description, commonly embedded in the compilers' internal algorithms, allows the compilation flow to determine the number and capacity, in terms of computing elements (e.g., configurable logic blocks or simple RAM modules) of existing reconfigurable devices. The knowledge of the relative capacity and speed of storage structures and their placement with respect to computing elements allows the compiler to perform judicious decisions about data and computation partitioning, as well as register versus memory caching.
- **Estimation of Mapping Decisions:** These estimates provide the compiler with an approximation in terms of resources and/or execution time for a specific mapping choice. Compilers use these estimates to adjust the aggressiveness of their mapping strategies. For instance, while applying *loop unrolling* a compiler can quickly exceed the available hardware resources. When back-end phases such as placement and routing require extremely long time, estimation provides a reasonable trade-off between hardware design accuracy and design exploration time.

Most, if not all, commercial tools rely on programmers to dictate the application of the supported transformations, either by use of directives or indirectly via constraints used in internal algorithms. Various research prototypes have shown the value of using estimates to effectively drive transformations and mapping algorithms (see, e.g., [96, 180]). Some design-space exploration algorithms use feedback from previous mappings in the form of estimates to backtrack and possibly undo several high-level transformations. By using estimates derived in a fraction of the time, that it would take for a compilation flow to derive the actual designs, tools can effectively explore a wide range of mapping choices that would be otherwise impractical.

3.1.3 Back-End

Lastly, the compilation flow includes a back-end for code generation and architectural synthesis. The architectural synthesis can be accomplished by a combination of two synthesis forms. In a first form, architectural synthesis is performed using a set of basic primitive blocks such as memories, registers, and predefined custom library blocks. The reconfigurable fabric implements those blocks and arbitrary topologies using its reconfigurable hardware resources. Once the target architecture is defined, the back-end schedules the execution of macro-operations and/or instructions alongside the generation of the concrete hardware architecture to carry out these operations. In a second form, a reconfigurable architecture natively supports a predefined, less flexible, set of operations. This is the case of coarse-grained reconfigurable arrays where the computations must be mapped to the underlying PEs (e.g., ALUs). A combination of the both forms is possible when the underlying fine-grained reconfigurable resources are used to combine high-level hardware templates that resemble the typical coarse-grained architectures, with the arbitrary blocks and topologies.

The back-end is thus responsible for the following concrete steps:

- **Code Generation:** This step is responsible for augmenting the source code, or the translation to intermediate format, with primitives to load the configurations in the RPU, synchronize their execution, and orchestrate the movement of data throughout the execution. Typically, it focuses on high-level scheduling and mapping abstractions, such as the mapping of data to global memories and synchronization between RPUs or the coarse-grained pipelining of the execution. The interaction with a host processor and the interface with a global memory are also addressed in this step.
- **Architecture Synthesis:** This step performs the synthesis of the specific hardware architecture to execute the computations assigned to each RPU. Typically, this synthesis performs the classical steps of allocation, scheduling and binding of low-level operations given the hardware and execution time constraints derived by the application of high-level transformations. The resulting bit-stream configuration (the set of bits that define the hardware design) is to be loaded on the appropriate RPU, which, and depending on the specific features of the RPU, can include classical instructions with a mix of programmable logic definitions.

The back-end code generation step outlined here commonly relies on system-level abstractions, such as the organization of the overall data streams and storage, and on the existence of a set of primitives for data communication, loading of configurations, and execution synchronization reminiscent to operating systems' services. These primitive services are typically very specific to the overall system organization of each reconfigurable system, such as address space organization, data consistency, and distributed control. The variety of system organizations using RPUs has, we believe, led to the lack of the definition of a de facto standard Application Programming Interface (API) to provide a common interface to a wide variety of systems.

The architecture synthesis step is also very dependent on the target reconfigurable fabric. In many instances, the fabric explicitly defines the internal and external organization characteristics of data-paths, FUs, and the corresponding execution controllers and address generation units designed to carry out the execution of the computation assigned to each RPU. In hybrid reconfigurable devices, such as emerging FPGAs with *hardcores* or *softcores* and programmable logic, compilation and synthesis can be truly mixed in the same step. While in many cases these steps are accomplished by the integration of commercial synthesis tools using target-specific component library modules, other efforts have developed their own approaches to map their computations onto the RPU using specific techniques that take advantage of particular architectural features.

3.2 Hardware Compilation and High-Level Synthesis

We now outline the main phases of hardware compilation and synthesis approaches as they provide the interface to the high-level hardware compilation flow depicted in Fig. 3.2. This high-level hardware compilation flow is organized into three major phases, namely, High-Level Synthesis (HLS) [114], RTL and Logic Synthesis [210], and Placement and Routing [266]. Still in the same flow, the compiler can internally generate an architecture using specific optimizations and including the required high-level synthesis steps. In this scenario, the flow usually outputs a behavioral RTL–HDL (Register Transfer Level–Hardware Description Language) hardware description as the input to RTL/logic synthesis. In this approach, the architecture is completely tuned to the application and it is built aware of the characteristics of the fine-grained resources of the target architecture.

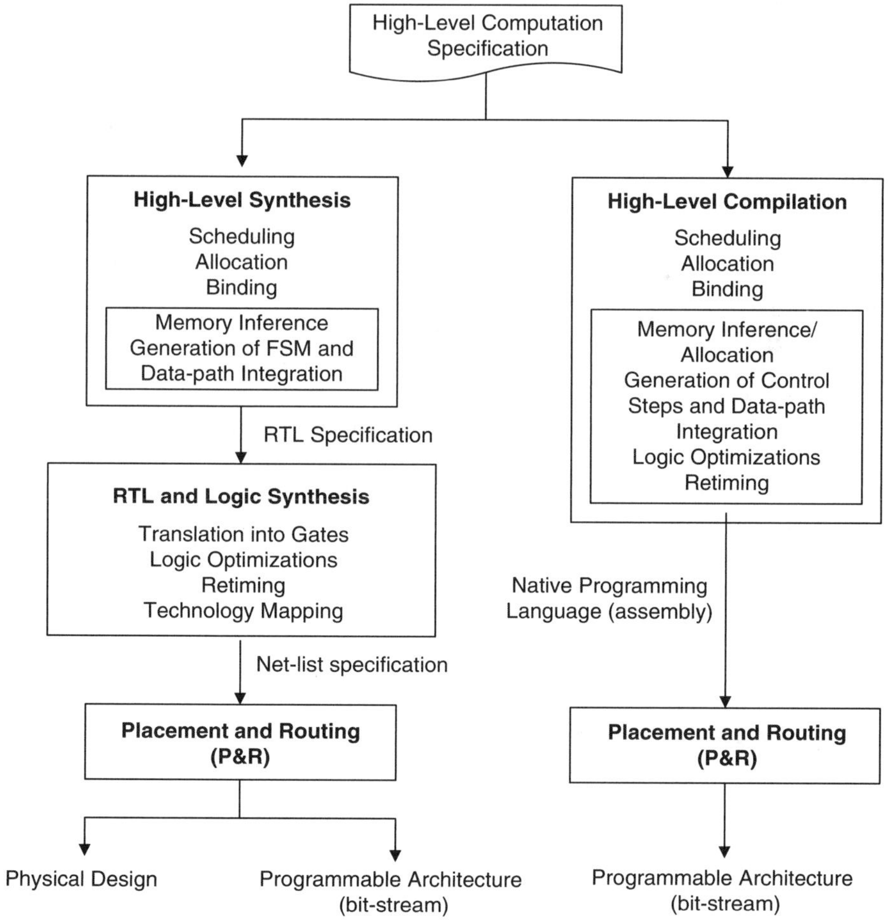

Fig. 3.2 Hardware compilation and high-level synthesis

Overall the granularity of the target reconfigurable architecture drives the kind of hardware compilation approach. When targeting fine-grained reconfigurable architectures, the compilation and synthesis flow may use high-level synthesis [114] tools for generating the application-specific architecture and then use RTL/logic synthesis [51, 210] tools for mapping this architecture to basic logic components. The input to this flow consists of a high-level representation of the computations using a common HDL, such as VHDL [162] or Verilog [163]. This specification is usually referred as behavioral at algorithmic level,[1] as the binding in time and space of its basic operations is not explicitly defined. A possible approach for the compilation flow, used for example in the DEFACTO compiler [96], relies on the compiler to generate the input HDL algorithmic representation required by this high-level synthesis flow from the computation's intermediate representation. The flow then leverages the capabilities of high-level synthesis tools to generate a feasible hardware implementation that meets the required performance and architecture resources constraints.

In the variant of the flow targeting coarse-grained reconfigurable architectures, the compiler translates high-level input operations into sequences of macroinstructions to be executed by each of the coarse-grained PEs. While the compiler now has a lesser role in architecture definition (as it relies on the existence of well-defined building blocks of the underlying architecture), it still needs to generate a mix of assembly and reconfigurable instruction descriptions. This compilation does not eliminate the need for data and computation partitioning as each PE typically performs ALU operations and has very limited local data storage. Despite the coarser granularity of the target architecture, the compiler still needs to engage in a form of placement and routing to assign operations to physical PE resources and to channel the data through the physical interconnection resources.

In both these compilation and synthesis flows variants, the output is a very precise specification of the execution of the input computations taking into account the hardware resources and time allocated for the execution. This very low-level specification can take on many forms depending on the precise nature of the target architecture. Compared to an ASIC (Application-Specific Integrated Circuit) design, where the flow must generate, possibly with the help of a library of standard cells or custom cell macros, a mask specification for fabrication, the flow for a programmable architecture must generate a bit-stream with the precise configuration of its many programmable points.

3.2.1 Generic High-Level Synthesis

High-level synthesis, also commonly referred to as behavioral synthesis and architectural synthesis, performs the three basic high-level functions or steps of allocation, scheduling, and binding [114], possibly carried out in this order. These basic

[1] We adopt here the widely accepted taxonomy presented in [320].

functions typically use a library of components consisting of hardware resources such as registers, multiplexers, and basic arithmetic and logic operators. Before these steps, however, the flow translates the input HDL description to an internal representation form commonly using a control/data-flow graph (CDFG) representation [114]. After this translation, the high-level synthesis flow performs allocation in which it determines which operations in the CDFG are to be allocated to what kind of FUs. Based on the allocation decisions and possible timing and/or resource constraints, the flow determines the scheduling of the operations, i.e., which operations are executed at each control step (commonly corresponding to a clock cycle). In the following step, binding, the flow determines, based on the previous allocation and scheduling steps, which operations are executed by each FU instance. Lastly, the flow derives, from the schedule and binding of operations, a finite-state machine (FSM) to control the underlying data-path that consists of the FU instances, registers, and additional routing logic.

Although conceptually simple, high-level synthesis hides many challenging aspects. For instance, the scheduling is highly dependent on the mapping of data to memories and the number of data ports they offer as well as the use of pipelined components as are the cases with multipliers and RAMs. Many commercial high-level synthesis tools provide an interface that allows users, and in their absence compilers, to define the number and kind of resources available (e.g., FU types and instances) as well as the mapping of array variables to RAM modules. In addition, the input language allows for users to specify which loops should be unrolled and in some case by how much. These facilities allow designers to explore a wide range of hardware implementations for a variety of resources and memory mapping settings.

To illustrate the variety of design choices possible in high-level synthesis, we depict in Fig. 3.3 a hardware synthesis example for a loop construct in VHDL that manipulates several array variables. The figure depicts three alternative design choices, denoted as implementations `A`, `B`, and `C`, high-level synthesis may consider, based on the use of pipelined execution techniques and on the number of hardware multipliers available. For each of the three implementations we illustrate the corresponding execution schedule for a sample choice of memory access latency of three clock cycles and considering an array variable mapping where each array is mapped to a distinct RAM module. Mapping various array variables to the same RAM module would lead to different schedules given the potential RAM contention issues. We further assume that multipliers have a latency of four clock cycles and when pipelined have an initiation interval of one clock cycle. Addition/subtraction operators are nonpipelined with a latency of two clock cycles.

3.2.2 Customized High-Level Synthesis for Fine-Grained Reconfigurable Architectures

In this variant of high-level synthesis, the compilation flow targets a fine-grained reconfigurable architecture that is organized as a set of highly parameterized and

```
FOR i IN 0 TO N LOOP
  x(i) := (a(i) * b(i)) - (c(i) * d(i)) + f(i);
END LOOP
```

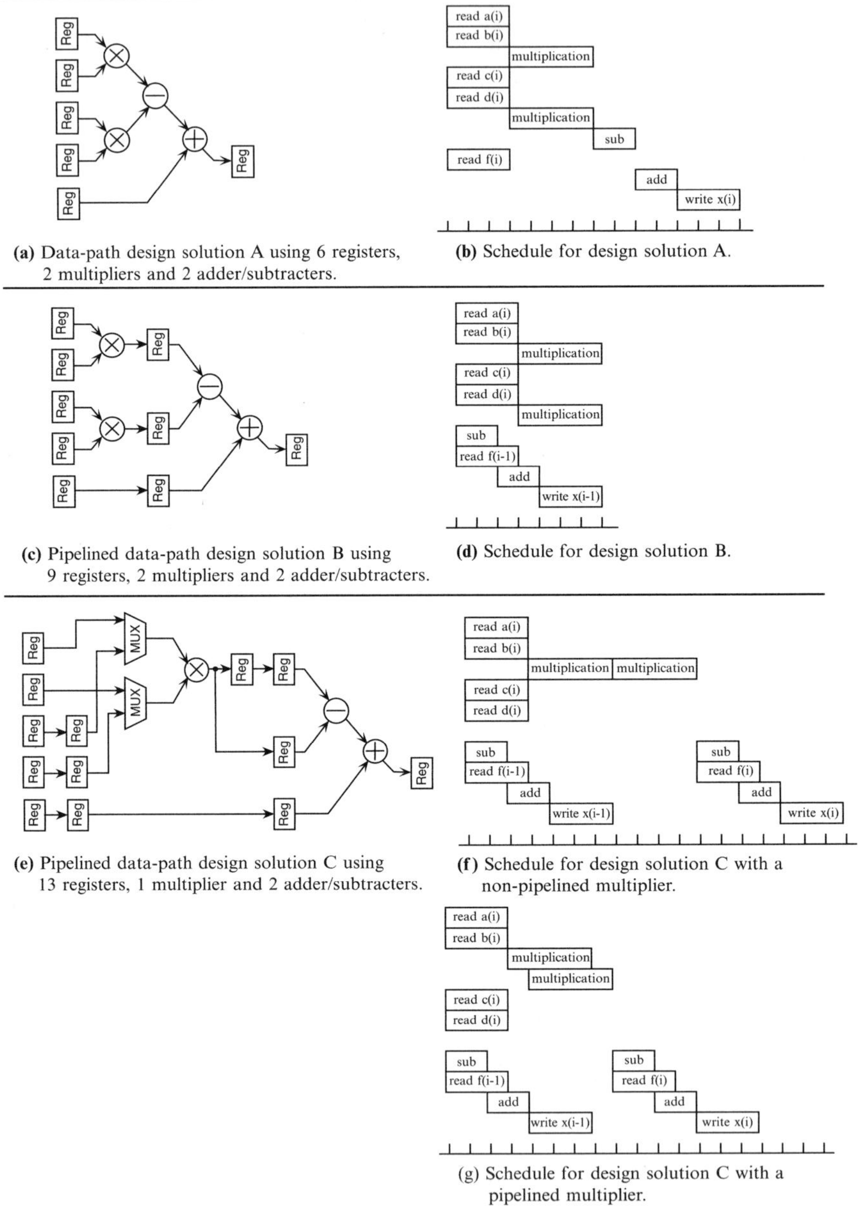

(a) Data-path design solution A using 6 registers, 2 multipliers and 2 adder/subtracters.

(b) Schedule for design solution A.

(c) Pipelined data-path design solution B using 9 registers, 2 multipliers and 2 adder/subtracters.

(d) Schedule for design solution B.

(e) Pipelined data-path design solution C using 13 registers, 1 multiplier and 2 adder/subtracters.

(f) Schedule for design solution C with a non-pipelined multiplier.

(g) Schedule for design solution C with a pipelined multiplier.

Fig. 3.3 Illustrative high-level synthesis examples

programmable structures. Thus, this customized flow generates application-specific architectures aware of the particular features supported by the target RPU, e.g., the vast number of distributed registers, local memories, distributed multipliers or DSP blocks, hardware virtualization schemes by time-sharing reconfigurable hardware resources among multiple configurations, etc. Another important characteristic of this flow is the fact that it targets an architecture with a predefined layout of configurable hardware structures and not an open layout present when designing ASICs. This aspect leads to high-level synthesis steps typically not strongly driven by resource sharing schemes as with in generic high-level synthesis tools.

As with the previous high-level synthesis approach, the compiler engages in some form of architecture design exploration to determine the best parameters values for each hardware structure. Once this selection is made the compiler relies on synthesis tools, such as RTL synthesis, to generate the concrete solution. Unlike the previously described generic high-level synthesis flow, this flow leverages the structure of the target fine-grain reconfigurable devices which might in some cases impose various space and timing constraints in the characteristics of the generated hardware implementations.

To illustrate this hardware compilation approach we use a sample C code segment that computes the integer values for several hypotenuses as depicted in Fig. 3.4a. Figure 3.4b depicts the corresponding instruction-level CFG. By forming a DFG corresponding to the computations, a compiler can easily generate the architecture shown in the block diagram of Fig. 3.4c.

As with generic high-level synthesis flow, the generated architecture consists of a control and a data-path unit, where the data-path does not consider sharing of hardware components and assumes the existence of the instantiated FUs from a library of synthesizable VHDL components (e.g., multiplier, adder, square root). In this case, we consider that each array variable is mapped to a specific local memory and thus the calculations of the addresses correspond to values of the variable `i`. The control unit can be generated directly from the control-flow graph (CFG) representation [9] where each CFG node, corresponding to a statement in the code, is directly assigned to a state of a FSM controlling its execution.

This simple translation between the CFG representing the computation and the corresponding FSM does not exploit several opportunities for concurrent operation execution. We depict in Fig. 3.5a a modified CFG for the example code where instructions to be executed in parallel were merged in the same CFG node as are the cases of memory loads for arrays `A` and `B`. The state transition graph (STG) depicted in Fig. 3.5b represents the FSM for the corresponding control unit. From this FSM description and the data-path structure depicted in Fig. 3.4b, a compiler can directly generate the VHDL code depicted in Fig. 3.6 implementing both the data-path and the control unit.

An alternative translation to behavioral RTL-VHDL is depicted in Fig. 3.7. This translation relies on the joint representation of a Finite-State Machine with Datapath (FSMD) [115] for the overall computation. This joint representation allows for a simpler translation to RTL-VHDL as it does not require an explicit structural

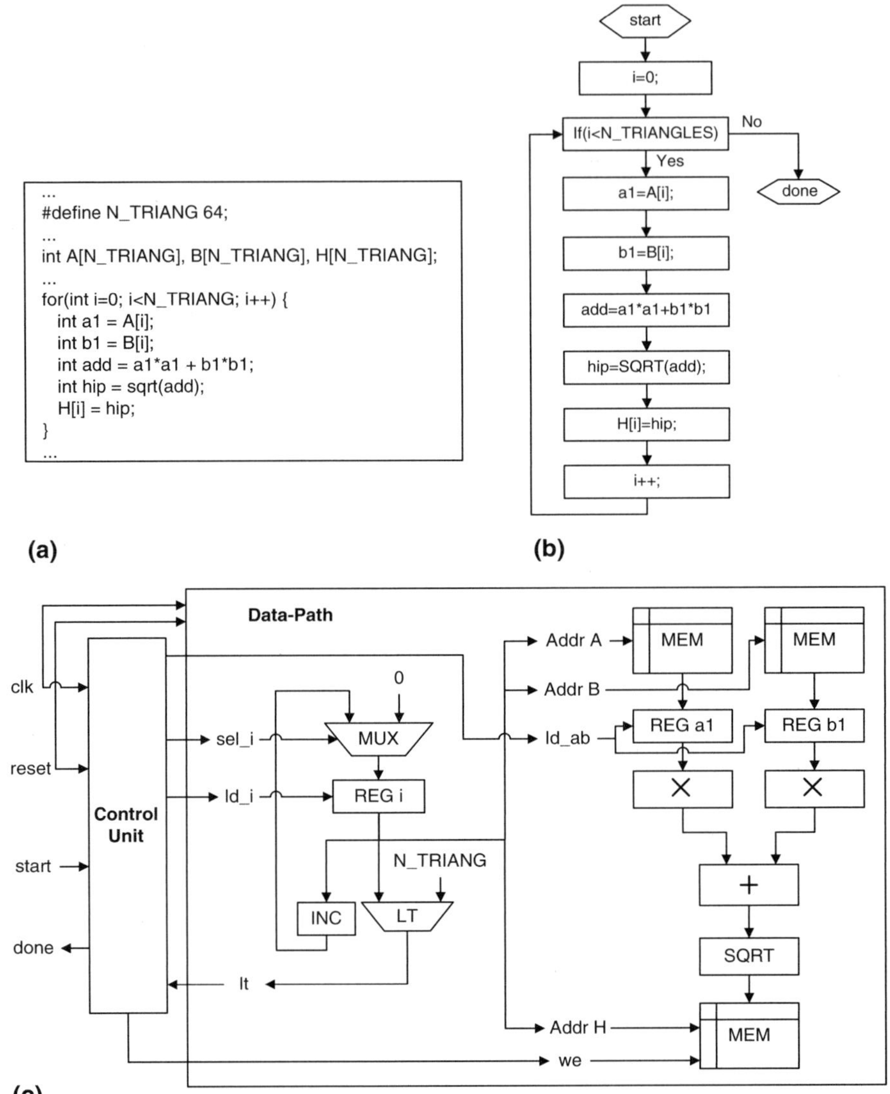

Fig. 3.4 Hardware compilation example: (**a**) high-level description (C code); (**b**) instruction-level CFG; (**c**) block diagram of data-path and control units

data-path definition. It does not, however, directly support multicycle operations. To support these multicycle operations, compilers either decompose the original operations in stages and assign the different stages to distinct FSM states, or abstract multicycle components as structural components.

Both these approaches for the generation of data-path and control units create VHDL specifications that directly use RTL and logic synthesis to create complete

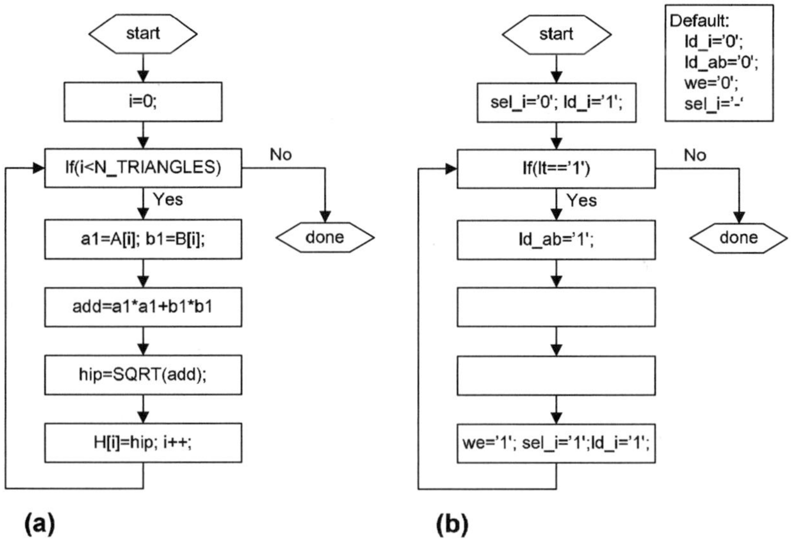

Fig. 3.5 Control unit generation example: (**a**) modified CFG; (**b**) state transition graph

hardware design specifications. Other approaches that generate algorithmic VHDL code, as illustrated by the example in Sect. 3.3, rely on the capabilities of an external high-level synthesis tool.

As with generic high-level synthesis tools, most compilation approaches use a repository of FUs. Typically, each FU and the corresponding control unit are described at behavioral RTL-HDL level and require logic synthesis for the generation of its logic structures. Alternatively, compilers can generate specifications for control units as microprogrammed units, or simple *one-hot* encoding FSMs, thus possibly requiring simple mapping steps or even avoiding the use of logic synthesis tools. In some extreme cases, the FUs can be represented as circuit generators [36,79,209] of the hardware structures of the target reconfigurable architecture, eliminating the need for logic synthesis. Leveraging logic synthesis for hardware generation offers, nevertheless, the advantages of better portability, as HDL input descriptions may not explicitly use specific components of the target architecture.

3.2.3 Register-Transfer-Level/Logic Synthesis

RTL/logic synthesis translates hardware specifications in RTL, possibly generated by high-level synthesis, into equivalent circuit specifications in terms of logic gates. The input to RTL synthesis consists of a description of the operations implemented by a hardware design specifying the inter-clock behavior of each operation. RTL/logic synthesis translates these operations into gate-level descriptions,

```
library IEEE;
use IEEE.STD_LOGIC_1164.ALL;...

entity pitagoras is
  Port (clk : in  STD_LOGIC; reset : in  STD_LOGIC;
        start : in  STD_LOGIC; done : out  STD_LOGIC;...);
end pitagoras;

architecture Behavioral of pitagoras is
  component add
  GENERIC (...); PORT (
    I0          : in   std_logic_vector(w_in1-1 downto 0);
    I1          : in   std_logic_vector(w_in2-1 downto 0);
    O0          : out  std_logic_vector(w_out-1 downto 0) );
  END component;
  ...
  component lt
   GENERIC (w_in  : INTEGER := 16); PORT (
    I0            : in   std_logic_vector(w_in-1 downto 0);
    I1            : in   std_logic_vector(w_in-1 downto 0);
    O0            : out  std_logic);
  END component;
  constant N_TRIANG : integer := 64;...
  signal reg_i, inc_i, mux_out: std_logic_vector(WIDTH-1 downto 0);
begin
  MEM1: MEM generic map(32,ADDR_WIDTH,N_TRIANG) port map(d_in=>in1,
  addr=>REG_i(ADDR_WIDTH-1 downto 0),we=>we1,clk=>clk,d_out=>a1);
  REG1: reg generic map(32) port map(clk=>clk,load=>ld_ab,D=>a1,Q=>a1_reg);

  MEM2: MEM generic map(32,ADDR_WIDTH,N_TRIANG) port map(d_in=>in2,
  addr=>REG_i(ADDR_WIDTH-1 downto 0),we=>we2,clk=>clk,d_out=>b1);
  REG2: reg generic map(32) port map(clk=>clk,load=>ld_ab,D=>b1,Q=>b1_reg);

  sqrt_out(31 downto 16) <= (others => '0');
  MUL1: mul generic map(32,32,32) port map(I0=>a1_reg,I1=>a1_reg,O0=>m1_out);
  MUL2: mul generic map(32,32,32) port map(I0=>b1_reg,I1=>b1_reg,O0=>m2_out);
  ADD1: add generic map(32,32,32) port map(I0=>m1_out,I1=>m2_out,O0=>add_out);
  SQRT1: sqrt port map(A=>add_out,SQRT_A=>sqrt_out(15 downto 0));

  MEM3: MEM generic map(32,ADDR_WIDTH,N_TRIANG)
     port map(d_in=>sqrt_out,
     addr=>REG_i(ADDR_WIDTH-1 downto 0),we=>we3,clk=>clk,d_out=>out1);

  MUX1: mux generic map(WIDTH)
     port map(sel=>sel_i,I1=>inc_i,I0=>ZERO, O0=>mux_out);
  REG3: reg generic map(WIDTH)
     port map(clk=>clk,load=>ld_i,D=>mux_out,Q=>reg_i);
  INC1: inc generic map(WIDTH,WIDTH) port map(I0=>reg_i,O0=>inc_i);
  LESS_THAN1: lt generic map(WIDTH) port
  map(I0=>reg_i,I1=>CONV_STD_LOGIC_VECTOR(N_TRIANG,WIDTH),O0=>lt1);

  FSM1: control_unit port map(clk=>clk,reset=>reset,lt=>lt1,start=>start,
  done=>done,sel_i=>sel_i,ld_i=>ld_i,we=>we3, ld_ab=>ld_ab);
end Behavioral;
```

(a)

```
library IEEE;
use IEEE.STD_LOGIC_1164.ALL;...

entity control_unit is
  Port ( clk : in  STD_LOGIC; reset : in  STD_LOGIC;
         lt : in  STD_LOGIC; start : in  STD_LOGIC;...);
end control_unit;

architecture Behavioral of control_unit is
  TYPE states IS (RESET_STATE,WAIT_START,INIT_STATE,...);
  signal CURRENT_STATE, NEXT_STATE: states;
begin
  PROCESS (CURRENT_STATE, start, lt)
  BEGIN
        done <=  '0'; sel_i <= '0';
        ld_ab <= '0'; ld_i <= '0';
        CASE CURRENT_STATE IS
        WHEN RESET_STATE =>
           NEXT_STATE <= WAIT_START;
        WHEN WAIT_START =>
          if ((start = '1')) then NEXT_STATE <= INIT_STATE;
          else NEXT_STATE <= WAIT_START ;
          end if;
        WHEN INIT_STATE =>
          sel_i<='0'; ld_i<='1';
          NEXT_STATE <= LOOP_HEADER;
        WHEN LOOP_HEADER =>
          if (lt = '1') then NEXT_STATE <= LOOP_BODY_1;
          else NEXT_STATE <= END_STATE;
          end if;
        WHEN LOOP_BODY_1 =>
          ld_ab <= '1';
          NEXT_STATE <= LOOP_BODY_2;
        WHEN LOOP_BODY_2 =>
          NEXT_STATE <= LOOP_BODY_3;
        WHEN LOOP_BODY_3 =>
          sel_i<='1'; ld_i<='1'; we <= '1';
          NEXT_STATE <= LOOP_HEADER;
        WHEN END_STATE =>
          done <=  '1';
          NEXT_STATE <= WAIT_START;
        END CASE;
        END PROCESS;

  PROCESS (clk, reset)
  BEGIN
    if (reset = '1') then
      CURRENT_STATE <= RESET_STATE;
    elsif (clk'event and clk = '1') then
      CURRENT_STATE <= NEXT_STATE;
    end if;
  END PROCESS;
end Behavioral;
```

(b)

Fig. 3.6 Behavioral RTL-VHDL ready for RTL and Logic Synthesis: (**a**) data-path structure with the control unit; (**b**) control unit description

resulting in a net-list output specification with logic gates and register components that comprise the data-path and its controller.

A technology mapping process is thereafter performed by logic synthesis taking as input a net-list specification and mapping the logic gates specification to the hardware resources supported by the target architecture or hardware library. In this mapping process, logic synthesis attempts to minimize the hardware resources and/or critical path delays by exploiting specific target architecture features as is the case of carry-chains in the implementation of adder circuits. For fine-grained reconfigurable architectures, this synthesis process maps gate-level specifications to pre-existing configurable logic elements in the target architecture [51]. In this case, the flow performs the mapping of gates (or sets thereof) to these configurable elements, a step known as mapping [210].

Advanced RTL/logic synthesis tools include various optimizations for speed and area, e.g., to increase operating clock frequency and/or to minimize hardware

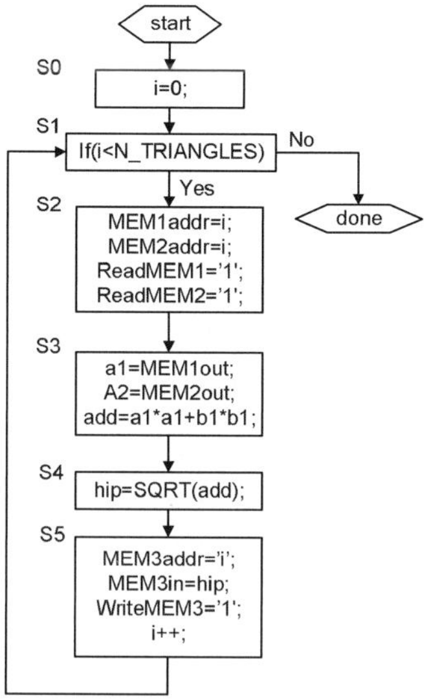

(a)

(b)

```
...
architecture Behavioral of FSMD is
  TYPE states IS (RESET_STATE, WAIT_START, S0, S1,...);
  signal CURRENT_STATE, NEXT_STATE: states;
  ...
begin
  PROCESS (CURRENT_STATE, start)
      variable i, ...
  BEGIN
      done <= '0'; ...
      CASE CURRENT_STATE IS
      ...
      WHEN S0 =>
        i := 0;
        NEXT_STATE <= S1;
      WHEN S1 =>
        if(i<N) NEXT_STATE <= S2;
        else NEXT_STATE <= END_STATE;
        end if;
      WHEN S2 =>
        MEM1addr := i;
        MEM2addr := i;
        ReadMEM1 := '1';
        ReadMEM2 := '1';
        NEXT_STATE <= S3;
      WHEN S3 =>
        a1 := MEM1out;
        a2 := MEM2out;
        add := a1*a1+b1*b1;
        NEXT_STATE <= S4;
      WHEN S4 =>
        hip := SQRT(add);
        NEXT_STATE <= S5;
      WHEN S5 =>
        MEM3addr := 'i';
        MEM3in := hip;
        WriteMEM3 := '1';
        i++;
        NEXT_STATE <= S1;
      WHEN END_STATE =>
        done <= '1';
        NEXT_STATE <= WAIT_START;
      END CASE;
  END PROCESS;

  PROCESS (clk, reset)
  BEGIN
    if (reset = '1') then
      CURRENT_STATE <= RESET_STATE;
    elsif (clk'event and clk = '1') then
      CURRENT_STATE <= NEXT_STATE;
    end if;
  END PROCESS;
end Behavioral;
```

Fig. 3.7 Behavioral RTL-VHDL using an FSMD description style: (**a**) algorithmic state machine (ASM) chart; (**b**) part of the corresponding VHDL

resources, respectively. One such important optimization is retiming [210], which aims at minimizing critical path delays by moving, and possibly inserting, registers throughout the circuit at the operation and/or gate level. Even though the overall latency of the implementation is unchanged, retiming may lead to faster executions as it enables the use of higher clocking rates, thereby increasing the throughput of its pipelined execution.

3.2.4 High-Level Compilation for Coarse-Grained Reconfigurable Architectures

A second variant of a high-level compilation flow targets coarse-grained reconfigurable architectures as depicted in Fig. 3.2. In this flow, the compiler constructs, using coarse-grained PEs such as ALUs and predefined interconnection blocks, a computing engine that offers a register-like instruction execution model. Given the constrained control and data-path structures at its disposal, the compiler has less freedom to match application-specific operations to the underlying architecture than with previous fine-grained reconfigurable architecture flows.

Besides the inclusion of common front-end and middle-end phases shown in Fig. 3.1, compilers for coarse-grained reconfigurable architectures have a back-end phase that generates an RTL description of the target code and typically do not require traditional logic synthesis or high-level synthesis. They still require, however, and often in a combined fashion, scheduling and placement and routing steps. The scheduling step is responsible for the generation of the execution control in each PE using either microcode (as in the RaPiD [101] architecture), or special control structures distributed in the reconfigurable array (as in the XPP [31] architecture). In the placement and routing step, the compiler assigns the register-like instructions to each PE and routes the results between them.

Regarding memory operations, there are two general scenarios. In one scenario, the architecture directly supports load/store memory operations in specific PEs that interface memory modules (memory accesses are performed as common processor load/store instructions). In a second scenario, all the data communications to/from memories are carried out by specialized memory interface units using customized address generation units. In this second scenario, the compiler may generate both control specifications and address generator units for selected PEs to synchronize the execution of the PEs with the memory interface units.

We illustrate this approach in Fig. 3.8 using the structure generated for the example in Fig. 3.4a, when targeting a coarse-grained data-driven reconfigurable architecture. We use as reference the XPP architecture [31] which directly supports a ready/acknowledge protocol between the PE components. The block diagram in Fig. 3.8 reflects a high-level data-flow organization of the original code. In this case, a counter (`CNT_UP`) is used to implement the original `for` loop behavior. One key aspect of this data-driven architecture, with a ready/acknowledge protocol, lies on its need not to delay the signals `wr` and `Addr_H`. A write access can stall the counter operation while waiting for the data from one PE to ensure the correct values are output to memory. To implement loop pipelining, the hardware implementation requires a sequence of registers to save the successive values of `wr` and `Addr_H`. The values for these signals are saved in a tapped-delay line until they reach the output memory while the counter is able to continue its operation. Although these details are very specific to a given architecture, they reflect the granularity of data and computation synchronization arising when compiling to coarse-grained architectures.

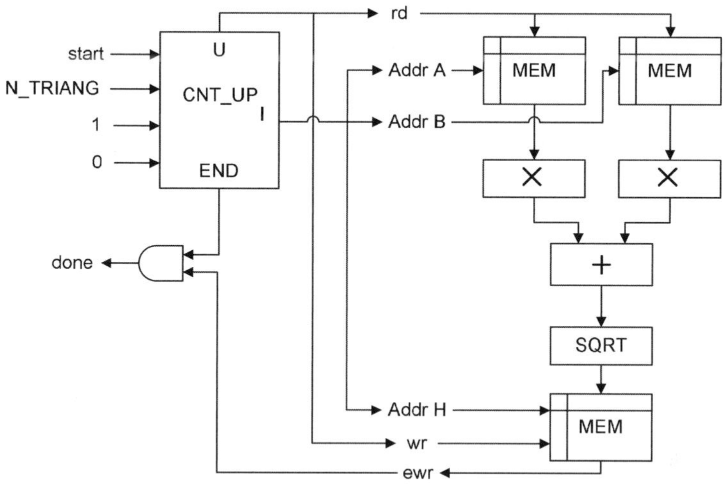

Fig. 3.8 Data-path organization example when targeting a data-driven coarse-grained reconfigurable architecture

In the case of the XPP, the hardware specification outlined above is output by the XPP-VC compiler [68] as an NML description, the XPP internal mapping language. The NML language represents XPP components, such as memories and operations (designated as XPP objects), to be mapped to the PEs of the array, and the interconnections between them to be routed through the physical interconnection resources. NML descriptions can include preplaced, or relatively placed, components/objects to ensure that a specific object is assigned to a specific physical resource in the array. NML descriptions are mapped and placed and routed by the `xmap` tool, responsible for satisfying timing constraints and balancing execution path delays imposed by the compiler. Figure 3.9 depicts a segment of NML generated by the XPP compiler.

3.2.5 Placement and Routing

It is common to both fine- and coarse-grained reconfigurable architectures to include a step of placement and routing (P&R) as the last step of a compilation and synthesis flow. This step takes a description of the configurable elements and their interconnections, and maps them to the physical hardware resources of the target reconfigurable architecture. After this placement and routing step, the tool generates a bit-stream specifying the configurations of each of the reconfigurable elements of the device. When loaded and programmed onto the reconfigurable device, this bit-stream will allow the device to implement the application-specific architecture. Depending on the granularity of the target reconfigurable architecture, the P&R process can be very time-consuming as it needs to map and interconnect each logic node to a physical node or configurable element in the target reconfigurable fabric. Due to

```
...
MODULE PITAGORAS {
 OBJ INTRAM5: IRAM @ $1,$0 {
  RD = N4.X
 }
 OBJ INTRAM6: IRAM @ $1,$1 {
  RD = N4.X
 }
 OBJ INTRAM7: IRAM @ $1,$2 {
  WR = N4.X
  IN = N13.X
  EWR = 0
 }
 OBJ N4: CNT_UP {
  STEP = Start.U EOR N29.R
  B =! 511
  A = 0
  A = N25.X
 }
 OBJ N13: MUL {
  B = INTRAM5.OUT
  A = INTRAM5.OUT
 }
 ...
 DELAY_CONSTRAINT(N21.R->CMPort0.IN == 0)
 ...
}
...
```

Fig. 3.9 A segment of NML code generated by the XPP-VC compiler

its inherent algorithmic complexity, most P&R tools resort to simulated annealing techniques [334] for the specific placement step, a proven robust approach for arbitrary designs [39].

Although it is common for compilation flow to carry out the steps of operation scheduling and placement and routing independently, there are, however, significant combined approaches. This is the case of the *modulo scheduling* technique based on congestion negotiation and simulated annealing. This approach is used by the DRESC compiler to map loop kernels to the ADRES coarse-grained architecture [207]. Another use of the module scheduling technique for mapping loops onto coarse-grained reconfigurable architectures is referred to as *modulo graph embedding* [240], and is based on a technique to map a guest graph into a host graph.

An alternative approach to compile-time placement and routing techniques, seldom explored in the context of reconfigurable architectures, is the use of hardware-assisted dynamic, run-time approaches [91, 335]. Generic run-time techniques can leverage placements in previous designs and/or rely on expensive first placement and routing of a computation amortizing these early costs in subsequent executions of the same computation. As with dynamic approaches in other compilation domains, run-time placement and routing techniques tend to sacrifice resource usage for speed, requiring in the case of the use of hardware-assisted techniques, additional specific hardware resources. As such, this dynamic P&R approach has not been adopted in an industry where device occupancy and resource use is a metric of great importance for end customers.

3.3 Illustrative Example

We now illustrate the various phases of the generic compilation flow described in Fig. 3.1 when mapping a computation specified using the popular C programming language to a reconfigurable architecture. The computation is translated to a behavioral algorithmic VHDL description or to a behavioral RTL-VHDL description ready for high-level synthesis or for RTL/logic synthesis, respectively. We opted for this particular example to show a translation from the C source code to an algorithmic VHDL description, highlighting the specific construct that resulted from the application of high-level compiler transformations. In this example, we target a generic FPGA device and omit for simplicity the output results regarding the actual synthesis process using commercial synthesis tools.

3.3.1 High-Level Source Code Example

The input computation for our example is depicted in Fig. 3.10 and is inspired in common image processing sliding-window kernels such as the ones used in edge-detection algorithms. The code is structured as an outer-loop in the body of which there are two loop constructs, respectively, `loop 1` and `loop 2`. The loops manipulate double-precision array variables `A`, `B`, and `C` and integer array variables `D` and `E`. The first loop computes the average of the elements of array `A` in a 2-by-2 window over consecutive rows and columns of the array (statements `s11` to `s13`)

```
#define DIM  16
#define N    DIM-2

double  A[DIM][DIM];
double  B[DIM][DIM];
double  C[DIM];
int     D[DIM];
int     E[DIM][DIM];

double  s1;
double  s2;
double  threshold;
```

```
Loop 0: for(i = 0; i < N; i++) {

Loop 1: for(j = 0; j < N; j++) {
S11:       s1 = A[i][j] + A[i][j+1]
S12:       s2 = A[i+1][j] + A[i+1][j+1];
S13:       u = (s1 + s2) /4.0;
S14:       B[i][j] = u;
S15:       if(u > threshold) {
               D[j] = D[j] + 1;
           }
       }

Loop 2: for(j = 0; j < N; j++) {
S21:       B[i][j] = B[i][j] * C[i];
S22:       if(D[j] != 0) {
               E[i][j] = 1;
           } else {
               E[i][j] = 0;
           }
       }
}
```

Fig. 3.10 Sample source C code

and saves the resulting values in array `B` (statement `s14`). It also records how many of these averages are numerically larger than an input threshold value (statement `s15`). The second loop, `loop 2`, scales the array `B` elements by the values in array `C` and uses the values of the `D` array accumulated in `loop 1` to indicate which of the columns of the two-dimensional `B` array has at least one value larger than the given threshold. This indication is recorded by the binary values 0/1 in the two-dimensional `E` integer array.

3.3.2 Data-Flow Representation

The compiler translates the C source code constructs and extracts data and control dependences between the various statements. Its internal representation can be abstracted as a sequence of data flows whose semantics is described by the sequence of basic instructions represented internally as Abstract-Syntax-Tree (AST) constructs or Data-Flow Graphs (DFGs). Figure 3.11 depicts a graphical representation of these data flows highlighting the flow of data between operation constructs such as adders and multipliers and indicating the source array variables for their inputs. In dashed boxes we indicate the statements in the C source code corresponding to each data flow. This representation reveals that, at the data-flow representation level, a possible implementation for the *if-then* construct in statement `s15` uses a multiplexer to

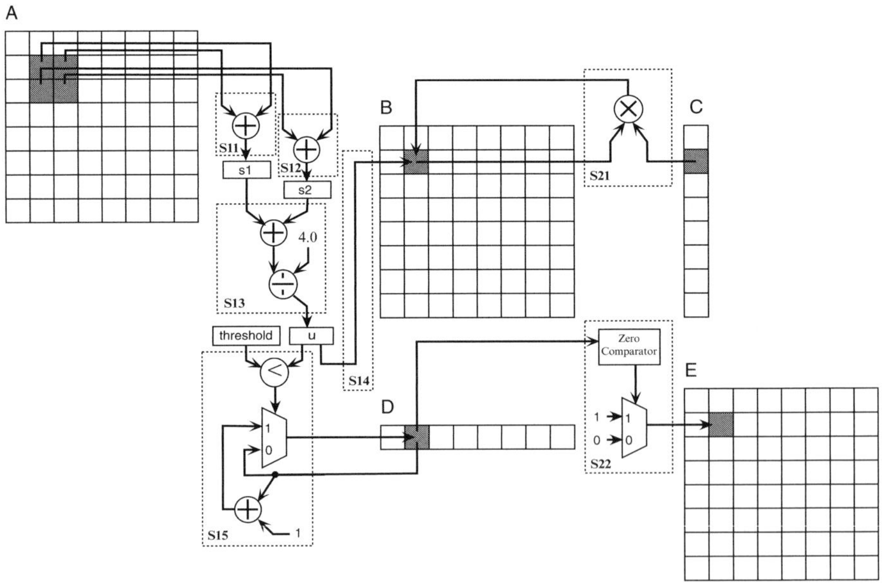

Fig. 3.11 Data flow and data dependences for sample computation

select if an element of the `D` array is updated using its previous value, thus resulting in a no-operation, or using the previous value incremented by 1. A similar representation is depicted for statement `s22`.

The compiler next determines an execution scheme for each of the loop constructs and/or for the overall computation. This scheduling depends on the available resources for the hardware units that will be responsible for carrying out the individual data-flow operations depicted in Fig. 3.11. The compiler must balance the existence of functional resources with the layout of the array data between the available storage resources and derive, at a higher level of abstraction, an execution and synchronization scheme before generation of the VHDL that once synthesized will produce a hardware implementation.

3.3.3 Computation-Oriented Mapping and Scheduling

When defining the overall execution scheme for the computation in the two loops, `loop 1` and `loop 2`, the compiler can exploit several alternatives. Figure 3.12 depicts four possible execution alternatives exploiting task-level and loop-level pipelining, indicating symbolically the execution of the C source code statements and their most significant data dependences. We assume for the sake of this illustration that the underlying hardware architectures consist of two FUs (FU1 and FU2) that execute the statements for each of the two loops.

In Fig. 3.12a we depict the schedule that would result should the compiler wish to explore task level pipelining. Here the compiler assigns the statements in `loop 1` to task `T1` and the statements in `loop 2` to task `T2`. It would then assign `T1` to `FU1` and `T2` to `FU2`. In this scheduling scheme both statements of each task execute sequentially without any loop pipelining. Figure 3.12b depicts the execution that would result by exploiting loop pipelining for each individual task while still executing the two tasks sequentially. At the top of this figure we depict all statements corresponding to tasks `T1` or `loop 1` executing in pipelined fashion with the assumption that each pipelined stage (at this level still abstract) is responsible for the execution of all the operations in each statement.

In Fig. 3.12c we depict a combined scenario of task- and loop-pipelining execution. Here the data dependences between the statements `S14` in `loop 1` and `S21` in `loop 2` prevent `loop 2` to be executed as quickly as would otherwise be possible. This is an important aspect as the analysis of dependences allows the compiler to evaluate the profitability of resource assignments. In this case, and rather than attempting to speed up the execution of the statements in `loop 2`, the compiler could opt for a slower hardware implementation, possibly without pipelined execution to match the execution rate of the statements in `loop 1`.

Another scenario, illustrated in Fig.3.12d, corresponds to the case where the available hardware resources are not enough to implement in a single partition all the computations corresponding to the statements `S11` through `S15`. In this scenario the compiler is forced to split `loop 1` into two loops, say `loop 1a`

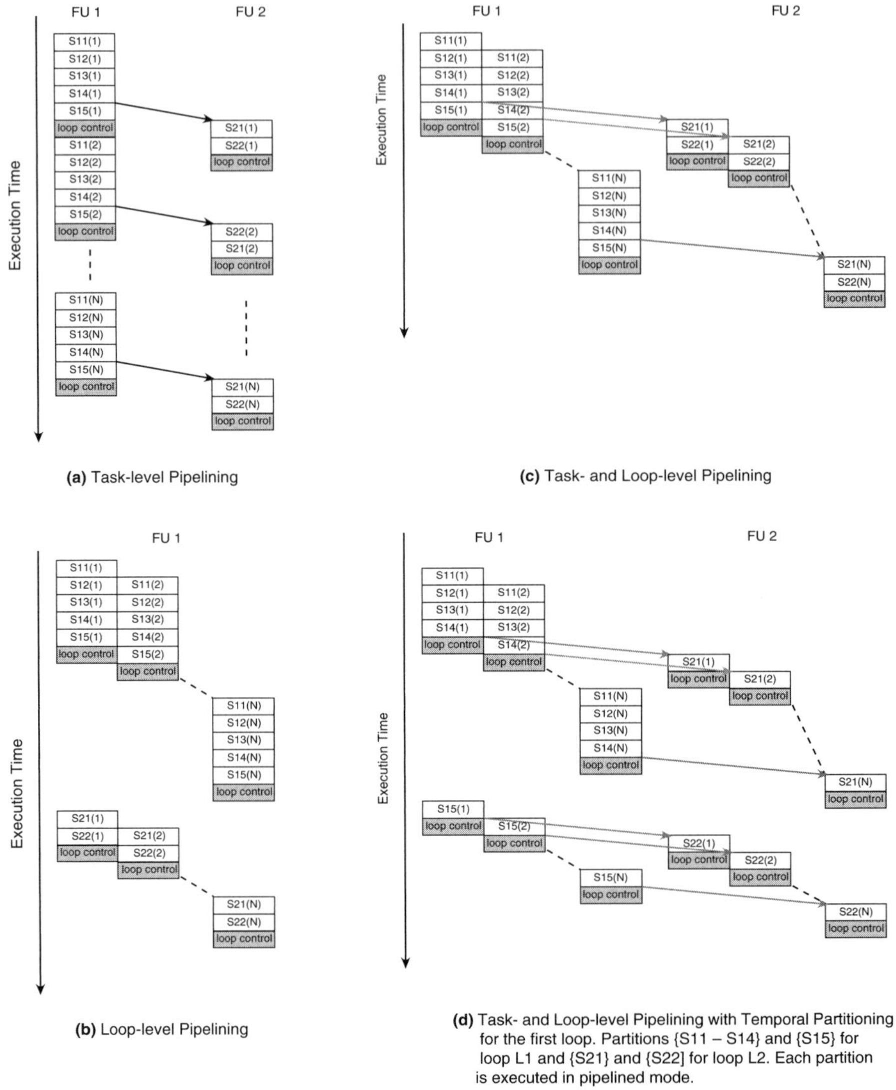

(a) Task-level Pipelining

(b) Loop-level Pipelining

(c) Task- and Loop-level Pipelining

(d) Task- and Loop-level Pipelining with Temporal Partitioning for the first loop. Partitions {S11 – S14} and {S15} for loop L1 and {S21} and {S22] for loop L2. Each partition is executed in pipelined mode.

Fig. 3.12 Task- and loop-level scheduling schemes for example computation

and `loop 1b`, where `loop 1a` retains the statements `S11` through `S14` and `loop 1b` consists of the statement `S15`. This partition transformation, depicted in Fig. 3.13, now requires the compiler to perform another data-oriented transformation called array expansion to promote the scalar variable `u` from a scalar to a four-dimensional array variable. At each iteration of `loop 1a`, the `j`th position of `u` records the value computed in that iteration of the original loop which is then used on the same iteration of `loop 1b`.

```
#define DIM  16
#define N     DIM-2

double A[DIM][DIM];
double B[DIM][DIM];
double C[DIM];
int D[DIM];
int E[DIM][DIM];

double u[DIM];

double s1;
double s2;
double tmp;
double threshold;
```

```
Loop 0: for(i = 0; i < N; i++) {

Loop 1b: for(j = 0; j < N; j++) {
s11:          s1 = A[i][j] + A[i][j+1]
s12:          s2 = A[i+1][j] + A[i+1][j+1];
s13:          tmp = (s1 + s2) /4.0;
              u[j] = tmp;
s14:          B[i][j] =tmp;
         }

Loop 1b: for(j = 0; j < N; j++) {
s15:          if(u[j] > threshold) {
                 D[j] = D[j] + 1;
              }
         }

Loop 2:  for(j = 0; j < N; j++) {
s21:          B[i][j] = B[i][j] * C[i];
s22:          if(D[j] != 0) {
                 E[i][j] = 1;
              } else {
                 E[i][j] = 0;
              }
         }
}
```

Fig. 3.13 Using loop fission and array expansion to support temporal partitioning

3.3.4 Data-Oriented Mapping and Transformations

We now turn our attention to data-oriented transformations and mapping steps, namely the mapping of array variables to RAM modules and data reuse in registers. For brevity we focus on the mapping of arrays `A`, `B`, and `D` to RAM modules for the pipelined execution of `loop 1`. We assume that memory accesses to RAM modules can be pipelined with an initiation interval of one clock cycle and exhibit an access latency of three clock cycles. For simplicity, we assume nonpipelined arithmetic operators such as adders and subtracters with a latency of four clock cycles. A division operation by a power-of-two (implemented as a shift-right operation) and an increment operation, even for 32-bit values, both execute in a single clock cycle. These latencies are for illustrative purposes only and do not represent any specific target architecture.

Figure 3.14a depicts a schedule for a single iteration of the `loop 1` where all arrays `A`, `B`, and `D` were mapped to the same `RAM 0` module. The shaded bars at the bottom of the schedule depict the intervals of activity for the adder/subtracter unit

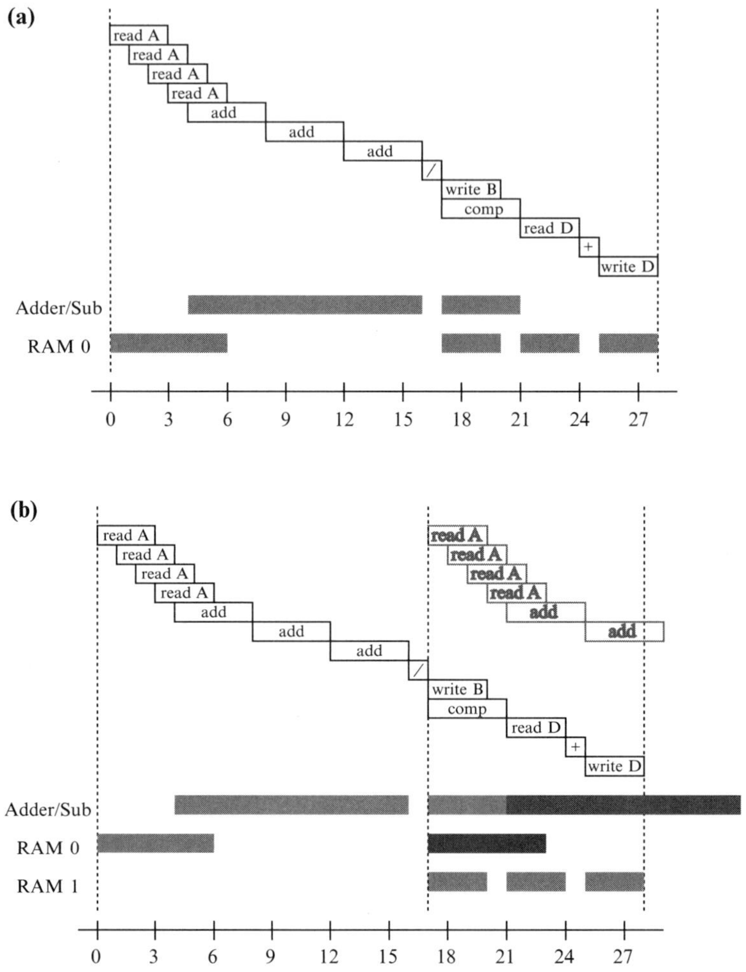

Fig. 3.14 Hardware scheduling under different array to memory mapping choices considering memory pipelined accesses and a single non-pipelined adder/sub unit: (**a**) Schedule for all data mapped to the same RAM 0 module; (**b**) Schedule for array A mapped to RAM 0 and arrays B and D mapped to RAM 1

and the `RAM 0` module.[2] These activity bars highlight that the schedule is limited by the dependences of the read/write RAM accesses and not by the contention at the adder/subtracter unit. The result is a schedule 28 clock cycles long which cannot be pipelined.

The schedule in Fig. 3.14b refers to a hardware implementation with two RAM modules. Here the arrays were mapped as follows: `A` to `RAM 0` and `B` and `D` to

[2] Here the subtracter is used to implement the comparison operation between the variables `u` and `threshold`.

`RAM 1`. The latency of a single loop iteration is still 28 clock cycles, but now it is possible to overlap the execution of consecutive loop iterations. The initiation interval is now 17 clock cycles and the limiting factor is the single adder/subtracter unit as revealed by the collision of the activity bars corresponding to two iteration executions (a light and a dark grey bar sets).

We now explore two additional hardware implementations mapping the array `D` to discrete registers. As depicted in Fig. 3.15a the latency of the execution of a single

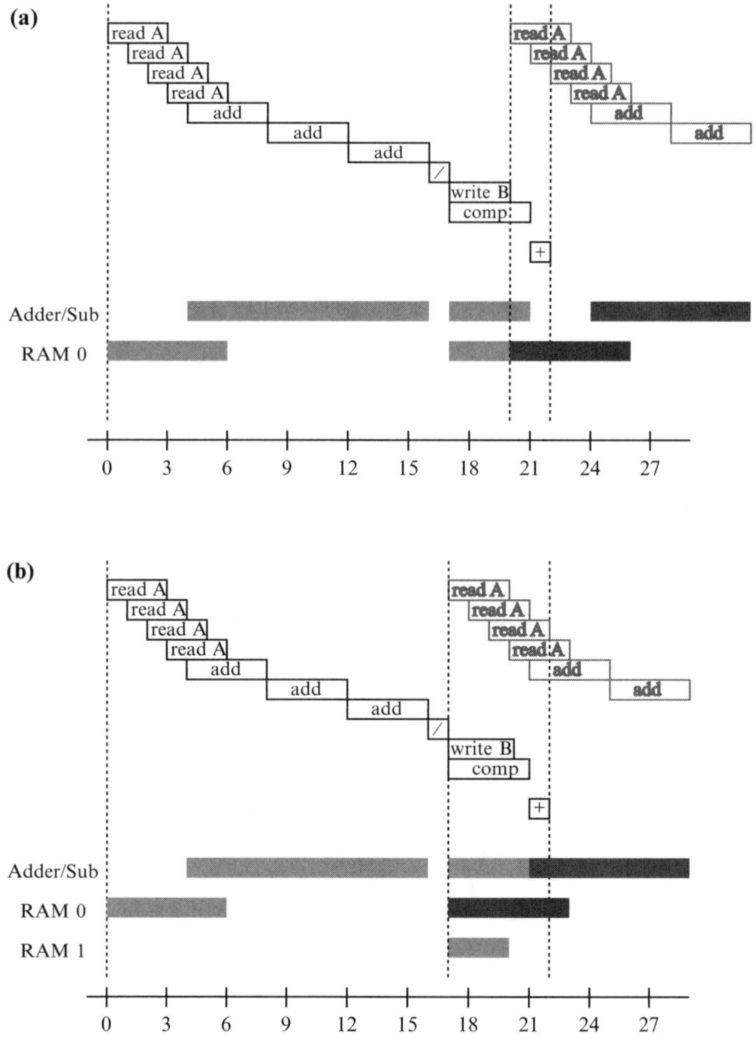

Fig. 3.15 Hardware scheduling under different array to memory and registers mapping choices considering memory pipelined accesses and a single non-pipelined adder/sub unit: (**a**) Schedule for arrays A and B mapped to RAM 0 and array D mapped to registers; (**b**) Schedule for array A mapped to RAM 0, array B mapped to RAM 1 and array D mapped to registers

iteration is reduced to 22 clock cycles as the read and write operations for array D have been incorporated as part of the increment operations directly using registers. Still, and because both arrays A and B are mapped to the same RAM 0 module, the initiation interval is 20 clock cycles as the last write operation on RAM 0 completes at that cycle. To alleviate this contention we augment the hardware implementation with a second RAM and map the array variables A and B to two RAMs. The resulting execution schedule is depicted in Fig. 3.15b. The latency of a single iteration execution is still 22 clock cycles but the initiation interval has been reduced to 17 clock cycles, now only limited by the existence of a single adder/subtracter unit.

The variety of the implementations illustrated above gives a glimpse of the complexity of an overall compilation approach in the presence of multiple loops and multiple arrays and RAM modules. In the four architectures whose schedules are depicted in Figs. 3.14 and 3.15 there are a range of choices for the number of RAM modules to be considered and an even larger number of possible array mappings. Each design choice means exploring a trade-off between execution time and hardware resources. Furthermore, as the examples revealed, in some cases the schedule exposes the bottleneck in the execution of the computation in terms of which resources limit the ability of the compiler to pipeline the execution of a loop. For instance, when all arrays A, B, and D were mapped to the same single-port RAM, even with pipelined accesses, this mapping decision was the limiting factor (see Fig. 3.14a). In this scenario, using more resources, e.g., two adder units, would not lead to any performance improvement thus wasting hardware resources. Conversely, when arrays A and B were mapped to distinct RAMs (see Fig. 3.14b and d) the limiting factor was the single adder/subtracter unit. In this scenario adding more RAM modules or increasing the number of ports would not improve the performance.

These hardware implementations corresponding to available compiler choices are summarized in Table 3.1 for the execution of the loop 1 in the code in Fig. 3.13. For each hardware implementation we present the hardware resources they require and the key pipelined execution metrics they exhibit, in terms of number of clock cycles for the pipeline latency and initiation interval.

3.3.5 *Translation to Hardware*

The translation of a computation to a hardware description language such as VHDL is commonly done from the compiler intermediate representation (IR). This translation can be done on a statement by statement basis (including loop constructs) after the compiler has selected an overall data and computation mapping strategy.

Irrespective of the translation approach, the compiler may leverage the capabilities of high-level synthesis tools to implicitly define the desired hardware implementations. In this approach, the compiler makes no effort to define the specifics of the architecture by not explicitly defining the structure of the control unit and the datapath. Instead, it specifies a set of hardware resources or timing constraints that will help the synthesis tools to define an appropriate hardware design that meets those

Table 3.1 Relative performance of hardware implementations for `loop 1` for several data mapping choices

Design	Storage resources: RAM mapping	Storage resources: Registers	Functional resources	Pipelined execution metrics: Initiation interval	Latency	Iterations	Total number clock cycles
1	RAM 0 A (2048 bytes) B (2048bytes) D (64 bytes)	s1 (8 bytes) s2 (8 bytes) u (128 bytes) Threshold (8 bytes)	1 64-bit adder/sub 1 Divisor by 4 1 32-bit incrementer	28	28	16	448
2	RAM 0 A (2048 bytes) RAM 1 B (2048 bytes) D (64 bytes)	s1 (8 bytes) s2 (8 bytes) u (128 bytes) Threshold (8 bytes)	1 64-bit adder/sub 1 Divisor by 4 1 32-bit incrementer	17	28	16	283
3	RAM 0 A (2048 bytes) B (2048 bytes)	s1 (8 bytes) s2 (8 bytes) u (128 bytes) Threshold (8 bytes) D (64 bytes)	1 64-bit adder/sub 1 Divisor by 4 1 32-bit incrementer	20	22	16	322
4	RAM 0 A (2048 bytes) RAM 1 B (2048 bytes)	s1 (8 bytes) s2 (8 bytes) u (128 bytes) Threshold (8 bytes) D (64 bytes)	1 64-bit adder/sub 1 Divisor by 4 1 32-bit incrementer	17	22	16	277

criteria. In some cases, the compiler can also be very specific about the number or type of operator implementations to be used by high-level synthesis thus, implicitly, controlling the final architecture the synthesis generates. The specifics of the actual synthesized architecture are totally hidden from the compiler and implicitly defined by architectural constraints imposed to the synthesis tools. When targeting an FPGA and after high-level synthesis, RTL/logic synthesis and placement and routing, the resulting net-list specification is translated to a bit-stream.

In Fig. 3.16 we depict an algorithmic VHDL description of the `loop 1` computation in the example C code in Fig. 3.4. In this description, arrays `A` and `B` are mapped to distinct RAMs, as highlighted as part of the VHDL description, and array `D` is mapped to registers. For brevity we have omitted the VHDL constructs for the initialization of the array variables. Notice also the linearization of multidimensional access functions and the registers declarations that support the mapping of array `D`.

3.4 Reconfigurable Computing Issues and Their Impact on Compilation

The flexibility and inherent spatial concurrency allowed by reconfigurable architectures exacerbate the complexity of compilation and synthesis flows for these architectures. We now outline three key aspects that contribute to this complexity and that are directly related to the three phases of the classic compilation flow, respectively, the front-end, the middle-end, and the back-end.

```
ARCHITECTURE behavioral OF ExampleCode IS
BEGIN
  -- reset_loop: omitted
  -- init_loop: omitted

  main_proc: PROCESS

    SUBTYPE resource IS integer;
    ATTRIBUTE map_to_module   : string;
    ATTRIBUTE variables       : string;
    ATTRIBUTE packing_mode    : string;
    ATTRIBUTE external_memory : boolean;

    VARIABLE s1: double_type;
    VARIABLE s2: double_type;
    VARIABLE u:  double_type;
    VARIABLE threshold: double_type;

    SUBTYPE  int_data_element IS signed(31 DOWNTO 0 );
    TYPE int_ram_type IS ARRAY (integer RANGE <>) OF int_data_element;
    TYPE int_array_type IS ARRAY (integer RANGE <>) OF int_data_element;

    SUBTYPE  double_data_element IS double_type;
    TYPE double_ram_type IS ARRAY (integer RANGE <>) OF double_data_element;
    TYPE double_array_type IS ARRAY (integer RANGE <>) OF double_data_element;

    VARIABLE ram_A : double_ram_type(0 TO 255);
    VARIABLE ram_B:  double_ram_type(0 TO 255);
    VARIABLE array_D : int_ram_type(0 TO 15);

    constant RAM_0 : resource := 0;
    attribute variables of RAM_0: constant is "ram_A";
    attribute map_to_module of RAM_0: constant is "singleport_ram_array";
    attribute packing_mode of RAM_0: constant is "compact";
    attribute external_memory of RAM_0: constant is FALSE;

    constant RAM_1: resource := 1;
    attribute variables of RAM_1: constant is "ram_B";
    attribute map_to_module of RAM_1: constant is "singleport_ram_array";
    attribute packing_mode of RAM_1: constant is "compact";
    attribute external_memory of RAM_1: constant is FALSE;

  BEGIN
    ...
    FOR i IN 0 TO 13 LOOP -- pragma dont_unroll
      ....
      -- Loop 1
      FOR j IN 0 TO 13 LOOP  -- pragma dont_unroll
        s1 := ram_A(i*16+j) + ram_A(i*16+j+1);
        s2 := ram_A(i*16+16+j) + ram_A(i*16+16+j+1);
        u := (s1 + s2)/ 4.0;
        ram_B(i*16+j) := u;
        IF (u > threshold) THEN
          array_D(j) := array_D(j) + 1;
        END IF;
      END LOOP;
      ....

    END LOOP;
  END PROCESS;
END behavioral;
```

Fig. 3.16 Algorithmic VHDL description for `loop 1` in example code

3.4.1 Programming Languages and Execution Models

It is widely believed that the major barrier for adoption of reconfigurable computing technology is the lack of adequate programming systems that offer a level of abstraction higher than currently provided by available HDLs [24]. Tools supporting high-level programming specifications would tremendously accelerate the development cycle of applications for reconfigurable systems and facilitate the migration of already developed algorithms to these systems, a key aspect for their widespread use and acceptance.

The main obstacle in offering a high-level programming abstraction, such as the imperative programming model of widely popular languages (e.g., C and Java), lies in the semantic gap between this imperative model and the explicitly concurrent models used to program hardware devices. Common hardware description languages such as VHDL or Verilog use an execution model based on Communicating Sequential Processes (CSP) [155] and thus far detached from the imperative models.

This semantic gap prompted the development of a wide range of approaches from the perspective of programming models. Theses approaches cover a wide spectrum of solutions, ranging from the easier approach where the input language already offers a concurrency execution model close to the hardware CSP model to the harder approach of automatic uncovering of concurrency from traditional imperative languages. Compilation of programs from the imperative paradigm to hardware has therefore to bridge this semantic gap by automatically extracting as much concurrency as possible. A popular alternative approach is to rely on library implementations where the notions of concurrent execution have been crystallized by library developers and openly publicized in application programmer interfaces (APIs).

The extraction of concurrency has been a long-standing and notoriously hard problem in the academic compiler and parallel computing communities. Constructs such as pointer manipulation in imperative languages, such as C or C++, hinder static analyses techniques that hamper a significant number of program transformations in the compilation and synthesis processes [276]. Compilation support for object-oriented mechanisms and dynamic data structures (e.g., memory allocation of linked lists) also requires advanced compiler analyses in the context of hardware synthesis [167, 249]. Alternative imperative execution models, such as languages with explicit support for data streaming (e.g., the Streams-C language [127]), alleviate some of the data disambiguation problems and substantially improve the effectiveness of the mapping to reconfigurable systems as they implicitly define concurrently execution processes. Intra-process concurrency, however, is still limited by the ability of the compiler to uncover concurrency from sequential statements.

Orthogonal to the general-purpose language efforts, other authors have developed their own target-specific languages. The RaPiD-C [84] and DIL [55] languages were developed specifically for pipelined-centered execution models supported by specific target architectures. While these languages have allowed programmers to close the semantic gap between high-level programming abstractions and the low-level implementation details, we strongly believe that they will ultimately serve as intermediate compilation languages a compiler tool can use when mapping higher level abstraction languages to these reconfigurable architectures.

Other research efforts have focused on the definition of languages with application-specific or domain-specific constructs explicitly exposing in some instances the computation concurrency. As an example, researchers developed the single-assignment SA-C language [44] geared toward image processing applications. SA-C has a number of attributes that facilitate its translation to hardware, namely, custom bit-width numerical representations, lack of pointer references, reduction operations with associative and commutative operators and loops with explicit index variables and window operators. The language semantic effectively relaxes the order in which imperative operations can be carried out and allows the compiler to use a set of predefined library components to implement them very efficiently. Other languages have opted for explicit mechanisms for specifying concurrency. In this class we see a wealth of efforts ranging from languages that expose concurrency at the operation-level (e.g., Handel-C [235]), task-level (e.g., Mitrion-C [217]), or thread-level (e.g., Java threads [310]).

The indisputable popularity of MATLAB [307], as a domain-specific language for image/signal processing and control applications, made it a language of choice when mapping to hardware computations in these domains. The matrix-based data model makes it very amenable to compiler analyses, in particular array-based data dependence techniques. However, the lack of strong types, a very flexible language feature, requires that effective compilation must rely heavily on type and shape inference (e.g., [141]), potentially limiting the applicability of more traditional analyses.

Lastly, there have also been compilation efforts using graphical programming environments such as the Cantata environment [229] and the Viva language [293]. Essentially, these graphical systems allow the concurrency to be exposed at the task level and are thus similar in spirit to task-based concurrent descriptions offered by CSP-like languages.

3.4.2 Intermediate Representations

Given the inherently parallel nature of reconfigurable architectures where multiple threads of control can operate concurrently over distinct data items, the intermediate representation a compiler uses for such architectures should explicitly represent this concurrency. Further, the intermediate representation should enable, rather than hamper, transformations that can take advantage of specific features of the target reconfigurable architecture.

An intermediate representation should also explicitly represent control and data dependences as in the traditional CDFG [114]. This representation uses the control-flow structure of the input computation representing each basic block with its DFG. Figure 3.17 illustrates part of a CDFG for the computation in `loop 2` of the example code in Fig. 3.10.

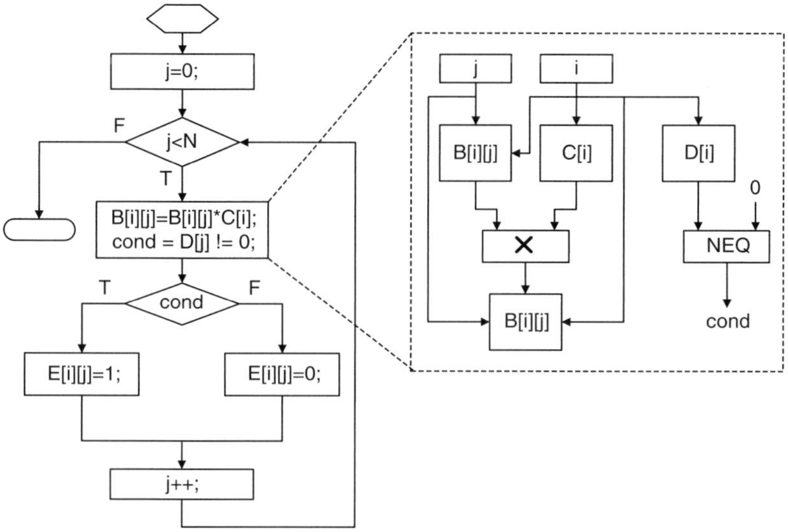

Fig. 3.17 Example of a CDFG

In this representation, however, the compiler is unable to exploit concurrency opportunities across multiple basic blocks. The hyperblock representation [200], mitigates this issue by aggregating a set of contiguous basic blocks with a single point of entry and possibly multiple exit points. This aggregation increases the amount of available concurrency in the representation [61] by enlarging the number of operations considered at the same time by a fine-grained scheduler [192].

A variant of the data-flow graph representation that captures more context nodes, adopted in the context of high-level synthesis when targeting ASICs (see, e.g. [140]), is the Hierarchical Task Graph (HTG) [120]. The HTG can represent efficiently the program structure in a hierarchical fashion and can explicitly represent functional parallelism exposed by an imperative programming language. The HTG combined with a global DFG, extended with program decision logic [22], has been argued to be an efficient intermediate model to represent parallelism at various levels, when exploiting speculative execution and multiple flows of control [222]. By exposing multiple flows of control it is possible to combine data-dependence graph (DDG) information and control-dependence graph (CDG) [85] information.

Also common in the co-synthesis community [212] is the use of task graph representations. An example representation is the Unified Specification Model (USM) [231], allowing the representation of task-level and operation-level control and data flow in a hierarchical fashion. Tasks are described at algorithmic level using a hardware description language. The USM graph-based representation explicitly captures data dependences between tasks and data sets (scalars and array sections) thus allowing compilers to explicitly manage the assignment of data sets to memories.

Regardless of the intermediate representation that exposes the available concurrency of the input program specification, still there is no clear, generic and efficient, migration path from common imperative programming languages to hardware-oriented representations as this mapping fundamentally relies on the ability of a compilation tool to uncover the data dependences in the input computation. In this context, languages based on the CSP abstractions are naturally more amenable to be mapped to hardware-oriented representations than state-full imperative languages such as C or C++.

3.4.3 Target Reconfigurable Architecture Features

As expected, the characteristics of the target reconfigurable architectures greatly affect the complexity of the compilation and synthesis process as it is apparent from the diversity of architectures described in Chap. 2. Furthermore, the compilation issues are exacerbated by the fact that these architectures can emulate, albeit at an appreciable performance loss, virtually any parallel architecture.

Besides the common aspects relating to address space and memory organization in parallel architectures (data partitioning and nonuniform accesses) alongside with the execution of control and synchronization, such as Single-Program-Multiple-Data (SPMD) or Single-Instruction-Multiple-Data (SIMD), we now highlight three aspects that are unique to reconfigurable architectures which directly impact the compilation and synthesis flow, namely:

- **Configurable Storage Structures:** Some architectures allow for their storage resources to be configured in terms of RAM modules with a variety of choices of capacity and data widths. These architectures can even offer a set of additional storage resources as discrete registers. Commonly, there is no notion of a unified address space and in the presence of data replication there is no provision for hardware-supported data consistency. These features place the burden of data mapping and management on the compiler when using data-oriented transformations such as caching (scalar replacement for array variables) or replication.
- **Configurable Functional Units:** Some architectures allow their execution units to be configured either by extending their ISA (e.g., Xtensa [134]) or by allowing the various functional elements to be customized for a specific application, thereby creating architectures that are truly heterogeneous. This heterogeneity can be visible as macrolevel FUs inserted in a flexible reconfigurable fabric as is the case with contemporary FPGAs [342]. This heterogeneity also creates an additional level of complexity as the execution models can now be distinct between FUs. For instance, it is possible to combine in the same architecture pipelined or systolic execution models [204] or VLIW [110] with thread-like execution. In this setting, the compiler must define a suitable communication and synchronization scheme to ensure data and control are preserved across execution domains, commonly achieved via hardware hand-shaking protocols or buffer synchronization using FIFO policies.

- **Trading Storage and Computational Resources:** Possibly the most notorious aspect of some reconfigurable architectures is their ability to trade storage resources for computing resources. This is the case with FPGAs where the Configurable-Logic-Blocks (CLBs) can be used as building blocks of either discrete registers, shift-registers, small memories, or combinatorial logic functions.

A possible approach to deal with the extreme flexibility, in terms of storage and computing resources reconfigurable architectures offer, is for compilers to engage in an exploration of alternative designs or design-space exploration (DSE) [96] created by the many code and mapping transformations at their disposal. The plethora of transformations, the wide range of architectural options, and the number of transformations and their interaction lead to huge design spaces. The various transformations, however, interact in nontrivial fashion exposing low-level issues such as contention for shared resources or bandwidth contention leading to possible execution bottlenecks.

To overcome the sheer dimension of these design-space researchers have developed various execution time performance modeling [242, 290] and resources estimation approaches [40, 180]. Using these modeling techniques, compilers can gage the pressure on resources for FUs and storage structures created by each sequence of transformations and thus select the transformations that lead to feasible and profitable hardware implementations. Although not completely accurate, some of these efforts have shown that even in the presence of inaccurate estimates a compiler can still make correct decisions about which transformations to use [288]. These early experiences suggest that indeed compilers must and can rely on simple, but effective modeling and estimation approaches to effectively explore a wide range of design options that would otherwise simply be unfeasible to explore.

3.5 Summary

Typical compilation flows for reconfigurable computing architectures translate the input computations (in a program) into data-path and control structures which define a computing engine specific to the input computations. Depending on the granularity of the target reconfigurable architecture, different back-end phases might be needed.

When targeting fine-grained reconfigurable architectures, traditional high-level synthesis and RTL/logic synthesis steps are needed. When targeting coarse-grained reconfigurable architectures, usually consisting of arrays of ALUs or other more complex PEs, the compiler has to create the computing engine, possible based also in data-path and control structures, using the PEs and interconnection topologies present in those architectures. In either these cases, the compiler has ample potential for optimizations, from specialization of data and operations to different pipelined execution forms.

Chapter 4
Code Transformations

In this chapter we describe various code transformations for reconfigurable architectures. We focus on transformations for which the ability of the architectures to provide custom/specialized hardware implementations increases their effectiveness in reducing, for example, execution time or hardware resource use.

We distinguish between very low-level code transformations which can exploit the fine-grained customization of reconfigurable architectures such as FPGAs, to coarse-grained instruction-level and loop-level transformations that are suitable when targeting fine- or coarse-grained reconfigurable architectures, such as the ADRES [206] and the XPP [31] architectures. While many of these transformations are not specific to reconfigurable architectures, they expose concurrency and data locality that can be exploited at various levels. For example, data reuse analysis and scalar replacement allow a compiler to define specific storage structures in number and capacity to save data that are reused throughout computations, either in registers or in internal RAM blocks. Loop distribution and loop unrolling allow a compiler to exploit both task- and instruction-level parallelism. An effective compiler for reconfigurable architectures must, therefore, uncover and leverage the great diversity of the interactions between these transformations to match the opportunities for customization enabled by the underlying architecture.

4.1 Bit-Level Transformations

We begin with three common bit-level transformations, namely, bit-width narrowing, bit-optimizations, and conversion between floating-point and fixed-point data formats. Overall, these bit-level transformations aim at exposing to the implementation the amount of bit-level resources strictly needed to carry out the arithmetic or logical operations at hand. While these transformations are also applicable to coarse-grained reconfigurable architectures, they are more suitable when targeting specialized functional units (FUs) in fine-grained reconfigurable architectures, as these architectures can leverage the bit-level information through customization

J.M.P. Cardoso, P.C. Diniz, *Compilation Techniques for Reconfigurable Architectures*,
DOI 10.1007/978-0-387-09671-1_4,

and specialization to deliver implementations with substantially fewer hardware resources than direct and naive implementations. In many cases, these implementations may exhibit faster clock rates as the critical path of the generated data-paths is shortened.

4.1.1 Bit-Width Narrowing

In many programs, the declared precision and range of the numeric data types used are overly-defined. This over-definition occurs when the bit-widths of the data types are much larger than the bit-widths required to store the data for the observed values during the execution of the computations [71, 295].

An illustrative example of this over-definition occurs by direct implementation in hardware of the arithmetic and logic operations used in loop control variables as depicted in Fig. 4.1. In this example, the native 32-bit two's complement integer representation for the loop's control variable `i` allows for a range of integer values of $[-2^{31}, 2^{31}-1]$, whereas in reality only 3 bits are required to span the range of values $[0,7]$.

A naive direct implementation of the controller for the execution of the loop would use the default 32-bit adder in the hardware solution depicted in Fig. 4.1b where the `(i<=7)` comparison relies on a comparator. Given the information about the range of values assumed by the variable `i`, a compiler could generate an hardware solution using a single 3-bit unsigned adder operator instead. Figure 4.1c depicts an even more aggressive hardware implementation variant where the carry-out signal (`cout`) of the 3-bit adder is used to indicate if the value of the variable `i` is less than 8 resulting in an extremely compact hardware design solution.

While there are high-level programming languages that allow programmers to explicitly define the bit-width of variables (e.g., Valen-C [161], NAPA-C [125], DSP-C [4]), this language feature still presents a challenge to programmers. First, some of the languages only allow for each variable a fixed bit-width to be declared

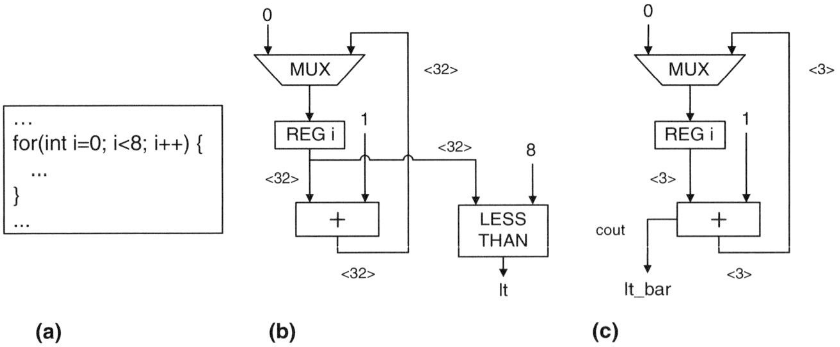

Fig. 4.1 Bit-width narrowing example in loop control variables: (**a**) original source code; (**b**) naive hardware implementation; (**c**) aggressive hardware implementation

for the entire program. This limitation precludes the use of distinct bit-widths in distinct locus of the program where the requirements may clearly be different. Second, in some cases, the definitions of bit-widths are restricted to type declarations and not variable declarations. This forces the programmer to use a higher number of user-defined data sets to accommodate the various bit-width requirements anticipated in the program. This second aspect is exacerbated by the potential need to have structured (e.g., nested) data types, given the increase of the number of combinations of the various bit-width variants of the nested data types. Although in some specific cases the use of declared data types and variables with predefined bit-widths is advantageous, it may lead to poor programming practices.

An alternative approach is to rely on compiler techniques for bit-width and type inference analyses [8]. Using these analyses, a compiler may estimate the type, shape, and the number of required bits for representing the underlying variables the program manipulates at all program points [143, 296]. For example, in a MATLAB program the compiler can determine that at specific program execution points a given variable, *e.g.*, `mat_a` is a two-dimensional array of binary values, whereas at a distinct program point, the same symbolic name `mat_a` is used as a one-dimensional double-precision vector.

Bit-width analysis relies on data-flow analyses techniques. As with any static analysis, bit-width analysis is naturally conservative given the undecidability limitations of fully static analyses. To circumvent this limitation, researchers have considered two alternative approaches to static bit-width analysis, namely, run-time profiling (while still relying on an off-line analysis technique) and truly dynamic run-time approach.

In approaches based on run-time profiling, the compiler combines static analysis results with assembled run-time profiling data. The compiler relies on execution traces to learn about the actual values being stored in each variable and the type and results of the operators that manipulate them. With this knowledge, the compiler derives actual observed and/or estimated bit-widths for each variable. These profiling-based approaches require an off-line execution of the program using test vectors (data sets) which can be either set up by programmers or automatically generated by the compiler to attempt to cover a wide range of internal control-flow path executions [227]. As with any profiling-based approach the validity of the results is very dependent on the relationship between the tested input data sets and the observed program behavior in actual production runs. In addition, and to increase the coverage of the observed data set, these approaches incur non-negligible profiling costs.

In the presence of loops, a compiler, using a combination of profiling and static analyses techniques, can generate precision adaptation strategy, where it determines for ranges of loop iteration counts the required precision of the variables the loop manipulates [48]. For example, for the first k iterations of the loop, the compiler can ensure a specific required bit-width for all the variables, whereas if the loop iteration count exceeds k, different bit-widths must be used instead. Based on the results of such analysis, the compiler generates a sequence of configurations where each one defines a specialized circuit, or partial changes to the previous circuit, to be loaded at specific loop iteration counts. To be practical, this approach requires hardware support for fast dynamic reconfiguration (possibly also including partial reconfiguration).

It is possible to envision a more radical, but expensive approach relying entirely on dynamic, run-time techniques, i.e., a true dynamic precision management approach. In such an approach, the compiler would gather, using a static analysis, some knowledge about types and required bit-widths, and then would postpone to run-time the completion of key steps of the analysis. Alternatively, it could also rely entirely on monitoring and adapting the required precision of the computations at run-time invoking a reconfiguration whenever the precision would warrant it. Naturally, this approach would have nontrivial execution time costs, not only for the monitoring of the precision but also for reconfiguration. We are not aware of any such approach.

As static bit-width analysis is the most commonly used, we now describe some of its approaches reported in the literature. With respect to mapping of computations to reconfigurable architectures, one of the first static bit-width analyses was presented by Razdan and Smith [258], developed strictly for acyclic program constructs. More recently Budiu et al. [56] described and evaluated a static bit-width analysis, named *BitValue* analysis, that handles loops. In *BitValue* analysis, the compiler attempts to determine the possible individual bit values for the binary representation of each variable in the program. Each bit can have a definite value, either 0 or 1, an unknown value, or can be represented as a "don't care." The authors formulate *BitValue* analysis as a data-flow analysis problem with forward, backward, and mixing steps. Data-flow analyses are used to propagate those possible bit values based on propagation functions dependent on the operations being analyzed. The backward analysis is used to propagate "don't care" values, and the forward analysis is used to propagate both defined and undefined values. Forward and backward analyses are done iteratively through bit-vector representations until a fixed point is reached.

At a simple operator level, the analysis relies on specific bit setting properties of the operations. For example, in the statement `b=a<<2`, and as a result of the "shift-left" operation by 2 bits, a compiler could determine that the two least significant bits after this shift operation are 0. Propagating this information, the compiler can determine similar properties for other variables leading to possible simplifications of arithmetic or logic implementations in subsequent instructions. For statements involving more operations, the analysis is more sophisticated and requires the two backward and forward steps as depicted in Fig. 4.2. For simplicity, we consider in this case that all the variables are of the unsigned byte type. In the example shown in Fig. 4.2a, the mask operation `a&&0xf` allows a compiler to determine by forward propagation that variable `d` only requires 4 bits and by backward propagation that variable `a` only requires 4 bits. Thus, the multiplication can be performed by a simple 4×4 hardware multiplier. In the example depicted in Fig. 4.2b, the mask operation `b&&0xf` limits the bit-width of `a` to 4 bits and thus allows the compiler to derive a 4×8 bits hardware multiplier to calculate the value of `c`. Backward propagation in this example can be used to derive that variable `b` only requires 4 bits. These steps are illustrated graphically in Fig. 4.2, where the inputs for each operator

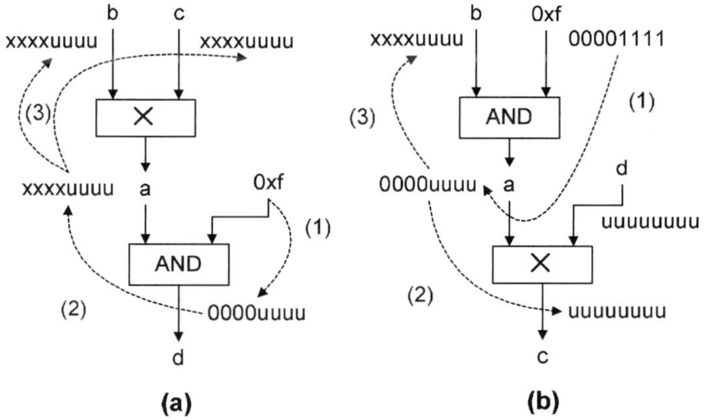

Fig. 4.2 Examples (**a**) and (**b**) of forward and backward bit-width information propagation considering variables of type unsigned byte. Annotations (1), (2), and (3) indicate the order in which the steps are executed

have been annotated with bit-vector representations resulting from *BitValue* analysis, along with the sequence of propagation of the results of this analysis. In Fig. 4.2, u represents an *unknown* bit value, whereas x denotes a "don't care" logic value.

A simpler case of bit-width analysis, referred here as *bit-width propagation*, consists in the propagation of bit-width values through the operations in a DFG. In this case, the propagation of bit-widths in the presence of an addition operator results in a number of bits equal to the maximum bit-widths of the two operands plus 1 bit. This analysis, however, does not find bit values as the *BitValue* analysis presented previously.

Range propagation analysis, also known as value range analysis, is a variant of bit-width analysis, where the compiler tracks the range of values each operand can assume [296]. The use of value range analysis allows a compiler to derive narrower bit-width requirements than by direct bit-width analyses, with the exception of the bounding bits (i.e., the LSBs and the MSBs). However, range analysis does not allow the determination of which bits in the operand's representation can be eliminated. To complement value range analysis, compilers can use auxiliary information, such as the bounds in each array dimension, to infer the values of scalar variables used in the array indexing functions, under the assumption of safe-bound array accesses.

In the presence of loop constructs, forward and backward propagation analyses either need to use analytical models that represent the increase in the number of bits when operations are repeated a specific number of times or need to iterate until a fixed point is reached, which in itself is a possibly very time-consuming process. When the loop bounds are not known at compile-time, the analysis must consider loop upper bounds (possibly derived indirectly by array bounds) or, more conservatively, does not perform bit-width narrowing and assume worst-case precision requirements.

Table 4.1 presents illustrative examples of three static bit-width narrowing techniques. The rightmost two columns of the table present the result of applying each

Table 4.1 Examples of bit-width narrowing techniques

		Examples (A, B, C, and D are unsigned variables)	
Analysis technique	Potential	A, B, C: 8 bits D: 16 bits D = ((B<<2)+(A<<3))+(C<<2);	A: 8 bits B: 6 bits C: 5 bits D: 16 bits D=(A+B)+C;
Bit-width propagation	Only eliminates most significant bits	(B<<2) ⇒ 10 bits; (A<<3) ⇒ 11 bits; (C<<2) ⇒ 10 bits; (B<<2)+(A<<3) ⇒ 12 bits (11-bit adder with carry-out) D: (B<<2)+(A<<3)+(C<<2) ⇒ 13 bits (12-bit adder with carry-out)	A+B ⇒ 9 bits (8-bit adder with carry-out) D=(A+B)+C ⇒ 10 bits (9-bit adder with carry-out)
BitValue	Can find bit information in every position of the bit representation	(B<<2): <uuuuuuuu00> ⇒ 10 bits (A<<3): <uuuuuuuu000> ⇒ 11 bits (C<<2): <uuuuuuuu00>⇒ 10 bits (B<<2)+(A<<3): <uuuuuuuuuu00> ⇒ 12 bits (8-bit adder with carry-out) D: <uuuuuuuuuuu00> ⇒ 13 bits (10-bit adder with carry-out);	A+B: <uuuuuuuuu> ⇒ 9 bits (8-bit adder with carry-out) D=(A+B)+C: <uuuuuuuuuu> ⇒ 10 bits (9-bit adder with carry-out)
Value range	Only reduces on the extremities (most and least significant bits), but can lead to more minimized implementations than the previous two analyses	B: [255:0] ⇒ (B<<2): [1,020:0]; ⇒ 10 bits A: [255:0] ⇒ (A<<3): [2,040:0]; ⇒ 11 bits (B<<2)+(A<<3): [3060:0] ⇒ 12 bits (11-bit adder with carry-out) C: [255:0] ⇒ (C<<2): [1,020:0]; ⇒ 10 bits D: [1,020:0]+[2,040:0]+[1,020:0]=[4,080:0] ⇒ 12 bits (12-bit adder)	A: [255:0] B: [63:0] C: [27:0] A+B: [318:0]; ⇒ 9 bits (8-bit adder with carry-out) D=(A+B)+C: [345:0]; ⇒ 9 bits (8-bit adder with carry-out)

of the techniques to the simple expressions depicted in the first row of the table. As can be seen in this example, the propagation of value ranges determines the minimum number of required bits. In the case shown in last column, value range analysis infers 9 bits for the variable `D`, instead of the 10 bits which would be required when using either bit-width or the *BitValue* technique. Note, however, that the propagation of bit vectors can find bit positions whose values are known statically. Such information can be used to simplify the FUs needed to perform the operations.

Although orthogonal to bit-width narrowing, bit precision information can be used at run-time to improve performance by shortening the execution time of operations. When an FU, capable of handling operands of a specific bit-width, is presented with operands with lower bit requirements, it can internally bypass some of its hardware resources and derive a correct output result quicker [53].[1] These dynamic execution techniques, however, require additional hardware resources to determine if operands have bit-width requirements below a specific level at run-time.

4.1.2 Bit-Level Optimizations

Bit-level optimizations refer to optimizations of logic functions, possibly performed at gate-level. In the example of program decision logic [22], a compiler may

[1] When presented with input operands requiring only precision in the lowest 3 bits, a 16-bit adder can very quickly generate a valid 4-bit output result.

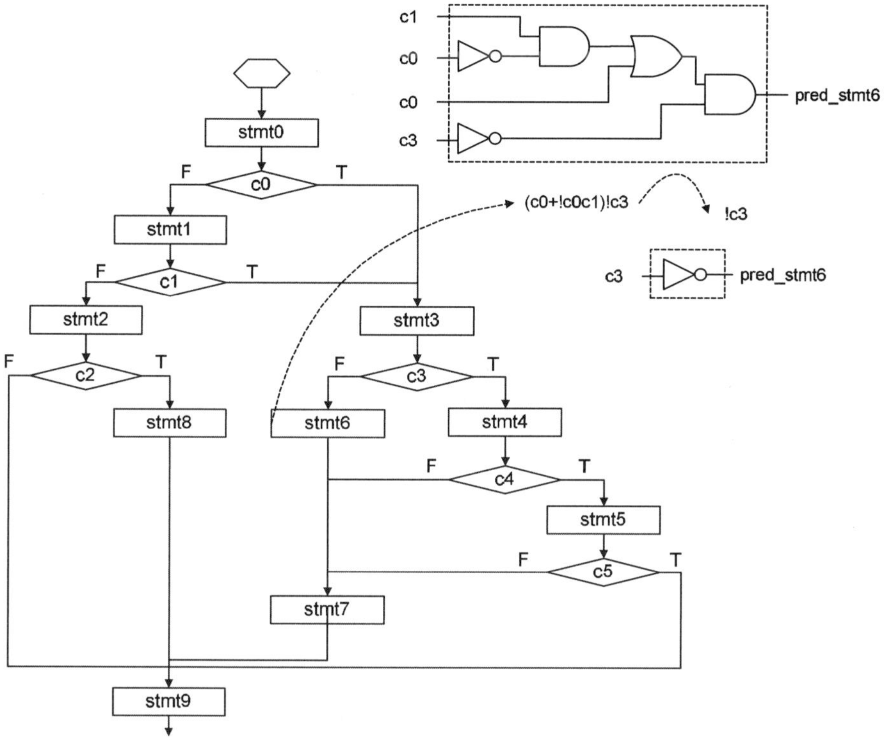

Fig. 4.3 Control-flow intensive example (based on [22])

try to simplify this logic by performing traditional boolean minimization techniques typically used in logic synthesis [210]. We present in Fig. 4.3 an example inspired by a section of code of the UNIX utility *wc* described in [22]. In this example, the labels `c0` to `c5` represent branch conditions. For this code, a compiler can determine, by inspecting the predicate logic for the execution of statement `stmt6`, as `(c0+!c0c1)!c3`. As the expression `c0+!c0c1` is equivalent to `c0+c1`, the compiler can simplify `(c0+!c0c1)!c3` as `(c0+c1)!c3`. By inspecting the conditions used in this expression, which are `c0: (32>=r4)`, `c1: (r4>=127)`, and `c3: (r4!=10)`, a compiler may further simplify the expression `(c0+c1)!c3` to `!c3`, given that `!c3` implies `c0` and excludes `c1`. These simplifications allow the compiler to generate an implementation for the program decision logic with fewer logic gates and lower execution delay. These simplifications may have a different impact when targeting fine- or coarse-grained RPUs. For example, when targeting an FPGA with basic configurable blocks consisting of 4-LUTs, i.e., lookup tables with four inputs, the predicated logic for `stmt6` will use the same number of FPGA resources as both circuits presented in Fig. 4.3 can be mapped to a single 4-LUT. When targeting coarse-grained RPUs, the simplifications may lead to implementations using only one FU than the five FUs required for the nonoptimized predicate logic for `stmt6`.

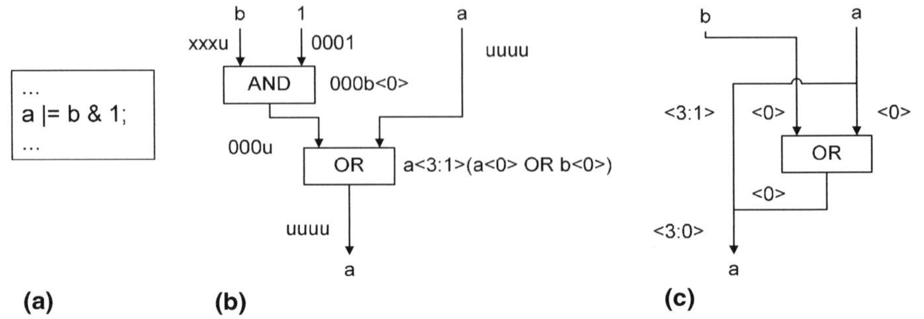

Fig. 4.4 A bit-level optimization example: (**a**) input statement; (**b**) naive operator translation and bit-value analysis results; (**c**) simplified implementation

```
int Reverse(int Word) {
  int WordRev = 0;
  for(int i=0; i<32; i++) {
    WordRev |= (Word & 1);
    WordRev << 1;
    Word >> 1;
  }
  return WordRev;
}
```

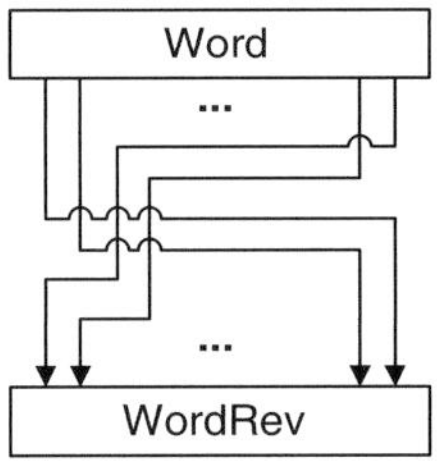

(a) (b)

Fig. 4.5 Bit reversing (32-bit word): (**a**) coded C programming language; (**b**) optimized implementation in hardware using wires

Bit-level optimizations may also use the bit-value results, gather by bit-width related analyses described in the previous section, to simplify, or even eliminate, arithmetic and logic operations. Figure 4.4 illustrates an example of these simplifications considering for simplicity 4-bit data representations. The initial 4-bit `&&` and `||` operations in Fig. 4.4a can be directly translated to 4-bit logic AND and OR gates as depicted in Fig. 4.4b. Using the information about the bit-values of the integer constant `1`, the compiler converts the 4-bit logic AND and OR gates to a single wire and a 1-bit logic OR gate, respectively as depicted in Fig. 4.4c.

Bit optimizations can even allow a compiler to eliminate the hardware that, in other case, would be associated with a given statement, as is the case of `if((ans&0x8000)==0x8000)` which can be implemented in hardware using a simple wire connected to the 15th bit of `ans`. Similarly, the evaluation of predicates of the form `(a<0)` and `(a>=0)` can be performed by inspecting the logic value of the most significant bit of `a` assuming the sign of the representation identified by that bit. A more elaborate example is depicted in Fig. 4.5. In this example, and after performing loop unrolling, the compiler can use bit-value analysis to determine that each bit in the result is a specific bit of the input word value, leading to an implementation that only uses hardware interconnections (wires). For coarse-grained reconfigurable architectures, however, this reversal would have to be accomplished by a combination of word-level routing (e.g., using 8-bit word reversal in the case of an 8-bit architecture), and bit-level operations such as masking and shifts by constants.

Applying bit-width narrowing and bit-optimizations to examples with intensive bit-manipulations, as are for example bit-masking, shift by constants or bit concatenation operations is likely to lead to significant improvements in size and execution time of the resulting hardware implementations. For instance, the simplification of the statement `c=(a.b)[7, 0]` in DIL [55], where `b` is an 8-bit variable, "." denotes the concatenation operator, and square brackets represent the bit-range of an expression, reduces it to `c=b[7, 0]`. The implementation of this statement only has to connect via wires the eight least significant bits of `b` directly to `c`.[2]

As these last two examples illustrate, applying bit-level optimizations earlier in the compilation flow, albeit depending critically on the ability of the compiler to apply other transformations, is important to improve the overall hardware resources and timing. A dramatic example is the bit-reversal example in Fig. 4.5. If the compiler does not fully unroll the loop, it is forced to generate a fairly ineffective hardware implementation that would reflect the control structure of the original computations without exploiting the embarrassingly bit-parallel interconnection nature of the optimized solution.

4.1.3 Conversion from Floating- to Fixed-Point Representations

Floating-point data representation is a commonly used format to represent real numbers in almost all computing domains. In the IEEE 754 [158] single precision floating-point standard each floating-point value is represented as: $(+/-)1.\mathtt{f} \times 2^{(\mathtt{exp}-127)}$, where `f` represents the fraction (mantissa) using 23 bits and `exp` represents the 8-bit exponent. The costs associated to the arithmetic operations in floating-point formats, however, are much higher than using an integer representation in terms of logic gates and timing. An alternative representation, commonly used in digital signal/image processing algorithm implementations, are the fixed-point data types. The fixed-point data types allow the arithmetic operations to be done by integer operations and scaling factors implemented by shifting the operands and/or the result of the operations.

In some cases the trade-off between precision and efficiency of computations in fixed-point format is acceptable given the substantial reduction of the costs of the arithmetic operations. Figure 4.6 shows the output of a function when using floating- and fixed-point representations. We can see in this simple example the different results achieved and the increase in the accuracy when using more bits for the fixed-point representation.

---

[2] This same DIL expression is equivalent to the C or Java statement `c=(0xff)&((a<<8)||((0xff)&b))` which requires a more aggressive analysis to expose the optimized circuit.

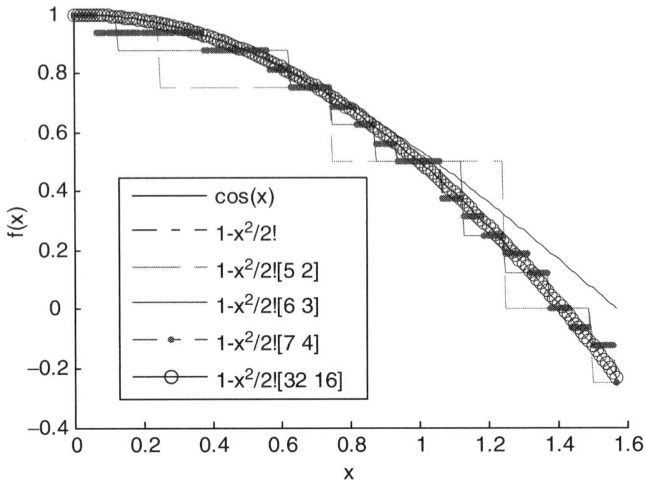

Fig. 4.6 Values obtained when approximating $\cos(x)$ by the function $1 - x^2/2!$ using floating- and fixed-point representations. Labels $[ab]$ represent fixed-point data types with word-length of a bits and including b bits for the fraction part

Given that most algorithms have been developed on computers natively supporting floating-point data types, porting floating-point based codes to use fixed-point data types requires an error-prone, tedious, and time-consuming conversion process. This floating-point to fixed-point conversion has been the focus of several research projects that compile C programs onto DSP (digital signal processor) architectures [1, 324]. Most, if not all of the approaches reported in the literature, use profiling and/or programmer annotations to assist the automatic phases of the conversion. It is common that whenever the tools are unable to find a translation for a specific variable, they prompt the user to provide additional information. Other tools rely on profiling techniques or interpolation analyses [300].

Floating- to fixed-point conversions have also been addressed when mapping computations to fine-grained reconfigurable architectures. Leong et al. [190] describe a conversion method based on profiling and on the minimization of a cost function. Nayak et al. [225] describe an automatic type analysis approach divided into two main steps. The first step seeks the minimum number of bits of the integer part of the fixed-point representation using range propagation analysis with forward and backward phases as described in the previous section. In the second step, the approach searches for the minimum number of bits in the fractional part of the fixed-point representation. It starts by using the same number of fractional bits for all the variables and then refines the representation via an error analysis technique.

In addition to the conversion of noninteger numeric data types, compilers also engage in a transformation or minimization of the hardware logic that carries out the numeric computations. The main objective of these transformations is the reduction, or even elimination, of shift operations used in adjusting of the exponents and mantissas. When targeting coarse-grained architectures, with or without barrel-shift hardware support, the compiler can attempt to reduce the number of scaling operations. This reduction can have a great impact on the overall performance of the implementation as a trivial translation can produce a large number of such shift operations. In addition, elimination of shift operations is also possible when the operands that need to be aligned (e.g., in additions) are represented with the same number of fractional bits. When targeting fine-grained architectures and when the amount of shifting is known at compile-time, shift operation can be implemented by simple redirection of the bits of the fractional part of the representation.

4.1.4 Nonstandard Floating-Point Formats

It is possible to improve the performance of arithmetic operations and/or reduce the amount of hardware resources used for specific applications by the adoption of nonstandard floating-point formats. These formats are used for variables that require more precision than the precision offered by fixed-point formats, but much less precision than offered by standard floating-point formats, as they only require specific numbers of bits for exponent and mantissa representations according to specific application accuracy requirements.

A nonstandard floating-point format is referred to as *block* floating-point number representation [252] , whose key idea is to split the value of a variable between two components. One component is defined for a set of variables as an implicit and common exponent *exp*. The second component is defined for each variable by an integer value denoted here by `int`. The value of each variable in this block of variables is thus defined as $\texttt{int} \times 2^{(-exp)}$.

Block floating-point formats can be profitably used in the context of fine- or coarse-grained reconfigurable architectures and are an important representation transformation when compiling DSP applications to reconfigurable architectures [177].

4.2 Instruction-Level Transformations

At a coarser level of granularity in code transformations, we include many instruction-level transformations that increase performance and/or simplify or reduce the hardware resources allocated for a given computation using a combination of algebraic simplification or circuit specialization. As instructions are translated into specific hardware operators such as adders or multipliers, the simplification or even elimination of operations (in the absence of resource sharing) directly corresponds to the elimination of hardware resources in the circuit that implements the desired computation.

Simple algebraic transformations, *common subexpression elimination*, *constant folding*, and *constant propagation*, have been extensively studied and used in the context of compilation for traditional architectures and have, often, a positive impact on the generated code. Examples of such transformations include the classical algebraic strength reduction and simplification cases such as replacing $-1 \times a$ by $-a$, $-(-j)$ by j, or $0+i$ by i. Other algebraic transformations, as is the example of replacing a square operation with a multiplication (a^2 replaced by $a \times a$), are useful when an architecture does not natively support the original operation.

Many of these algebraic transformations are independent of the target architecture and have a positive impact both in terms of timing and used hardware resources. We focus here on three key transformations enabled or emphasized by the flexibility of reconfigurable architectures, namely *operator strength reduction*, *tree-height reduction* [222], and *code hoisting/sinking*.

4.2.1 Operator Strength Reduction

In operator strength reduction (OSR) the compiler replaces a specific operation with a sequence of less expensive operations. Strength reduction can achieve resource savings and reduce the delay of the operation, and is therefore well suited for compilers to fine-grained reconfigurable architectures given their ability to implement specific operations by direct manipulation of wires and the ability to customize and/or combine operators.

A first class of strength reduction is usually applied in the context of software compilers to induction variables [222], as is the example of replacing `j=i*2` with `j=j+2` for loops with `i` control variable and unit step.

A second class of strength reduction transformations contains simple bit-manipulation operations that can be trivially implemented by changing the meaning of the wires that carry the values of the variables, thereby eliminating altogether the "instructions" or operators. As an illustrative example, the operation $2 \times$ `i` can be replaced by the operation `i<<1` which in fine-grained reconfigurable architectures (i.e., with support to bit-level routing) can be implemented using wire connections. Also, the operation $3 \times$ `i` can be implemented by the combination of `i+(i<<1)`. Figure 4.7 depicts an illustrative implementation of the latter operation strength reduction example.

A third class of strength reduction specializes an operation based on the value of its operands. This is particularly relevant in the context of arithmetic operations given the computational weight and amount of resources needed to implement these operators. For example, when a constant of the form 2^N is added to an operand, an increment and a bit-level concatenation can be used instead of a full adder as depicted by the particular example in Fig. 4.8, where a 32-bit operand is added to the constant 2^{16}, thus only requiring a 16-bit increment unit rather than a 32-bit adder.

Generically, integer divisions and multiplications by compile-time constants can be transformed into sequences of shifts, additions, and subtractions [199]. Trivial cases occur when there is a multiplication or a division of an integer operand by a

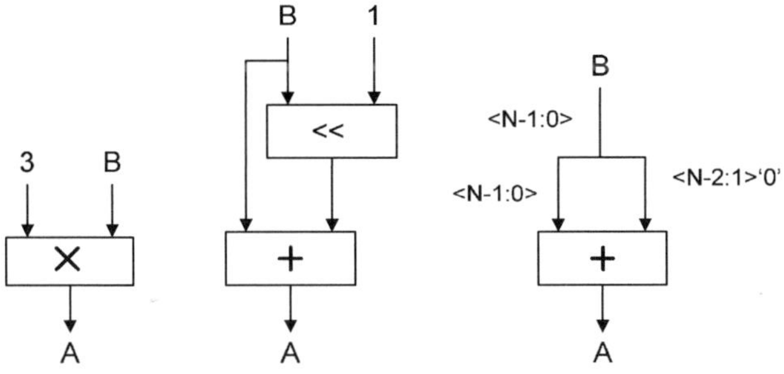

Fig. 4.7 OSR example: (**a**) implementation without OSR; (**b**) implementation with OSR; (**c**) simplified implementation

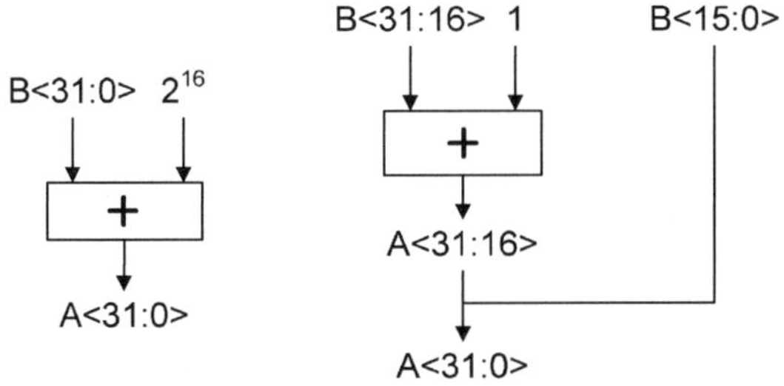

Fig. 4.8 Bit-level operation specialization example: (**a**) nonoptimized implementation; (**b**) implementation after specialization

power-of-two constant. For these cases, a multiplication is accomplished by a simple shift of the operand, which, in fine-grained reconfigurable architectures, requires only a hardware implemented with wire interconnections. The nontrivial multiplication cases require the use of other implementation schemes. Some authors have proposed arithmetic operations (e.g., factorization) to deal with the multiplications by constants, for which optimal algorithmic solutions described in the literature have exponential time complexity [38]. An efficient scheme for transforming multiplications by constants to less costly operations uses the Canonical Signed Digit (CSD) representation [150]. Using CSD a constant is uniquely represented with a minimum number of symbols -1, $+1$, and 0 such that no two consecutive bits are non-zero. This representation allows the use of a small number of adder/subtracter components for multiplications, which can be further reduced by the application of common-subexpression elimination (CSE) to the CSD representation. Table 4.2 presents three illustrative examples of the application of operator strength reduction to the sample arithmetic operation $231 \times A$. The binary case refers to the direct use of the binary representation, and corresponds to a hardware solution with the largest number of operations, and therefore of hardware resources required. The two other

Table 4.2 OSR example on integer multiplications by constants (shift operations are not included)

Operation	231×A		
Representation	Binary	CSD	CSD+CSE
	011100111	100-10100-1	Pattern: 100-1
Resources (not considering shifts)	5 adders	2 subtracters and 1 adder	1 adder and 1 subtracter

cases use the CSD representation without and with CSE revealing substantial reductions in the number of additions and subtractions used.

Although in much limited contexts, operator strength reduction can also be used when dealing with floating-point operations. For example, the implementation of the expression $x/2.0$ can be implemented by subtracting one unit to the exponent in the floating-point representation of x.

4.2.2 Height Reduction

Height reduction is an instrumental transformation when compiling arithmetic expressions to hardware. It rearranges the way operations are performed preserving the functionality of the original computations. By exploiting commutative, associative, and distributive properties of arithmetic operations, a compiler using height reduction can reduce the number of operations in an expression, or/and the critical path of the resulting hardware implementation. A special case of height reduction is *tree-height reduction* (THR) also known as *tree-height minimization* [210] which is applied to operations organized as a tree. By reducing the height of an expression tree, the technique exposes operator concurrency and consequently reduces the latency of the hardware circuit that implements the expression.[3]

Simple uses of tree-height reduction, such as in `t=a+b+c+d`, only require the application of arithmetic associativity to derive `t=(a+b)+(c+d)`. In other arithmetic expressions, distributivity is a key transformation that exposes a wide variety of hardware implementation trade-offs. For this reason we focus on distributivity in the remainder of this section.

Often, the distributive property leads to implementations with more operations and without lower latency, but in some cases distributivity can expose subexpressions common to other expressions in the program. For instance, the application of distributivity to the instruction sequence: `t1=a*(b+c+d); t2=a*b+a*d;` leads to the transformed instruction `t1=a*b+a*c+a*d;` which exposes the common subexpression: `a*b+a*d` resulting in the code sequence `t2=a*b+a*d; t1=t2+a*c;`. Without any resource sharing, direct hardware implementations of both sequences have the same latency. The transformed sequence, however, requires

[3] In the best case, THR reduces the height of an expression tree from $O(n)$ to $O(\log n)$ where n represents the number of nodes (operations) in the expression.

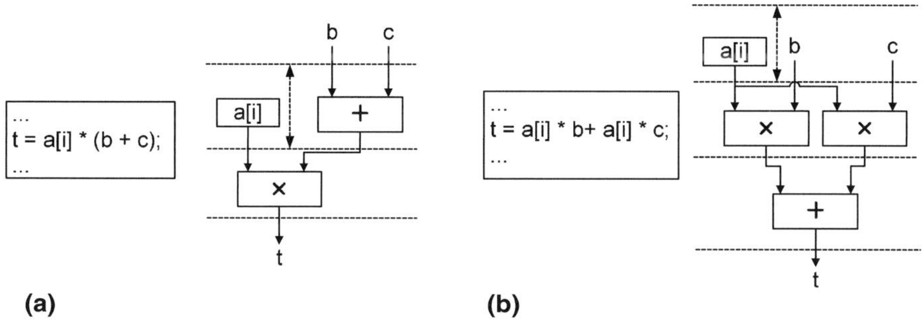

Fig. 4.9 Distributive transformation: (**a**) original code and possible implementation; (**b**) code after distributivity and possible implementation

only two additions and three multiplications whereas the original code would require three additions and three multiplications.

Distributivity can also be used to reduce the latency of a hardware implementation as illustrated by the statement `t1=a*(b*c*d+e);`. The transformed code after applying distributivity results in `t1=(a*b)*(c*d)+a*e;` which requires one additional multiplication. Its hardware implementation exhibits a latency of $2 \times \mathtt{Lat}(*) + \mathtt{Lat}(+)$ clock cycles rather than $3 \times \mathtt{Lat}(*) + \mathtt{Lat}(+)$ clock cycles for the hardware implementation of the original statement.

There are cases, however, where distributivity leads to performance degradation and an increase in the number of operations (i.e., and consequently hardware resources) as illustrated in the example in Fig. 4.9. Without distributivity the memory read, `a[i]`, can be performed in parallel with the addition `(b+c)`, which can result in a latency of two clock cycles, when considering one cycle to read data from memory. The implementation using distributivity does not allow this parallelism and the memory read for `a[i]` must be done before the additions. This results in a latency of three clock cycles.

Although distributivity does increase the number of operators in a given expression, its application may break dependences leading to shorter execution schedules when the number of hardware resources is limited. Figure 4.10 illustrates this scenario for the original code in Fig. 4.10a and for hardware implementations constrained to two hardware multipliers. The hardware implementation of the original code, depicted in Fig. 4.10a, would have to implement the multiplication in statement `t1=...` in a second cycle due to the dependence on the addition in the same statement. This would imply that in a second cycle one would have three multiplications, one corresponding to `t1= ...` and two multiplications corresponding to the statement `t2=...`. Given the implementation constraint of two multipliers, these three multiplications would have to be carried out in two additional steps, leading to a schedule with three overall execution steps as depicted in Fig. 4.10b. When applying distributivity, as depicted by the code in Fig. 4.10c, the multiplications corresponding to statement `t1=...` can be performed during a first execution step using the two available multipliers. The multiplications corresponding to statement

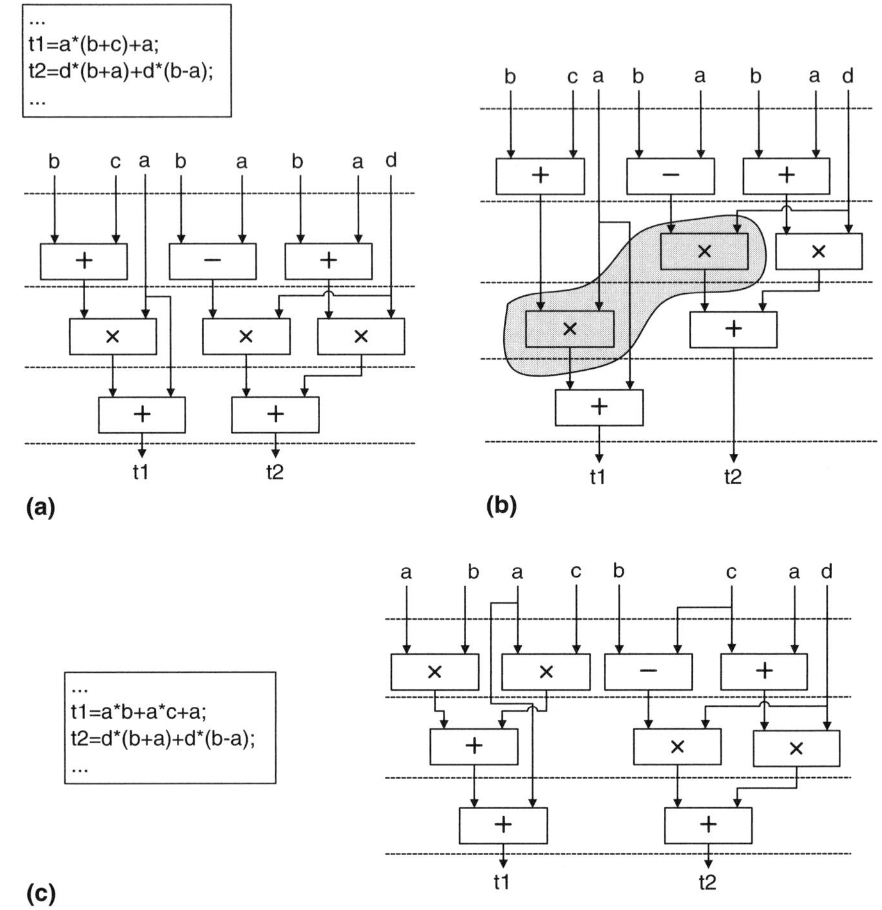

Fig. 4.10 Example of reduction in execution latency by using distributivity in the presence of limited hardware multipliers: (**a**) original code and correspondent data-path; (**b**) possible implementation when a maximum of two multipliers are available; (**c**) code after distributivity and corresponding data-path

`t2=...` can be carried out in a second execution step concurrently with the additions for statement `t1=...` resulting in an overall execution with two steps as depicted in Fig. 4.10d.

THR can be easily performed when the expression consists of operations of the same type. When expressions include operations of various types, THR can be executed by finding the best combination of the arithmetic properties of those operations and factorization techniques. A THR algorithm can exploit commutative and associative properties of the operators in an expression tree by subtree swapping and rotation (left or right) with the goal of minimizing the tree height.

Applying THR may, in some cases, worsen the hardware implementation results, when some operations in the expression tree share hardware resources as their

```
s = a[0] + a[1] + a[2] + a[3];
```

(a)

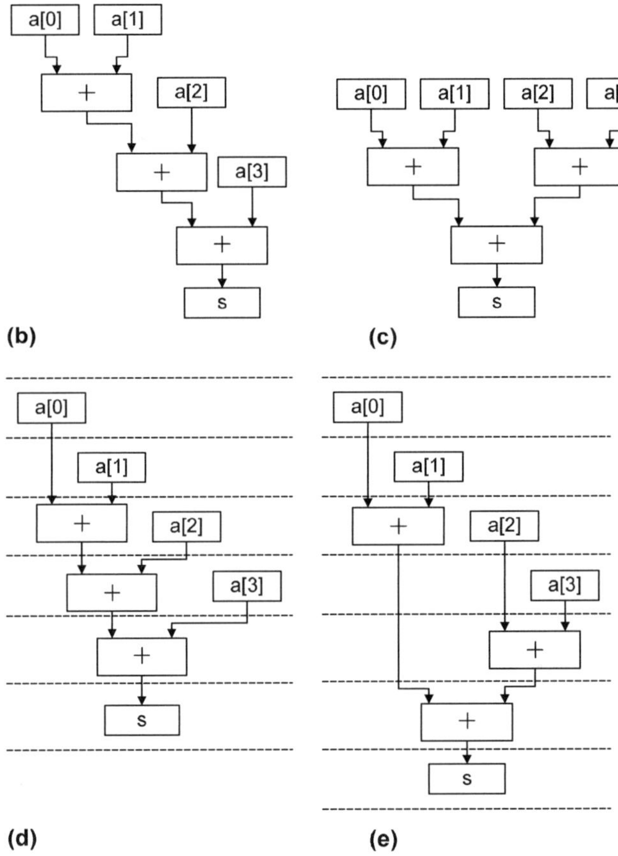

Fig. 4.11 THR: (**a**) a simple expression; (**b**) DFG with operations in cascade; (**c**) DFG after the application of THR; (**d**), (**e**) impact on the scheduling length considering the serialization of memory accesses when applied to the DFG in (**b**) and in (**c**), respectively

execution must be serialized. Figure 4.11e depicts a schedule length, obtained after THR, which is longer than the schedule length directly obtained from the original DFG (Fig. 4.11d). This example illustrates the need of a compiler to be aware of the overall execution schedule when applying THR.

Lastly, THR can also be applied in the context of selection points in control-flow intensive constructs. In this case, THR can be performed by reordering the various multiplexers that might be needed to select among values, possibly adapting the selection logic. Figure 4.12 illustrates this height reduction transformation for a simple code example with several nested *if-then-else* constructs depicting the corresponding hardware implementations before and after the application of THR.

```
if(c[i] == '*') {
  if(c[k] == '+') {
    oper = 1;
  } else {
    if(c[k] == '-') {
      oper = 1;
    } else {
      oper = 0;
    }
  }
} else {
  oper = 0;
}
```

(a)

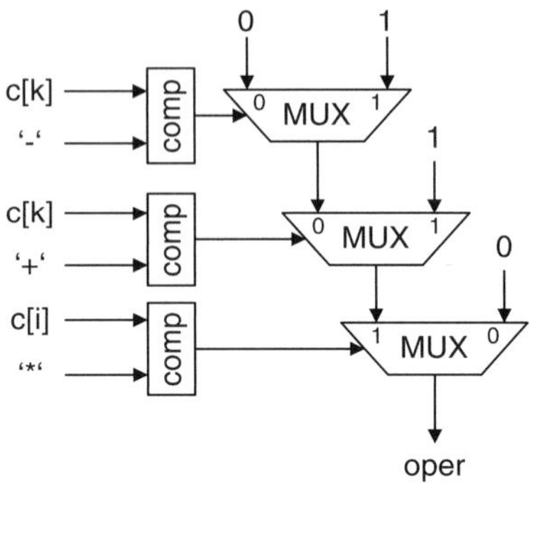

(b)

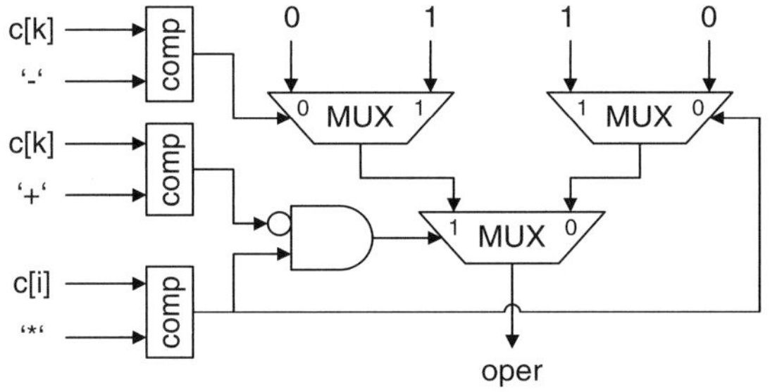

(c)

Fig. 4.12 Height reduction transformation for multiplexer-based implementation of control-flow intensive computations: (**a**) original code; (**b**) direct hardware implementation; (**c**) transformed hardware implementation

4.2.3 Code Motion

Code motion [222] is a technique that changes the order of the execution of instructions in a program by moving them either against the flow of control (hoisting) or along the flow of control (sinking).

Code motion is used extensively across control-flow branches [140, 271]. By moving an instruction in a shared section of the control-flow graph against the flow of control (hoisting) into disjoint sections of the control-flow graph, the compiler is trading off resources for concurrency. The two instances of the instruction are potentially realized by distinct hardware operators and the overall execution path is shortened. Figure 4.13 shows some examples of code hoisting and sinking (Fig. 4.13a–e) and an example of the application of code hoisting and THR to reduce the critical path of the computation (Fig. 4.13c,f). This code hoisting transformation results in one more adder unit, but decreases the critical path length by the delay/latency of one adder unit. Code sinking, the reverse code transformation,

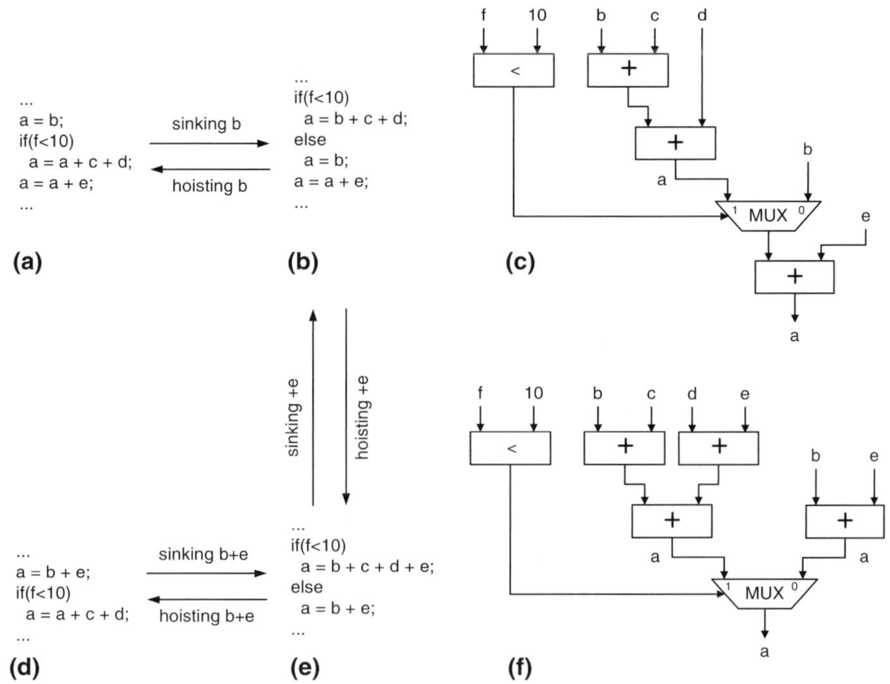

Fig. 4.13 Code hoisting in the presence of control flow: (**a**) original code; (**b**) transformed code sinking b; (**c**) DFG implementation of (**b**); (**d**) transformed code from (**a**) by hoisting a + e; (**e**) transformed code from (**d**) by sinking b + e; (**f**) DFG implementation of (**e**)

can be used to move the addition +e in the direction of the control flow. Using code sinking, the code in Fig. 4.13e would be transformed into the code depicted in Fig. 4.13b, in this case increasing latency but saving hardware resources. Other forms of code hoisting and code sinking can be applied to Fig. 4.13e to move upwards or downwards the subexpression b+e, respectively.

Conversely, when moving a common instruction or a common sequence of instructions along the control flow from two disjoint paths of the CFG into a shared section of the CFG, the required hardware resources are reduced, but the execution of the operations corresponding to the instructions is serialized.

In addition to its application within basic blocks or across control-flow constructs, code motion is also used in wider scopes. In the context of loops, loop invariant code motion hoists to the loop preheader instructions that are always executed when the loop executes and that evaluate to the same values on every iteration of the loop. This loop invariant code motion transformation has the same benefits than in traditional architectures as it reduces the number of times an instruction is executed. When compiling for reconfigurable architectures, loop invariant code motion leads, in general, to hardware implementations with fewer hardware resources for the execution of the computations of the loop body, as well as to a possible benefit in terms of the length of schedule of the execution of the loop body.

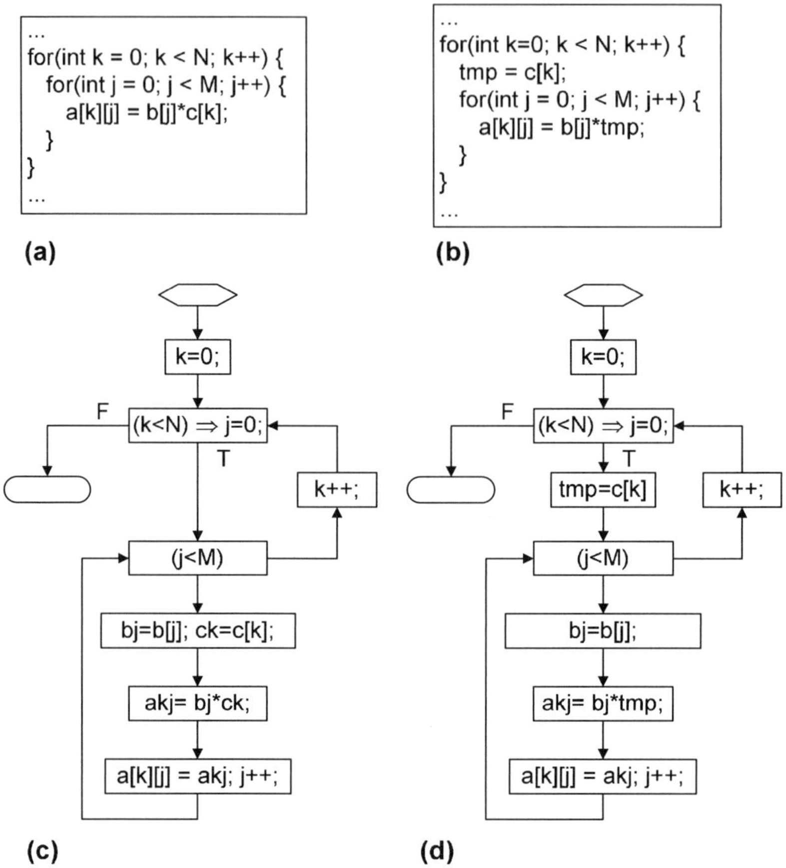

Fig. 4.14 Code hoisting example: (**a**) original code; (**b**) code after loop invariant code motion; (**c–d**) algorithmic state machine charts representing possible hardware implementations for the two code excerpts, respectively

The spatial nature of reconfigurable architectures leads, however, to particular applications of this transformation that degrade the performance of the hardware implementation as depicted by the example in Fig. 4.14. In Fig. 4.14b we depicted the application of loop invariant code motion for the source code depicted in Fig. 4.14a, where the loop-invariant statement `c[k]` (Fig. 4.14a) is moved outside `j` loop. In this example we assume that the target architecture has at least two independent memory modules to which the compiler can map distinct array variables `b` and `c`. In a direct hardware implementation corresponding to the original computation (not shown), the execution would be able to concurrently access the arrays `b` and `c` as depicted in the corresponding ASM chart in Fig. 4.14c. After the application of loop invariant code motion, the hardware implementation is forced to execute the memory accesses in disjoint steps as depicted in the ASM chart in Fig. 4.14d. Thus, and although there is a reduction of the number of memory accesses, as `c[k]` is only performed once for each iteration of `k` loop, the execution latency of the `j` loop increases.

4.3 Loop-Level Transformations

An important goal of the more complex and thus far-reaching code transformations is the matching of the instruction-level parallelism (ILP) in a given computation to the available resources in the target reconfigurable architecture. Many of these transformations expose the available concurrency in the input program, e.g., by unrolling, and/or increase the required data availability, e.g., by tiling. In addition to enabling transformations such as the ones described in the previous section and even other more generic code transformations, many of loop-level transformations enable and/or expose many opportunities for data management as described in the next section.

Tables 4.3 and 4.4 illustrate representative loop transformations [332] such as coalescing, collapsing, distribution (fission), jamming (fusion), unroll-and-jam, interchanging, peeling, reordering, reversal, strip-mining, tiling, splitting, and unrolling, whose application in the context of reconfigurable architecture exhibits various unique characteristics. A base loop transformation that simplifies the application of many other loop transformations is loop normalization. In this loop iteration-space transformation, the compiler sets the loop control variable to exhibit an initial zero value and a unity increment step adjusting accordingly all the uses of the control variable in the loop body as well as the loop's upper bound expression.

We now illustrate the use of three common loop transformations that focus on increasing the available parallelism, namely loop unrolling, loop tiling, and loop fusion.

4.3.1 Loop Unrolling

Loop unrolling is the most commonly used loop transformation when mapping loop computations to hardware. The body of the unrolled loop, usually the innermost loop of a nest, is replicated, and the index expression corresponding to each of the unrolled iterations is propagated to the statements in each instance of the loop body as illustrated in Fig. 4.15.

By replicating the statements in the body of the loop, loop unrolling exposes more opportunities for the concurrent execution of the multiple instances of arithmetic operators corresponding to the various instructions in the statements of the loop, only subject to data or hardware resource dependences. In addition to the increase in the potential for instruction-level parallelism, loop unrolling also decreases

Table 4.3 Sample loop transformations and illustrative examples (part I)

Loop transformation	Illustrative examples	
	Original source code	Transformed code
Normalization	for(i=2; i<N; i++) sum += A[i-2];	for(i=0; i<N-2; i++) sum += A[i];

Unrolling
(fully or by a factor *k*)
	for(i = 0; i < N; i++){
	sum += A[i];
	}
		for(i = 0; i < N; i+=2) {
		sum += A[i];
		sum += A[i+1];
		}

Unswitching	for(i=0; i<N; i++) {
	sum += A[i];
	if(b) A[i] = 0;
	}
		if(b)
		for(i=0; i<N; i++) {
		sum += A[i];
		A[i] = 0;
		}
		else
		for(i=0; i<N; i++)
		sum += A[i];

Reversal	for(i=0; i<N; i++) sum += A[i];	for(i=N-1; i>=0; i--) sum += A[i];

Interchange/reordering	for(j=0; j<M; j++)
	for(i=0; i<N; i++)
	sum += A[j][i];
		for(i=0; i<N; i++)
		for(j=0; j<M; j++)
		sum += A[j][i];

Strip-mining
(single nested loops)
	for(i=0; i<N; i++)
	sum += A[i];
		for(is=0; is<N; is+=S)
		for(i=S; i<min(N,is+S-1); i++)
		sum += A[i];

Tiling/blocking
(generic nested loops)
	for(j=0; j<M; j++)
	for(i=0; i<N; i++)
	sum += A[j][i];
		for(jc=0;jc<M; jc+=B)
		for(ic=0;ic<N; ic+=B)
		for(j=jc;j< min(M,jc+B-1); j++)
		for(i=ic;i<min(N,ic+B-1);i++)
		sum += A[j][i];

Fusion/merging	for(i=0; i<N; i++)
	sum += A[i];
	for(i=0; i<N; i++)
	prod += B[i]*B[i];
		for(i=0; i<N; i++) {
		sum += A[i];
		prod += B[i]*B[i];
		}

Fission/distribution	for(i=0; i<N; i++) {
	sum += A[i];
	prod += B[i]*B[i];
	}
		for(i=0; i<N; i++) sum += A[i];
		for(i=0; i<N; i++) prod += B[i]*B[i];

Splitting	for(i=0; i<N; i++)
	sum += A[i];
		for(i=0; i<N/2; i++)
		sum += A[i];
		for(i=N/2; i<N; i++)
		sum += A[i];

the iteration control overhead as the run-time tests used to determine if a given iteration of the loop is executed are partially or totally eliminated.

The increase in the required resources to meet the demands of the operators in the unrolled loop may require a slight increase in storage to accommodate the many temporary register values used in the evaluation of the various operations. Furthermore, the potential concurrent execution of many operators, and despite the potential for data reuse, increases the pressure on data bandwidth or data availability, measured on a per iteration basis. As such, in some instances, loop unrolling might not

Table 4.4 Sample loop transformations and illustrative examples (part II)

Loop transformation	Illustrative examples	
	Original source code	Transformed code

Peeling	for(i=0; i<N; i++)
	sum += A[i];
		sum += A[0];
		for(i=1; i<N; i++)
		sum += A[i];

Coalescing	for(j=0; j<N; j++)
	for(i=0; i<N; i++)
	sum += A[j][i];
		for(t=0; t<N*N; t++) {
		j = t/N;
		i = t%N;;
		sum += A[j][i];
		}

Collapsing (a special form of coalescing when loop limits match array bounds)	for(j=0; j<M; j++)
	for(i=0; i<N; i++)
	sum += A[j][i];
		for(i=0; i<N*N; i++)
		sum += A[i];

Alignment	for(i=1; i<=N; i++) {
	b[i]=a[i];
	d[i]=b[i-1];
	c[i]=a[i+1];
	}
		d[1]=b[0];
		for(i=2; i<=N; i++) {
		b[i-1]=a[i-1];
		d[i]=b[i-1];
		c[i-1]=a[i-1];
		}
		b[N]=a[N];
		c[N]=a[N+1];

Unroll and Jam	for(j=0; j<M; j++)
	for(i=0; i<N; i++)
	sum += A[j][i];
		for(j=0; j<M; j+=2)
		for(i=0; i<N; i++) {
		sum += A[j][i];
		sum += A[j+1][i]; }

Shifting	for(i=1; i<=N;i++) {
	a[i]=b[i];
	d[i]=a[i-1];
	}
		for(i=0; i<=N;i++) {
		if(i>0) a[i]=b[i];
		if(i<N) d[i+1]=a[i];
		}

Skewing	for(j=0; j<M; j++)
	for(i=0; i<N; i++)
	sum += A[j][i];
		for(j=0; j<M; j++)
		for(i=j; i<N+j; i++)
		sum += A[j][i-j];

```
...
#define W 3
...
int a[W][W], b[W][W], c[W];
...
for(x=0; x < W; x++) {
  sum = 0;
  for(y=0; y < W; y++) {
    sum += (a[x][y] * b[y][x]);
  }
  c[x] = sum;
}
...
```

(a)

```
...
#define W 3
...
int a[W][W], b[W][W], c[W];
...
for(x=0; x < W; x++) {
  sum = (a[x][0] * b[0][x]);
  sum += (a[x][1] * b[1][x]);
  sum += (a[x][2] * b[2][x]);
  c[x] = sum;
}
...
```

(b)

Fig. 4.15 Full loop unrolling transformation and opportunities for parallel execution: (**a**) original C source code; (**b**) full unrolling of inner loop

be profitable, or the corresponding performance gains might not justify the additional required resources.

A loop can be unrolled either partially or fully. In partial loop unrolling, the body of the loop is replicated only k times with k less than the number of loop iterations to be executed.[4] When the loop bounds are not known statically, loop unrolling requires the use of control-flow constructs to determine if given iteration should be executed. This overhead can be mitigated by the use of predicates that check, and thus validate, the execution of chunks of k iterations, allowing the unrolled k iterations to be executed without checks. In fully loop unrolling the loop is completely unrolled, i.e., the body of the loop is replicated as many times as the number of iterations of the loop. In this case, the loop bounds must be known statically, possibly by the use of constant propagation, as in the example depicted in Fig. 4.15.

After loop unrolling, the compiler can apply a wide range of other code transformations. For example, exploiting commutative and associative properties to the example of Fig. 4.15b, a compiler can rearrange the accumulations in the `sum` variable and apply THR while still exploiting the potential for concurrent execution of the three multiplications. Figure 4.16 depicts two illustrative hardware implementations corresponding, respectively, to the original source code in Fig. 4.15 and the transformed code using loop unrolling and THR targeting an architecture with multiple hardware multipliers.

4.3.2 Loop Tiling and Loop Strip-Mining

Loop tiling [332], or blocking, transforms the iteration space of the loop nest by structuring the execution of the loop into blocks/tiles of iterations of the original loop. A tilled loop is thus structured as two loops, where an outer loop, called *control loop*, determines which of the blocks of iterations the inner loop executes. Figure 4.17 depicts an example of loop tiling, where the iteration space of the original loop is split into blocks of size $B1 \times B2 \times B3$.

As highlighted in this example, loop tiling promotes locality, which is an important property to reduce cache hit misses when cache memories are used [205]. More importantly, in the absence of data dependences, invocations of the innermost loop in a tiled loop can be executed concurrently. After loop tiling, a compiler can distribute the computation associated with each iteration of the control loop (an invocation of the inner loop) across distinct FUs and distribute the corresponding data they manipulate between multiple distributed memories e.g., the block RAMs in FPGAs). A particular case of loop tiling is *loop strip-mining* [332], where tiling is applied to singly nested loops, creating an inner loop responsible for the computation on each strip and an outer loop to control or traverse the various strips.

[4] Common implementations of partial loop unrolling use an unrolling factor that evenly divides the number of loop iterations. Otherwise, the transformed code will have to include an epilogue or additional control flow in the body of the loop.

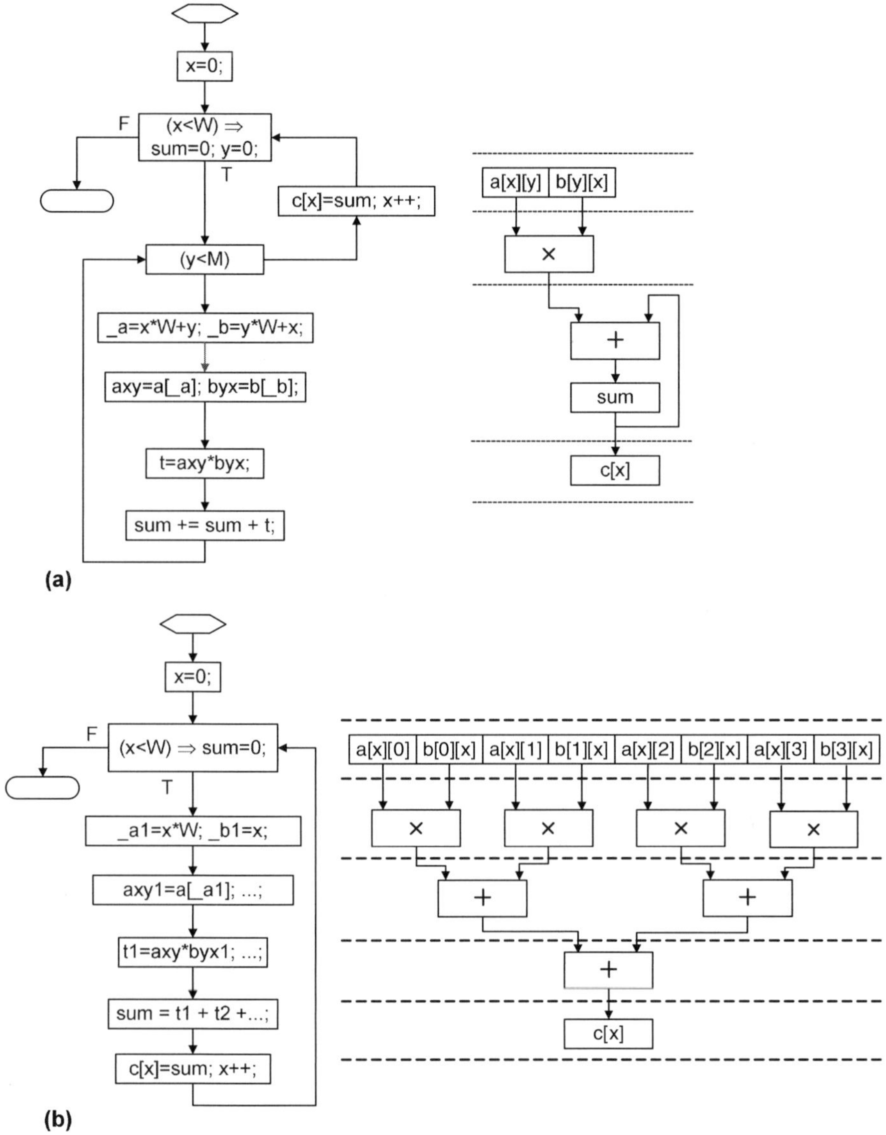

Fig. 4.16 Full unrolling hardware implementations: (**a**) from the original code depicted in Fig. 4.15a; (**b**) resulting from loop unrolling and THR (code presented in Fig. 4.15b)

The locality and coarse-grained concurrency make loop tiling or loop strip-mining particularly suited for either fine-grained or coarse-grained reconfigurable architectures as highlighted by the example in Fig. 4.18. Figure 4.18b depicts the application of loop strip-mining to the source code in Fig. 4.18a whose normalization of the innermost loop is depicted in Fig. 4.18c. The inner loop of the strip-mined

```
...
for(i=0; i<N; i++)
  for(j=0; j<N; j++)
    for(k=0; k<N; k++)
      C[i][j]+=A[i][k]*B[k][j];
...
```

(a)

```
...
for(ii=0; ii<N; ii+=B1)
  for(jj=0; jj<N; jj+=B2)
    for(kk=0; kk<N; kk+=B3)
      for(i=ii; i<min(ii+B1,N); i++)
        for(j=jj; j<min(jj+B2,N); j++)
          for(k=kk; k<min(kk+B3,N); k++)
            C[i][j] = A[i][k] * B[k][j];
...
```

(b)

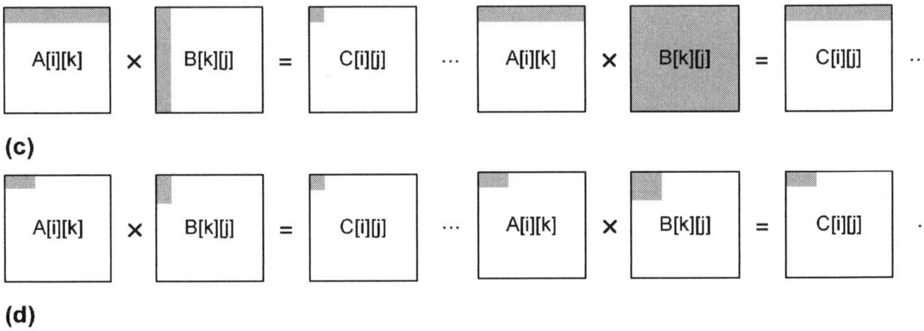

Fig. 4.17 Loop tiling applied to a matrix multiplication example: (**a**) original source code; (**b**) code after loop tiling; (**c–d**) layout of data being read/write using the (**c**) original source code and the (**d**) transformed code

```
...
for(i=0; i<512; i++)
  c[i] = a[i]*b[i];
...
```

(a)

```
...
for(is=0; is<512; is+=64)
  for(i=is; i<is+64; i++)
    c[i] = a[i]*b[i];
...
```

(b)

```
...
for(is=0; is<512; is+=64)
  for(i=0; i<64; i++)
    c[i+is] = a[i+is]*b[i+is];
...
```

(c)

```
...
for(is=0; is<512; is+=64) {
  for(i=0; i<64; i++)  { // L1: load block
    local_a[i] = a[i+is];
    local_b[i] = b[i+is];
  }

  for(i=0; i<64; i++)  // L2: compute over block
    local_c[i] = local_a[i]*local_b[i];

  for(i=0; i<64; i++) // L3: store block
    c[i+is] = local_c[i];
}
...
```

(d)

Fig. 4.18 Loop strip-mining example: (**a**) original code; (**b**) code after strip-mining with strips of 64 values; (**c**) normalization of the innermost loop; (**d**) distribution of the innermost loop

loop can then be split into three consecutive loops using loop distribution (described in the next section) resulting in the code in Fig. 4.18d. In the first of these three loops, the computations access data in the two arrays a and b mapped to local storage. In the second loop, the computations perform the multiplications using the data in internal storage and in the last loop the computation writes the results to the array c mapped to external storage. A hardware implementation based on the transformed

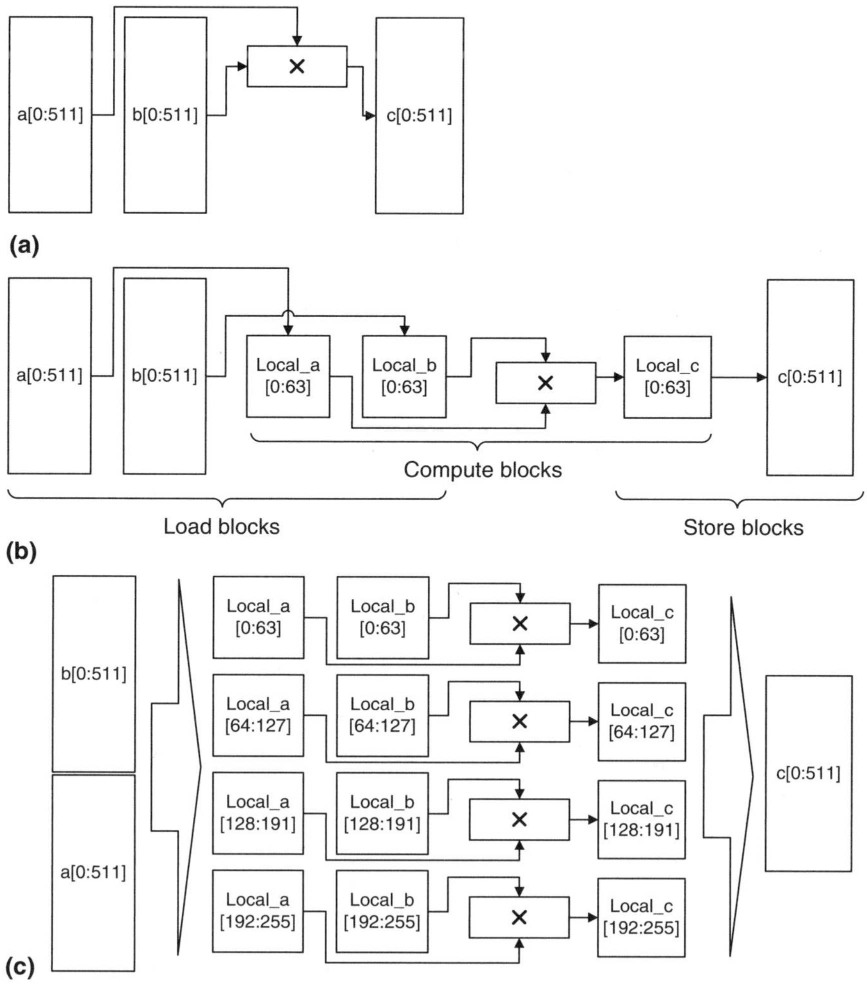

Fig. 4.19 Possible implementations for the example in Fig. 4.18: (**a**) based on the original code; (**b**) after loop strip-mining and loop distribution; (**c**) considering coarse-grained vectorization

code in Fig. 4.18d is depicted in Fig. 4.19b. It can take advantage of the use of distributed local memories and of the splitting of the computations in three stages corresponding to the three loops: loading of a block of data, computing over a block, and storing a block of results. The organization of the computation in stages suggests the application of coarse-grained pipelining execution, a technique described in Chap. 5.

An alternative compilation strategy is for the compiler to apply unrolling to the outer loops followed by strip-mining of the inner loops of the loop nest as depicted in Fig. 4.19c, resulting in a code that is easily vectorizable. As it is also apparent in Fig. 4.19c the data in the input arrays a and b can be easily partitioned across two internal/external RAMs thereby increasing the availability of the data, and thus improving the overall performance of the implementation, even without resorting to pipelining execution techniques.

Overall, loop tiling/strip-mining transformations potentially increase data locality and enable the application of coarse-grained parallelization and pipelining execution techniques, across iterations of the control loops. Loop tiling also exposes opportunities for array memory mapping (described in Chap. 5), as blocks of iterations of the tilled loops may access disjoint sets of data. If the compiler maps these sets to distinct physical memories, memory access contention is avoided.

4.3.3 Loop Merging and Loop Distribution

Loop merging or *loop fusion* [332] merges two loops into a single loop. The body of the fused loop consists of the concatenation of the loop bodies of the two original loops as depicted in the example in Fig. 4.20. This transformation is trivially implemented when the loop bounds of the loops are identical and there are no data dependences between the two loops, as in the transformed code the sequences of the statements of the two original bodies execute in an interleaved order.

When targeting reconfigurable architectures, loop fusion converts coarse-grained to fine-grained concurrency. As it is apparent in the example in Fig. 4.20, a compiler could easily identify that the two loops can be executed in parallel (coarse-grained concurrency) and generate an architecture with task-level parallelism with access to the shared data array a. Loop fusion may increase the pressure on memory bandwidth and on register usage, as the statements corresponding to the merged loop bodies can be concurrently executed (fine-grained concurrency), thus requiring more registers/operations and memory accesses per iteration.

The dual loop transformation to loop fusion is loop fission or loop distribution. Loop distribution splits a single loop into two loops with the exact same loop bounds but distributing the statements in the body of the original loop between the bodies of the two newly created loops. Excluding output- and antidependences, the transformation is always legal as the relative order in which the statements execute in the original loop is preserved in the transformed code. As this transformation is the dual of loop fusion, we omit another illustrative example here.[5]

```
for(i=0; i<N; i++)
   sum += a[i];
for(i=0; i<N; i++)
   prod += a[i]*a[i];
```
(a)

```
for(i=0; i<N; i++) {
   sum += a[i];
   prod += a[i]*a[i];
}
```
(b)

Fig. 4.20 Loop fusion example: (**a**) original source code; (**b**) code after loop fusion

[5] Loop distribution can be applied to the code of Fig. 4.20b to derive the code in Fig. 4.20a.

4.4 Data-Oriented Transformations

We now describe three basic data-oriented transformations that are particularly suited for reconfigurable architectures, given the flexibility of organization and configuration of storage structures they allow, namely, data distribution, data replication, and scalar replacement. Many, if not all, of the data-oriented transformations exhibit a strong synergy with loop-level transformations, in particular for computations that manipulate array variables using affine index access functions.

4.4.1 Data Distribution

Data distribution, commonly used for array variables, partitions each array into disjoint array subsets, each of which is then mapped to a distinct memory module. This transformation, when combined with loop unrolling, improves array data availability and allows the generation of hardware implementations that can concurrently access the data without contention.

Figure 4.21 illustrates the application of loop unrolling, and data distribution for the `img` array variable. The original `img` array is first partitioned into two distinct arrays, `imgOdd` and `imgEven`, which are then mapped to two different memories. This memory mapping of the two arrays allows the two memory load operations, corresponding to the unrolled statement in the code shown in Fig. 4.21b, to be executed concurrently.

Data distribution does not increase the required storage needs as the original data is partitioned into disjoint data sets. Other than a possible execution time overhead in reorganizing the data via distribution, data distribution increases the availability of data, provided the architecture has enough disjoint memory modules with adequate capacity to accommodate the partitions.[6]

```
...
type img[N][N];
...
for(j=0; j < N; j++) {
  ...
  for(i=0; i < N; i++) {
     ... = img[j][i];
  }
  ...
}
```
(a)

```
...
type imgOdd[N][N/2], imgEven[N][N/2];
...
for(j=0; j < N; j++) {
  ...
  for(i=0; i < N; i+=2) {
     ... = imgOdd[j][i/2];
     ... = imgEven[j][i/2];
  }
  ...
}
```
(b)

Fig. 4.21 Loop unrolling and array data distribution example: (**a**) original source code; (**b**) loop unrolled by 2 and distribution of `img`

[6] The use of distributed memories can be avoided when memory banks have enough memory access ports.

4.4.2 Data Replication

Data replication creates various copies, or replicas, of specific data items which are then mapped to distinct storage structures. This transformation thus increases the availability of the data by allowing concurrent data accesses at the expense of increased storage use. Figure 4.22 illustrates a combined application of loop unrolling and data replication for the `img` array in the original example code. The code is first unrolled by a factor of 2, generating two statements that access the `img` array. These accesses are then matched with two distinct array copies `imgA` and `imgB` of the original `img` array. For simplicity we omit here the additional code a compiler has to generate to support the initialization of the data replicas. In many reconfigurable architectures, however, the overhead of this setup phase can be mitigated by the support in hardware for concurrent memory operations and/or by overlapping this phase with other computations.

When applied to array variables, this transformation has to be exercised with caution as it increases the availability of data at the expense of potentially substantial increase in allocated storage. Its applicability may be therefore limited to small arrays that are immutable for a specific locus of computation. For example, while an array variable is modified throughout the entire program, in a specific loop nest it may only be read. This is a common case with algorithm parameters or computational coefficient loaded at the beginning of the program and never modified afterwards. In the presence of mutable data, replication raises the issue of consistency. The execution must ensure all replicas are updated with the correct values before the multiple copies can be accessed, and that any additional computation executed afterwards observes any possibly modified values [352].

4.4.3 Data Reuse and Scalar Replacement in Registers and Internal RAMs

In many computations, particularly in the context of digital image and signal processing, data values are often reused. Examples of this reuse occur when the

```
...
type img[N][N];
...
for(j=0; j < N; j++) {
  ...
  for(i=0; i < N; i++) {
     ... = img[j][i];
  }
  ...
}
```
(a)

```
...
type imgA[N][N], imgB[N][N];
...
for(j=0; j < N; j++) {
  ...
  for(i=0; i < N; i+=2) {
     ... = imgA[j][i];
     ... = imgB[j][i+1];
  }
  ...
}
```
(b)

Fig. 4.22 Loop unrolling and array data replication example: (**a**) original source code; (**b**) loop unrolled by 2 and replication of `img`

computation repeatedly uses coefficients of a signal transformation or reuses values when repeatedly accessing overlapped sections of an array.

A compiler can exploit this data reuse by selectively choosing which data values are reused in a given computation and saving or caching them in scalar variables, which are mapped to registers, in a transformation known as *register promotion*. The compiler transforms the code to save the reusable values in registers (or internal RAMs) the first time the computation accesses them. The values are then reused for the remainder of the computation. Storage allocated to this reusable data is reclaimed when the values are no longer needed.

As with traditional architectures this caching of data "locally" in registers or RAMs has the potential to improve the overall performance of the corresponding hardware implementation by two main factors. First, the use of registers substantially decreases the data access latency. In fine-grained reconfigurable architectures where registers and RAMs are distributed throughout the architecture, reusing data in discrete registers tremendously increases the amount of data bandwidth as all the registers can be accessed concurrently. Second, by reusing data internally, the implementation can drastically reduce the number of external memory accesses [289, 291].

The advantages of data reuse and scalar replacement come at the expense of increased storage requirements and the need for the compiler to explicitly manage the caching of data in internal storage resources. Given the common lack of support (most notably in fine-grained architectures) for hardware mechanisms that support high-level abstractions of virtual memory and memory coherency between external and internal storage, compilers for reconfigurable architectures must control precisely which data items are cached, where to allocate them, and when to discard them, as well as maintain coherency between internal and external data.

Figure 4.23 illustrates the application of scalar replacement to the `vec` and `coeff` array variables. In the original code, in Fig. 4.23a, the `N` locations of the `vec` array are repeatedly accessed on every iteration of the `j` loop. A way to capture this reuse is to peel the first iteration of the `j` loop (for `j=0`) and during the `i` loop corresponding to this first iteration, save the `N` elements of each row `k` of `vec` in the auxiliary vector `vec_sr`. The values in `vec_sr` are mapped to a set of N registers or an internal RAM module in the target architecture and reused through the remainder `N-1` iterations of the `j` loop. Similarly, the location `coeff[k]` is repeatedly accessed throughout the entire computation and can be saved (outside the `j` loop) into a scalar variable.

Data reuse analysis and scalar replacement can also be used in more sophisticated reuse cases. The example code depicted in Fig. 4.24a repeatedly accesses a set of three consecutive locations of the `y` array variable. Across all but the first two iterations of the `i` loop, two of the three array references have been already accessed in the previous iteration of the loop. Their values can thus be saved in registers. By organizing the registers in a tapped-delay line with *shifting* between the values of the line at every iteration of the `i` loop no explicit addressing is required [94]. The transformed code shown at the top of Fig. 4.24b can be synthesized using a tapped-delay line, where the various taps correspond to the scalar variables `D1`, `D2`, and

(a)

```
type coeff[M];
type vec[N];
...
for(k=0; k < M; k++) {
  ...
  for(j=0; j < N; j++) {
    ...
    for(i=0; i < N; i++) {
      ... = vec[k][i] * coeff[k];
    }
    ...
  }
}
```

(b)

```
type coeff[M], coeff_sr;
type vec[M][N], vec_sr[N];
...
for(k=0; k < M; k++) {
  ...
  /* i,j loop invariant */
  coeff_sr = coeff[k];
  /* iteration for j = 0 */
  for(i=0; i < N; i++) {
     vec_sr[i] = vec[k][i]; /* saving data */
     ... = vec_sr[i] * coeff_sr;
  }
  ...
  for(j=1; j < N; j++) {
    ...
    for(i=0; i < N; i++) {
       ... = vec_sr[i] * coeff_sr;
    }
    ...
  }
}
```

Fig. 4.23 Scalar replacement using loop peeling: (**a**) original source code; (**b**) scalar replacement of `vec` and `coeff` using loop peeling

```
...
for(int i=3; i<N; i++) {
  y[i] = y[i-1]*w1+y[i-2]*w2+y[i-3]*w3;
}
...
```

```
...
int d3, d2=0, d1=0;
...
for(int i=1; i<N; i++) {
  d3 = d2; /* shifting */
  d2 = d1;
  d1 = y[i-1];
  if(i>2)
    y[i] = d1*w1+d2*w2+d3*w3;
}
...
```

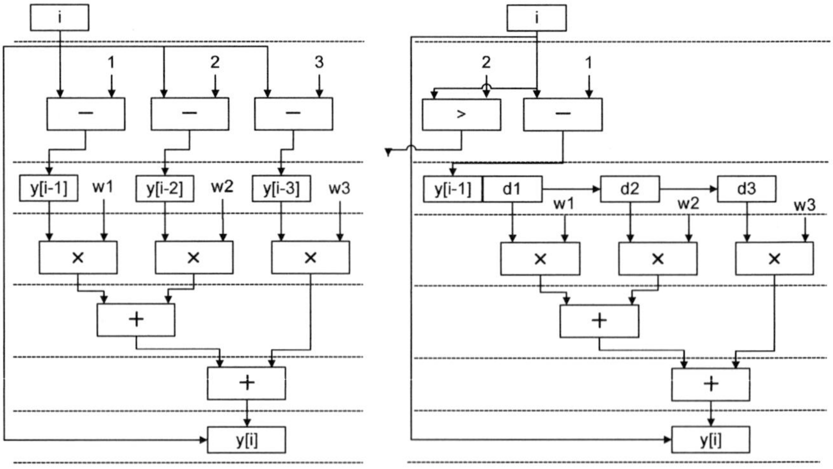

(a) (b)

Fig. 4.24 Data replacement and scalar replacement example using a tapped-delay line: (**a**) original code and partial implementation; (**b**) transformed code and partial implementation

D3.[7] For this particular reuse case, the data transformation allows the implementation to reduce the number of memory reads from $3 \times \mathtt{N} - 3$ to N-1, which can be a substantial reduction for large values of N. This reduction has a potential substantial impact on the length of the schedule for the hardware implementation, in a setting where the implementation does not have enough memory bandwidth (or simply available ports) to fetch three simultaneous data items corresponding to the 3 reads to the y array variable.

While in this example we have chosen to exploit the reuse in scalar variables with a tapped-delay line, it is also possible to reuse the data using a local RAM module. In this latter case, the delay line is conceptually implemented using *read* and *write* RAM operations. This implementation typically uses much fewer resources, but all the data elements of the tapped-delay line are not immediately available which can be a substantial disadvantage. The work by Baradaran et al. [29] explores the space and time trade-offs for these alternative implementations.

This data transformation is simple to understand and apply when, in the context of the execution of a given loop, the reused data is only read. However, scalar replacement is fairly complicated to implement, when in a given loop data that is reused is both read and written, in particular in the presence of multiple data references that reuse the same array location [28]. In these more complex scenarios, care must be taken to ensure that the cached data in the scalar replaced register is copied back into the original array so that future instantiations of the transformations can use the correct value.

Data-reuse is also exploited in temporal common subexpression elimination. In this technique, a compiler identifies expressions already computed in previous iterations of a loop, replacing them with the registered values. This variant of data reuse is commonly used in the compilation of window-based image processing applications [44], as illustrated in Fig. 4.25.

4.4.4 Other Data-Oriented Transformations

We now briefly describe various less commonly used, data-oriented transformations that arise naturally in the context some of the loop transformations previously described.

As an example, when performing loop fission or loop fusion is often needed to perform scalar expansion or array contraction. Scalar expansion uses an array to store the successive values of a scalar variable accessed for each iteration of the loop. Array contraction refers to the opposite transformation. Figure 4.26 illustrates the need for scalar expansion when applying loop distribution between the statements 6 and 7 in the loop in Fig. 4.26a. This loop distribution requires the implementation to save the value of the max variable at each iteration of the first loop, as each of these

[7] This use of a tapped-delay line is similar to the approach used in VLIW (Very Long Instruction Width) [110] and EPIC (Explicitly Parallel Instruction Computing) [272] architectures known as rotating registers [86, 98].

```
...
int sum1, sum2;
...
for(i=0; i<N_COLS-1; i++) {
  int sum1 = 0;
  int sum2 = 0;
  for(j=0; j<N_ROWS; j++) {
    sum1 += A[j][i];
    sum2 += A[j][i+1];
  }
  B[i] = (w1*sum1 + w2*sum2)/2;
}
...
```

(a)

```
...
int sum2 = 0, sum;
...
for(i=0; i<N_COLS-1; i++) {
  sum1 = sum2;
  sum2 = 0;
  for(j=0; j<N_ROWS; j++) {
    if(i==0) {
      sum1 += A[j][i];
      sum2 += A[j][i+1];
    } else {
      sum2 += A[j][i+1];
    }
  }
  B[i] = (w1*sum1 + w2*sum2)/2;
}
...
```

(b)

Fig. 4.25 Temporal common subexpression elimination: (**a**) original code; (**b**) possible transformed code

```
...
max = MIN_INT;
for(i=0; i<N; i++) {
  t1 = a[i]*b[i];
  c[i] = f1(t1);
  if(t1>max) max = t1;
  d[i] = f2(max);
}
...
```

(a)

```
...
max = MIN_INT;
for(i=0; i<N; i++) {
  t1 = a[i]*b[i];
  c[i] = f1(t1);
  if(t1>max) max = t1;
  array_max[i] = max;
}
for(i=0; i<N; i++) {
  max = array_max[i];
  d[i] = f2(max);
}
...
```

(b)

Fig. 4.26 Loop distribution requiring scalar expansion: (**a**) original code; (**b**) code after loop distribution

specific values is required in the same iteration of the second loop. To save these values of the scalar variables, the transformation creates the array `array_max` variable as depicted in the transformed code in Fig. 4.26b. The opposite transformation, loop fusion, can be applied to merge the two loops in Fig. 4.26b and in this case *array contraction* is used to remove the array variable `array_max`.

Another common data-oriented transformation consists in the reorganization of the data-layout of array variables. The classic example is the transposition of an array from column-major to row-major data-layout organization (and vice versa) to best match the data access patterns of a specific loop nest. This alignment of data layout with data access patterns allows a computation to improve its data locality and data reuse, possibly eliminating many redundant address calculations as described in Sect. 5.5.2. Another data-layout transformation is *array padding*. Array padding increases the length of array dimensions in order to change the distances between consecutive array elements (known as intra-array padding) or between arrays (known as inter-array padding). This transformation can be useful in the context of fine-grained reconfigurable architectures, as it may reduce the complexity of the address generation units by allowing the same address generator to be used when addressing different arrays in the same loop [275]. In addition, arrays can be allocated and padded at specific address boundaries such that the corresponding addresses are calculated by concatenating a base address value with the index value of the element being accessed, thereby avoiding the need for the addition of the base address of the array to the index value.

Lastly, and closely related to loop-level transformations, are the data strip-mining and data-permutation transformations. Data strip-mining transforms a single-dimensional array into a two-dimensional array and is used in combination with data-layout techniques commonly when compiling for multi-processor architectures with distributed memories [18]. Data-permutation preserves the dimensionality of an array but substitutes the original array indexing, say `a[i]` with a generic mapping function of the enclosed loop indices, say `a[f(i)]`. The last technique is used to transform array access patterns in a given loop, according to different data layout organizations, and is used when explicit data-reorganization is impractical.

4.5 Function-Oriented Transformations

We now describe several function-oriented transformations used when compiling to hardware procedure/function constructs in imperative languages,[8] namely, function inlining/outlining and recursive functions.

4.5.1 Function Inlining and Outlining

Function inlining and *outlining* are dual source code transformations with complementary effects. *Function inlining* (also known as *function unfolding* and *inline expansion*) replaces a call instruction or function invocation statement with the statements in the body of the invoked function [251]. In the context of hardware compilation, this transformation instantiates the hardware corresponding to the implementation of the function, at the portion of the hardware implementation that corresponds to the call instruction. *Function outlining* (also known as *inverse function*

[8] Although similar in spirit, the techniques described here are not to be confused with specific research work on compilation to hardware of programs specified using functional programming languages.

inlining, *function folding*, and *function exlining* [313]) abstracts two or more similar sequences of instructions replacing them with a call instruction or function invocation of the abstracted function. While *function inlining* increases the amount of potential instruction-level parallelism by exposing more instructions in the function call-site, function outlining reduces it.

We now illustrate the application of these transformations for the implementation in hardware of C program functions and segments of code. Figure 4.27b illustrates the hardware implementation of the `func` function with two input arguments as depicted in Fig. 4.27a. A noninlined hardware implementation is depicted in Fig. 4.27c where the function hardware is shared by the two call sites. In this case multiplexers are used to select the appropriate input argument values and registers are used to store return results corresponding to each call site. A truly inlined implementation of the `func` function is depicted in Fig. 4.27d where instantiations of the hardware corresponding to each function call site do not share resources and have taken advantage of the specific value for the argument in the first call site. In addition to increasing the opportunities for resource sharing [253], function inlining also allows the hardware specialization corresponding to the inlined code for each specific

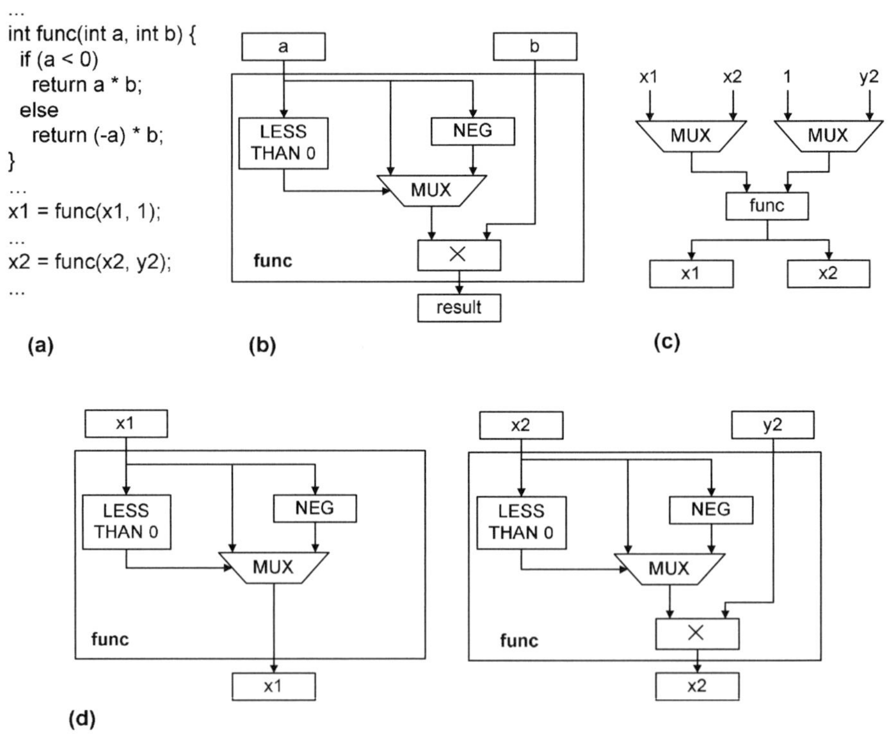

Fig. 4.27 Example with *function inlining*: (**a**) source code; (**b**) hardware block for the function; (**c**) hardware block for sharing the function hardware; (**d**) hardware implementation without sharing

```
...
x = a + b;
y = x + 1;
...
z = k + t;
w = z + 1;
...
```

(a)

```
...
void func(int *v1, int *v2,
            int p1, int p2) {
  int temp;
  temp = p1 + p2;
  *v1 = temp;
  *v2 = temp + 1;
}
...
func(&x,&y,a,b,);
...
func(&z,&w,k,t);
...
```

(b)

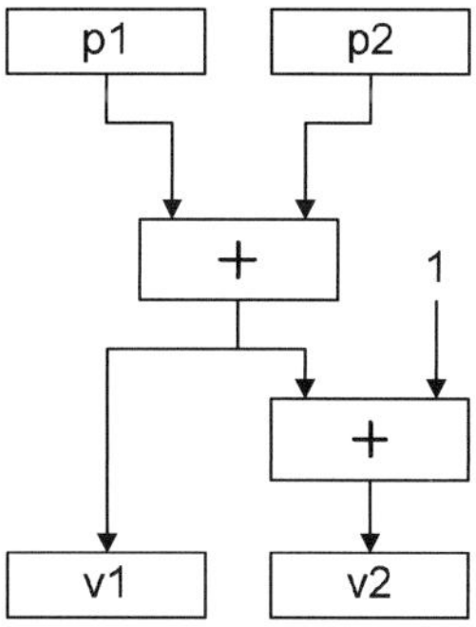

(c)

Fig. 4.28 Example with function outlining: (**a**) source code; (**b**) code after outlining; (**c**) shared hardware block

call site. Typical examples of specialization include the use of constant parameters, leading to constant propagation, type specialization as well as bit-width and operator specialization.

Figure 4.28 depicts the application of function outlining. For the code segment in Fig. 4.28a the compiler recognizes a similar computational pattern for the two sequences of instructions. Figure 4.28b depicts the transformed code using software function outlining where the two sequences are now replaced by call instructions to the abstracted `func` function whose hardware implementation is depicted in Fig. 4.28c. Function outlining therefore improves the amount of resource sharing as all invocations use the same hardware for implementing the original functionality. The advantages of resource sharing come at the expense of constraining the potential instruction-level parallelism in the hardware implementation as the various function invocations now need to have their execution serialized by the shared hardware resources.

When performing function inlining or outlining a compiler can strike a balance between concurrency and resource sharing, as depicted in the example in Fig. 4.29 for function outlining. In the code depicted in Fig. 4.29a the compiler can readily recognize the same computational patterns across the two sets of statements {`s1`,`s2`} and {`s3`,`s4`} with the exception of a subtraction operation in `s1` and an addition operation in `s3`. Still, the compiler can generate the combined hardware implementation depicted in Fig. 4.29b, that implements both structures. This hardware implementation uses a multiplexer to select the intermediate value that corresponds to each function while sharing all hardware resources corresponding to common operations in the two sequences of instructions in the original code. When using pipelined execution techniques, the implementation can effectively time share the resources corresponding to the multiplication by `c0`, the addition by `c1`, and the shifting by `c2` operators and thus exploit instruction-level parallelism.

```
...
s1: q0a = h3 -g3;
s2: q0  = (q0a * c0 + c1) >> c2;
s3: t0a = h3 + g3;
s4: t0  = (t0a * c0 + c1) >> c2;
...
```

(a)

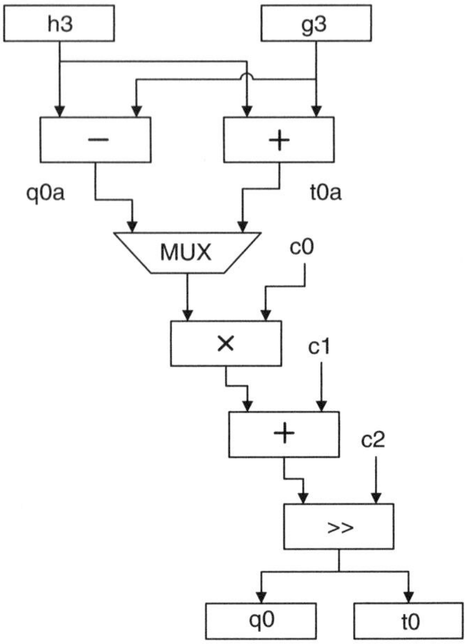

(b)

Fig. 4.29 Example of abstraction of highly similar code sequences: (**a**) original segment of code taken from a real implementation; (**b**) hardware block abstracting code sequences {`s1,s2`} and {`s3,s4`}

4.5.2 Recursive Functions

The compilation to hardware of recursive functions presents a serious challenge, as in a strict sense it would require dynamic hardware replication on recursive invocation. An obvious alternative is to generate specific hardware implementations with auxiliary storage for a call-stack and argument stack. Upon invocation, the implementation would have to save the relevant execution state, i.e., internal register data and overall execution points, onto the call-stack and invokes the called function. On a return, the state of the hardware resources would have to be restored so that execution would proceed. Clearly saving and restoring the state of a concurrent hardware execution that possibly exploits pipelining and other execution schemes is far from being trivial.

Another possible implementation transforms first the recursive function to an iterative implementation. A simple transformation is possible with tail-recursive functions as the recursive call is the last operation in these functions. However, automatic translation of nontail recursive functions is still nevertheless a challenge to perform automatically.

4.6 Which Code Transformations to Choose?

While the code transformations described in this chapter are well known in the realm of compilation for traditional architectures targeting either uniprocessor or multiprocessor machines, they expose hardware resources and execution time trade-offs that are specific to reconfigurable architectures. Despite the possibility of a synergetic combination with many other loop transformations and the instruction-level transformations described here, many of these transformations interfere with each other. The choice of which code transformations to use, which transformation parameters to select, and what transformation sequence to apply are fundamentally hard problems.

In the context of reconfigurable architectures the possibility of exploiting various execution schemes (see Chap. 5) both spatially and temporally and the inherent limitations of the target hardware devices exacerbate the difficulty of this selection process. Invariably, and given the pressure for fast compilation times, compilers use predefined and empirically established combinations of transformations to deliver effective hardware implementations.

Ultimately, the application of the transformations is constrained by the characteristics of the target architecture. When using an internal compilation algorithm, the compiler may rely on the perceived impact of each of these transformations in specific target architecture metrics such as the amount of storage, operator resources, or memory bandwidth. To illustrate such process we present in the Table 4.5 a set

Table 4.5 Selected transformations and their qualitative metric impact

	Concurrency		Resource pressure		
Transformation	Coarse-grained parallelism	Fine-grained parallelism	Operator	Storage	Data availability
Bit-level transformation					
Bit-level operator specialization	n/a	n/a	↓	↓	↓
Bit-width narrowing	n/a	n/a	↓	↓	↓
Floating- to fixed-point conversion	n/a	n/a	↓	↓	↓
Instruction-level transformation					
OSR	n/a	↓	↓	↓	↓
THR	n/a	↑	↑	—	↑
Code motion (hoisting/sinking)	n/a	↑			
Loop transformation					
Unrolling	—	↑	↑	↑	↑
Tiling	—	—	—	—	↓
Fusion	↓	↑	↑	↑	↑
Distribution	↑	↓	↓	↓	↓
Function transformations					
Inlining	↓	↑	↑	↑	—
Outlining	↑	↓	↓	↓	—
Recursive Functions into iteration	n/a	n/a	—	↓	—

Table 4.6 Applicability and potential for performance impact of compilation techniques to fine- and coarse-grained reconfigurable architectures

	Architecture granularity	
Transformation	Coarse-grained	Fine-grained
Bit-level transformations		
Bit-level operator specialization	•	•••••
Bit-width narrowing	••	•••••
Floating- to fixed-point conversion	•••	•••••
Instruction-level transformations		
OSR (Operator strength reduction)	••	•••••
THR (tree-height reduction)	••••	•••••
Code motion (hoisting/sinking)	•••••	•••••
Loop transformations		
Unrolling	•••••	•••••
Tiling	•••••	•••••
Fusion	•••••	•••••
Distribution	•••••	••••
Function transformations		
Inlining	•••••	••••
Outlining	••	••
Recursive to iteration conversion	•••••	••

of code transformations and a set of qualitative evaluation metrics compilers can use to gage the application of these transformations. In this table we describe two concurrency metrics, coarse-grained parallelism and fine-grained parallelism. For each transformation we qualitatively represent the impact either as positive (as an increase of the metric represented by the symbol $\uparrow$) or as negative (as a decrease of the metric represented by the symbol $\downarrow$), or even as neutral when no significant impact is, typically, observed.

In this description, we have indicated as nonapplicable (n/a) the impact of the bit-level transformations in both the coarse- and fine-grained concurrency as these transformations tend to eliminate resources in the form of less bit-width required, and tend to change little the nature of the operations.

Finally, we present in Table 4.6 the applicability of each of the techniques described in this chapter as the potential for performance impact when targeting either coarse- or fine-grained reconfigurable architectures. In this table a high applicability, meaning that there is potentially a high impact on the transformed code for that target architecture, is indicated by five bullets whereas a very low impact is indicated by a single bullet. While it is evident that loop transformations are equally applicable in both classes of reconfigurable architectures, the gains in fine-grained reconfigurable architectures are possibly larger than in coarse-grained architectures as fine-grained architectures are more sensitive to variations of the input program specification. For example, the bit-level transformations are a better match to fine-grained reconfigurable architectures.

4.7 Summary

In this chapter we described code transformations used when mapping computations to reconfigurable architectures, illustrating the application of these transformations for specific source code examples and generic hardware implementations. We categorized and described various code transformations, respectively, as bit-level optimizations, conversions between data representations, instruction-level transformations, loop-level and data-oriented transformations, and finally function-level transformations. As with many source code transformations used in the context of compilation and hardware synthesis, they interact, in many cases, synergetically. We addressed this interaction by organizing the transformations described here in terms of their impact on generic architectural performance metrics such as operator, storage, and bandwidth pressure. In addition, and given that different transformations expose different levels of concurrency, some transformations are more suitable to fine-grained than to coarse-grained reconfigurable architectures. The extraordinary variety of choices of transformations and their application sequences pose a huge challenge for any effective compiler and synthesis tools for contemporary and future reconfigurable architectures.

Chapter 5
Mapping and Execution Optimizations

This chapter describes important aspects related to the mapping of computations to reconfigurable architectures. The inherently spatial nature of these architectures, their heterogeneity and the invariable limitations of its physical resources, makes this mapping an extremely challenging task. Compilers and tools must judiciously balance the use of different kinds of resources in space and time, engaging in algorithmic and mapping techniques similar to the ones used in the context of low-level hardware synthesis, albeit with mapping choices that can be leveraged at much higher levels of abstraction.

We begin this chapter with control-flow mapping techniques enabled by the spatial nature of the target reconfigurable architectures. Next, we address spatial and temporal partitioning of computations within a single or multiple devices, respectively, followed by high-level techniques to map scalar variables and operations to hardware resources. We then describe memory mapping techniques for high-level data abstractions such as multidimensional arrays or data streams. Finally, and given their importance, we describe pipelining execution schemes at either fine- or coarse-grained levels.

5.1 Hardware Execution Techniques

The natural parallelism in many reconfigurable architectures allows them to exploit various sources of concurrency, either by parallel execution of independent operations, or by the speculative execution of multiple control-flow branches. While these techniques are also exploited in traditional architectures for increased performance, reconfigurable architectures offer the additional possibility of customization of the parallel execution by defining the number, and structure, of each of the parallel execution units, thus better matching the specific needs of the computation at hand.

J.M.P. Cardoso, P.C. Diniz, *Compilation Techniques for Reconfigurable Architectures*,
DOI 10.1007/978-0-387-09671-1_5,

5.1.1 Instruction-Level Parallelism

The ability of reconfigurable architectures to implement multiple hardware datapaths and control units allows them to execute multiple instructions in a truly concurrent fashion. A compiler uncovers these opportunities for instruction-level parallelism (ILP) by data-dependence analysis [26] commonly at two levels, respectively, at a fine level within each statement and at a coarse-level across multiple statements.

At a fine level of granularity, the compiler examines a sequence of high-level program constructs, such as statements, to determine which operations or instructions in each statement can be safely executed in parallel. It then schedules these instructions onto different execution units for increased performance. Figure 5.1 illustrates a simple example where a compiler exploits concurrency between the operations of a given statement for a reconfigurable architecture with two nonhomogeneous execution units, respectively, `FU1` and `FU2`. For the statement depicted in Fig. 5.1a, the compiler uncovers the data-flow graph (DFG) depicted in Fig. 5.1b and then schedules the execution of the operations in this DFG onto the two functional units (FUs). This execution schedule must respect the data dependences between the operations

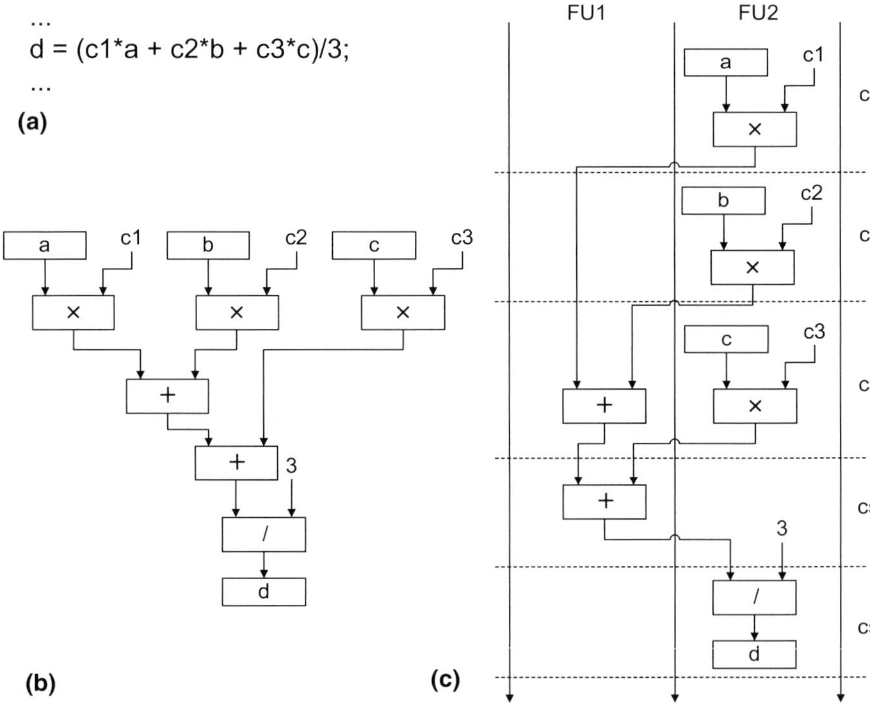

Fig. 5.1 Example of mapping: (**a**) single-statement source code; (**b**) data-flow graph; (**c**) possible scheduling organized in control steps (cs)

as well as the availability of FUs. For this specific example, we assume that all the operations execute in a single clock cycle and execution unit `FU1` cannot handle either division or multiplication operations. Under these FU constraints the schedule of the execution is five clock cycles long as depicted in Fig. 5.1c.

At a higher level of granularity, the compiler can also exploit ILP across multiple statements, possibly inside the same basic block,[1] thus expanding the range of instructions that it can schedule for parallel execution. When considering the various statements, the compiler will again rely on the two basic constraints of data dependence between instructions and the availability of FUs.

A common strategy for a compiler to increase its ability to uncover ILP opportunities relies on loop transformations, most notably, *loop unrolling*. With *loop unrolling*, a compiler creates a long sequence of statements in the body of the loop corresponding to the execution of successive loop iterations, thereby increasing the likelihood of finding data independent instructions.

Figure 5.2 illustrates the application of loop unrolling for a loop with a single statement in its body. The original loop is depicted in Fig. 5.2a, which is then executed using a simple schedule as depicted in Fig. 5.2d. This schedule reveals no opportunities for exploiting ILP due to the data dependency imposed by the accumulation in the `sum` scalar variable. By fully unrolling this loop, the compiler

```
...
sum = 0;
for(i=0; i<4; i++) {
  sum += x[i]*x[i];
}
...
```

(a)

```
...
sum = 0;
sum += x[0]*x[0];
sum += x[1]*x[1];
sum += x[2]*x[2];
sum += x[3]*x[3];
...
```

(b)

```
...
x0=x[0];
x1=x[1];
x2=x[2];
x3=x[3];
sum = x0*x0 + x1*x1 + x2*x2 + x3*x3;
...
```

(c)

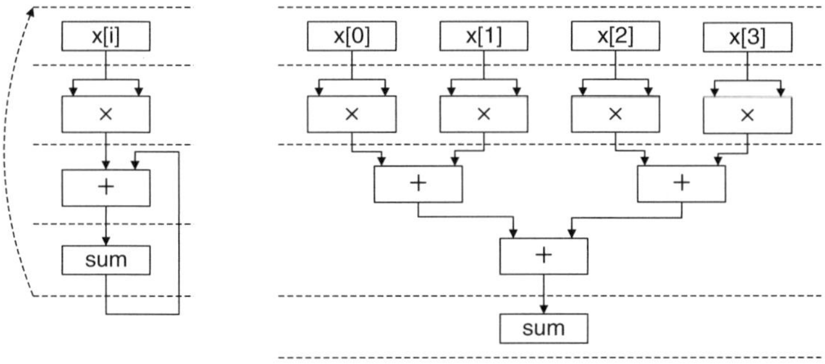

(d) **(e)**

Fig. 5.2 Applying loop unrolling to exploit ILP: (**a**) original code; (**b**) code after loop unrolling; (**c**) code after scalar replacement (see Sect. 4.4.3); (**d–e**) possible schedulings for hardware implementations

[1] A basic block [9] is the maximal sequence of program instructions with a single entry and a single exit point.

creates a sequence of four statements as depicted in Fig. 5.2b, enabling it to exploit a second transformation – associativity. By rearranging the accumulation as depicted in Fig. 5.2c, the compiler can now aggressively exploit ILP by performing the various, memory read accesses, multiplications, and additions concurrently as depicted in Fig. 5.2e and only subject to the availability of FUs. After unrolling the overall schedule length is now only four clock cycles, whereas the schedule depicted in Fig. 5.2d would yield, respectively, 4×4 and nine clock cycles, for the entire execution of the loop without and with loop pipelining.

This example illustrates the performance gains a compiler may attain by exploiting the potential of ILP. In addition to loop unrolling, compilers can also leverage a wealth of data-dependence analyses developed in the context of automatic parallelizing compilation for shared and distributed memory multiprocessors [12]. These dependence analyses focus on loop-based computations that manipulate array variables [26], allowing compilers to uncover concurrency at coarser granularity levels in what is commonly known as loop-level parallelism or task-level parallelism. The application of these analyses techniques in the context of reconfigurable architectures is entirely analogous to their use in multiprocessors, with the added benefit of exploiting FU and interconnection customizations, as well as native support for high levels of customized parallelism and pipelining.

5.1.2 Speculative Execution

Reconfigurable architectures can support the speculative execution of instructions by allowing FUs to concurrently execute mutually exclusive control-flow computation branches. If the control flow of a speculatively executed instruction is valid, the outcome of the instruction is committed as part of the state of the execution. Otherwise, the results of the execution of the mis-speculated instructions are discarded along with possible state restoring.

High-level control-flow constructs, such as *if-then-else* statements, present compilers with common scenarios for exploiting speculative execution techniques. As illustrated in Fig. 5.3, the compiler can use available resources to concurrently execute, in spatially distinct FUs, the instructions corresponding to the two control-flow branches of an *if-then-else* construct. It then uses hardware multiplexers to select which of the outcomes of the two branches is to be selected to update the storage values involved in the execution. As depicted in Fig. 5.3b, the result of the evaluation of the condition `(f<10)` dictates which of the computed values at the two inputs of the multiplexer will be assigned to the `a` variable.

Hardware speculation using spatial execution is particularly beneficial when the instructions are free of side-effects and there are ample hardware resources available. When the hardware resources are scarce, the hardware implementation may need to share hardware operators between the speculative execution paths, thus reducing the performance advantages of speculative execution.

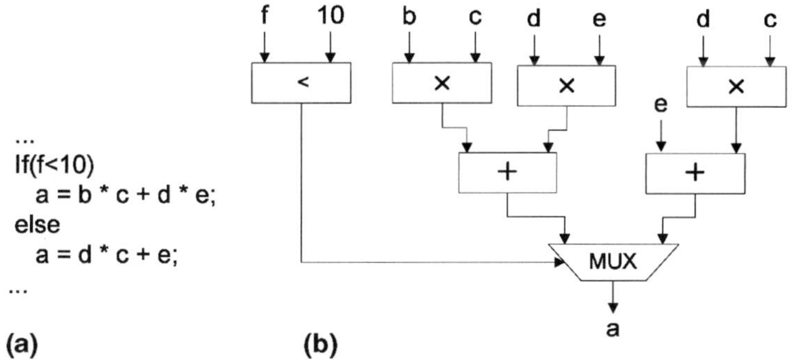

Fig. 5.3 Concurrent evaluation of branches: (a) source code; (b) data-path

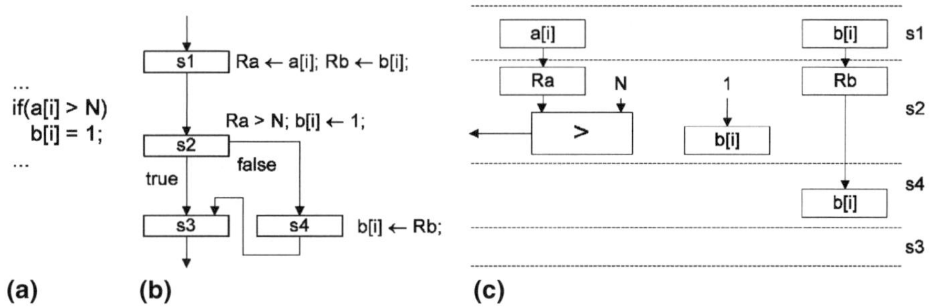

Fig. 5.4 Speculative execution of operations with side-effects and the restore mechanism when in the presence of mis-speculation: (**a**) simple example; (**b**) state transition graph; (**c**) a schedule of the operations in the data-path

As with traditional architectures, speculation can also lead to an increase in memory accesses when the speculatively executed instructions involve memory operations. While this increase can be considered benign in the case of memory read operations, the presence of memory write operations is more problematic. Although the latency of a memory write operation can be hidden by the use of a *write buffer*, the penalty of having to recover from a mis-speculated memory write operation is substantial. The overwritten value would have to be restored, for which the original value would need to have been initially read. Figure 5.4 illustrates this scenario.

For instructions with side-effects, speculation also raises the issue of implementation correctness. A speculative execution can execute an instruction that raises an exception, such as an arithmetic exception or a memory access violation, where no exception ever existed in the nonspeculative variant of the execution. A common approach to deal with this issue is for the compiler to generate code that records, for the speculatively executed instructions, any possible internal exceptions, for example via an additional hardware bit-register. Should the exception correspond to a legitimately executed instruction, the hardware will handle it, discarding it otherwise.

5.1.3 Predication and if-conversion

The spatial nature of reconfigurable architectures allows compilers to exploit predicated execution techniques as hardware implementations concurrently execute multiple flows of control from disjoint control-flow paths in the input program. Rather than allowing these flows to execute speculatively, an architecture can use predicates associated with each control-flow path to enable or disable the corresponding operators from producing output results [32].

To enable this execution technique, compilers can rely on the *if-conversion* transformation [11]. This transformation associates to instructions in a control-flow a predicate that reflects the condition under which the instructions should be executed. In traditional processors branch instructions are eliminated and the instructions converted to predicated instructions, thus avoiding common pipelining stall issues related to mispredicted branches.

In reconfigurable architectures, *if-conversion* and predication can be naturally exploited by translating the input control-flow graph (CFG) representation of the computation into a data-flow representation[2] amenable to direct hardware implementation. Mutually exclusive updates to variables are naturally captured by hardware multiplexers whose selection logic determines at run-time the particular variable definition. In architectures where variables can be bound to discrete and spatially distributed registers, the hardware corresponding to the computation of mutually exclusive data-flow branches proceeds concurrently without the concern for the updates to the registers in case some of them correspond to invalid predicates. In some instances, it is even possible for the implementation to omit some predicates as operands and results are stored in local registers or simply translated to wire connections between operations.

The logic to calculate predicates and to select between different inputs in each multiplexer and/or activate the outcomes of specific operators is known as program decision logic [22]. Fine-grained reconfigurable architectures can directly support the implementation of predication by directly implementing as hardware circuits the program decision logic. The definition of the program decision logic may rely on boolean expression minimization to reduce the amount of operations required [22]. Although the impact of this minimization may not be significant for fine-grained architectures, for coarse-grained architectures, where each logic operation typically requires an FU, the minimization of the program decision logic may thus lead to a substantial reduction of the number of required resources. When targeting coarse-grained architectures, however, the transformations described here are only employed if the architecture includes support for predicated execution or when side-effect-free operations in branches do not require predication.

A key aspect in the implementation of this technique is the determination of the program selection points for the insertion of predicates associated with each updated program variable. As with software predication, this information is easily determined by transforming the input program into an SSA-form [85], where the selection points are explicitly represented as ϕ-function statements.

---

[2] Not to be confused here with a data-flow architecture execution.

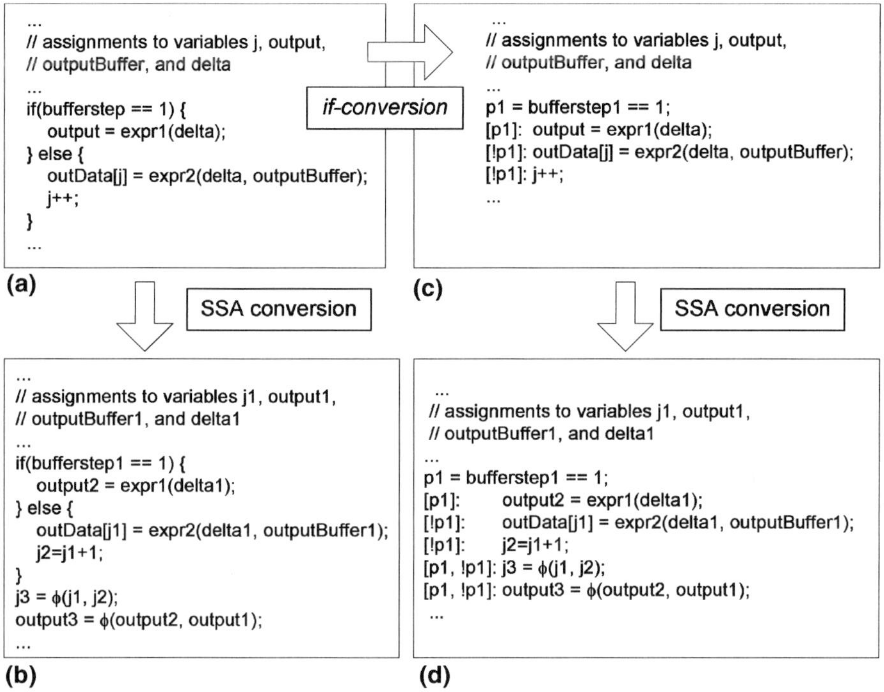

Fig. 5.5 From an *if-then-else* statement to SSA form and predicates: (**a**) original source code; (**b**) code after SSA conversion; (**c**) code after if-conversion; (**d**) code after if-conversion and SSA conversion

In Fig. 5.5, we illustrate the application of *if-conversion* and predication execution using an SSA representation for an example computation. For the code in Fig. 5.5a, the compiler can generate a control unit directly reflecting the structure of the control-flow graph (CFG) of the code. The CFG ensures the activation of the operations in the branches of the *if-then-else* structures as those branches are also reflected in the control unit. A more aggressive implementation of this simple scheme uses a control unit based on the latencies of regions of instructions (e.g., the hyperblock [200]). In this case, the control unit orchestrates the execution of the regions of code relying on a fully predicated SSA representation as depicted at the bottom of Fig. 5.5d. Figure 5.6a depicts a straightforward translation to hardware of this predicated SSA representation for the example code in Fig. 5.5d. A relaxed implementation of predicated execution is depicted in Fig. 5.6b which relies on the fact that some updates to registers are local and will not be used if the corresponding predicates are false.

In data-driven reconfigurable architectures, such as the XPP, the predicated SSA representation forms the base for the mapping of predicates to assignments to variables as the predicates (guard or selection signals) are associated to hardware events that enable/disable the operations in each PE. In architectures, where each PE includes a data-path and a control unit, however, the predicates must be

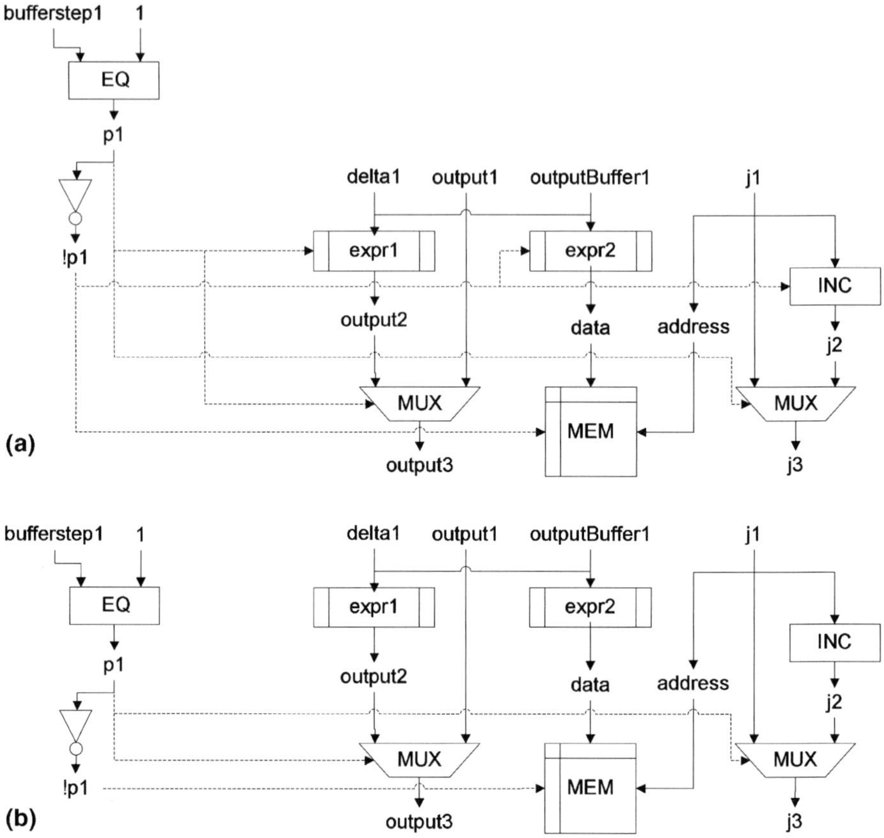

Fig. 5.6 Possible data-path implementations: (**a**) considering full predication; (**b**) considering partial predication

routed through the control unit, so that they can generate the signals needed to enable/disable operations (e.g., writes to memory).

Besides *if-conversion*, other techniques can transform control-flow constructs to simple data-flow representations suitable to be mapped to hardware. For instance, the statement `if((a&1)==1)a++;` can be implemented by adding 0 to `a` and connecting the least significant bit of `a` to the carry-in (`cin`) of the adder as depicted in Fig. 5.7. Although seldom applicable, the resource savings of this transformation are substantial.

5.1.4 Multi Tasking

By supporting spatial computations, reconfigurable architectures allow multiple flows of control to exist simultaneously as a form of spatial multitasking. A form of

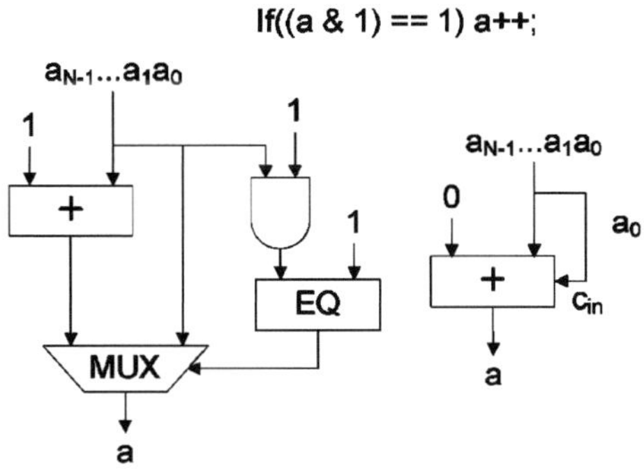

Fig. 5.7 Two possible hardware implementations for a given computation

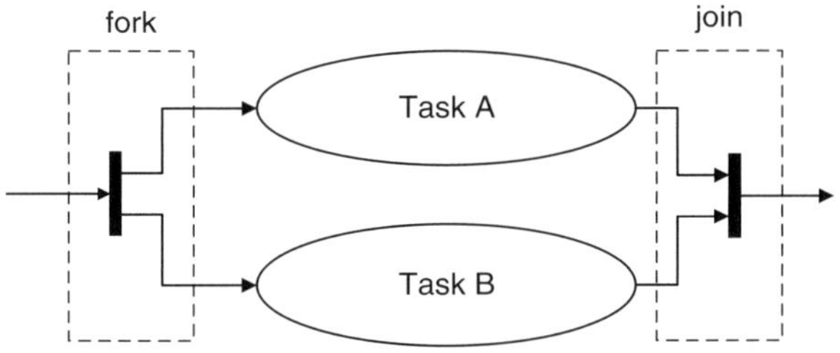

Fig. 5.8 Illustrative implementation of hardware fork and join synchronization

fine-grained multitasking with limited scope,[3] occurs when a hardware implementation evaluates in parallel, using distinct resources, disjoint branches of control-flow programming constructs. A coarse-grained multitasking, with a much wider scope, occurs when the architecture implements data-path structures that execute sequences of instructions or tasks with much longer execution spans. These tasks can correspond to high-level concurrent programming constructs such as parallel threads defined as part of the input language semantics (e.g., as in Java) or uncovered by the compiler using sophisticated data-dependence analyses [26]. Distinct resources are allocated to each task and synchronization of the many flows of control can be achieved by hardware *fork/join* points. In a direct implementation of this synchronization, illustrated in Fig. 5.8, a *fork* point consists of a wire signal activating each of the threads. A *join* point is more elaborate as it needs to capture in time the fact that two or more activities have completed.

In multitasking, the access to shared resources, e.g., access to shared memory structures, either internal or external, must be subject to arbitration, unless a predefined scheduling of accesses to such resources is imposed. In addition, the definition of a controller for multitasking execution schemes poses serious challenges to a compiler, given the many possible execution interleaving scenarios between tasks (see, e.g., the work presented by Lakshminarayana et al. in the context of concurrent

[3] This form of fine-grained multitasking can be see as a form of multithreading.

execution of distinct loops [184]). An alternative approach is to rely on the notion of *tokens* and allow shared resources to manage the requests submitted by the various tasks. The *token* allows the controllers of the shared resources to identify to which task a specific request should be directed to. Each task has its own controller which now needs only to coordinate the submission of requests to the shared resources in the pursue of the completion of its computation. This conceptually elegant approach has been used in the context of pipelined multitasking execution of data-dependent loops where different iterations that may have very distinct execution pathsaccess shared resources [298].

In the context of high-level synthesis for ASICs, there have been various efforts focusing on the generation of specific hardware implementations able to execute concurrently loops without dependences. Lakshminarayana et al. [184] describe a static scheduling algorithm that generates control units to coordinate the parallel execution of such concurrent loops. Ouaiss et al. [232] present an arbitration scheme to deal with concurrent accesses to the same hardware resources at run-time.

5.2 Partitioning

Partitioning for reconfigurable architectures deals fundamentally with two different problems, respectively, temporal partitioning and spatial partitioning. Temporal partitioning deals with the time multiplexing of hardware resources for distinct computations, whereas spatial partitioning splits a computation between multiple hardware resources. Figure 5.9 depicts an example illustrating the difference between spatial and temporal partitioning for a computation represented by its DFG where nodes denote either fine-grained instructions or coarse-grained tasks. The partitions depicted in Fig. 5.9b correspond to a feasible spatial partitioning but an infeasible

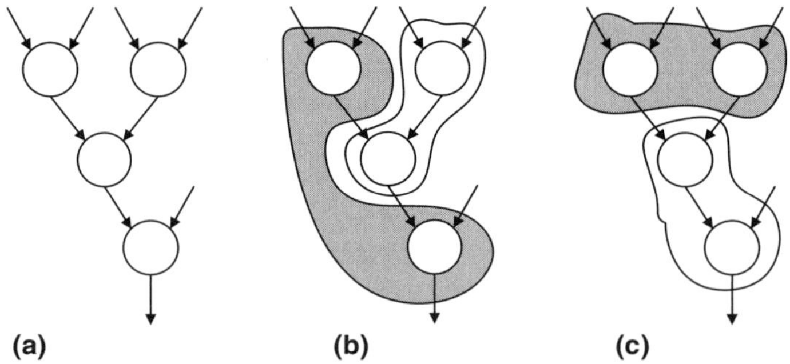

Fig. 5.9 Examples of partitions where the graphs represent a DFG or a task graph: (**a**) original graph; (**b**) possible spatial partitions but impossible temporal partitions; (**c**) possible spatial and temporal partitions

temporal partitioning, as the partition in the shaded region is nonconvex.[4] The partitions depicted in Fig. 5.9c, however, correspond to a feasible spatial and temporal partitioning.

These two forms of partitioning may be performed on computations described either at a structural or at a behavioral level, being the latter also known as functional partitioning. Given the focus of this book on compilation for high-level computation descriptions, we describe in this section the main partitioning techniques for behavioral descriptions.

5.2.1 Temporal Partitioning

There are two possibilities to map computations requiring a number of hardware resources larger than the available resources in the target reconfigurable architecture: resource sharing and temporal partitioning. Temporal partitioning exploits the reuse of hardware resources by distinct configurations in a time-multiplexing fashion. In cases where the original computations cannot be implemented as a single partition, compilers may aggressively exploit resource sharing within or across partitions.

Although the goal of temporal partitioning is to split the input computation so that each partition meets the target architecture hardware resource limitations, this technique offers other possible advantages. First, and foremost, it enables the use of smaller area/devices (with lower-cost) to implement complex applications. Second, by overlapping configuration and computation phases of subsequent hardware configurations, the implementation may even be able to amortize configuration times across partitions. Third, by partitioning computations in time, each of the implementations is simpler, possibly leading to better overall performance/power/energy results. Lastly, it allows more aggressive hardware implementations as each partition can exploit all the available hardware resources, rather than competing with all other partitions for the same resources. This individual partition optimization, leveraging the many code transformations and ignoring reconfiguration costs, can even lead to overall better performance implementations, than an implementation where the computation is aggregated in a single partition constrained to the physical hardware resources available.

While the minimization of the number of overall partitions is important, and often the most significant metric, the minimization of the data that needs to be communicated and thus saved between the execution of subsequent partitions is also important, as it directly relates to the amount of required temporary storage and communication costs during execution. The example in Fig. 5.10 illustrates two different temporal partitions with distinct amount of required data to be communicated, given the different number of edges in each computation's data-flow graph bisected by the partition cuts.

---

[4] A convex partition does not have data-flow edges that momentarily traverse nodes outside it.

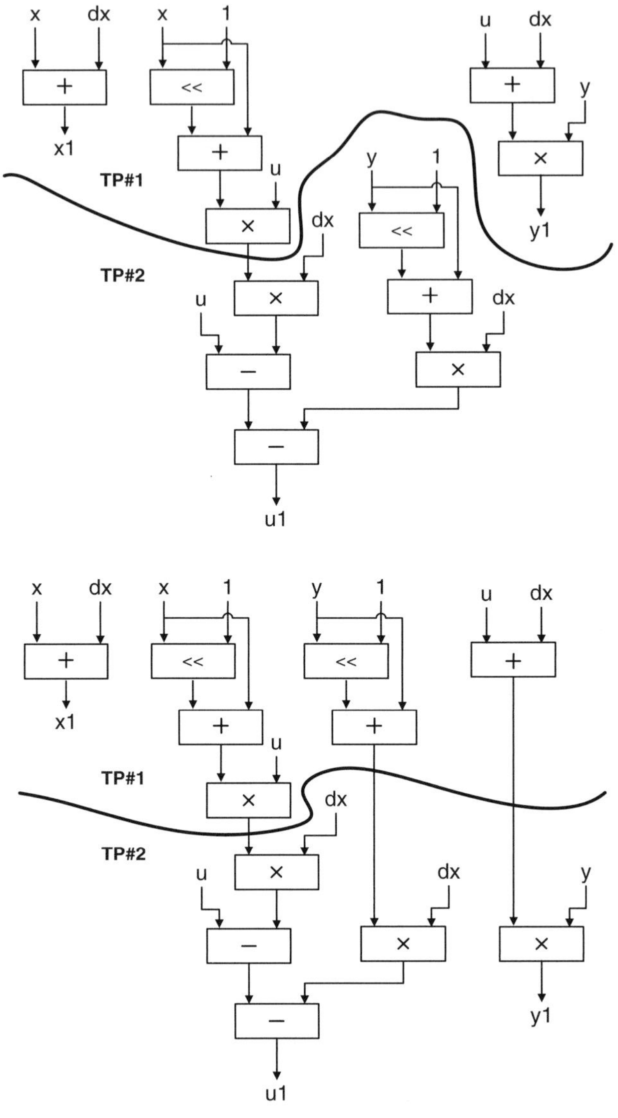

Fig. 5.10 Temporal partitioning examples with different communications costs

Temporal partitioning has been traditionally geared for two main applications, namely, rapid prototyping of large hardware circuits and program compilation. For rapid prototyping of hardware circuits, temporal partitioning methods (e.g., [196, 309]) have used net-list representations of circuits and can thus be considered a gate-level structural temporal partitioning. When compiling programs, a common internal representation (IR) is used for temporal and spatial partitioning which relies on the use of task graphs, control/data-flow graphs (CDFGs) or data-flow graphs

(DFGs). For any of these representations, temporal partitioning amounts to its decomposition into (mostly) disjoint parts attempting to minimize specific performance metrics subject to the underlying architecture resources constraints. Given a temporal partition, the compiler is still responsible for scheduling the execution of the various partitions such that the data and control dependences of the original representations are respected.

The application of temporal partitioning in high-level compilation was possibly first described in the literature by Gokhale and Marks [124]. Their compiler performed temporal partitioning at source code function boundaries thus mapping one function to a single configuration. The users resorted to function encapsulation to directly control the application of temporal partitioning. Only recently was temporal partitioning at the operation level transparently explored in compilers such as the Nenya [65] and the XPP-VC [68] compilers.

The similarities between High-Level Synthesis (HLS) scheduling and temporal partitioning have allowed researchers to leverage a wealth of approaches from scheduling to temporal partitioning of computations described at behavioral level (e.g., [230]). A common approach in temporal partitioning makes extensive use of simulated annealing techniques with diverse objective function minimization [176]. This algorithmic approach, however, has been deemed very computationally expensive despite its proven robustness.

As a result, researchers have developed newer temporal partitioning algorithms by augmenting known HLS scheduling algorithms, e.g., list-scheduling, relying on greedy algorithmic solutions for implementation expediency. Naturally, the simplest approaches have neither exploited the sharing of FUs nor the ability of architectures to support partial, dynamic reconfiguration. Purna and Bhatia [248] developed an algorithm that uses the information from an As-Soon-As-Possible (ASAP) scheduling of the computation's DFG to greedily assign operations to each partition. The selection of operations in each scheduling level is arbitrary and the algorithm creates a new temporal partition when the current partition exceeds the available resources. This approach neither considers communication costs between distinct partitions nor resource sharing. A refinement of this basic approach is described by Takayama et al. [302] where nodes are selected to be included in a temporal partition by decreasing communication costs for the same scheduling level. The work by Cardoso and Neto [64] considers both the latency of each tentative temporal partition and the communication costs among partitions. Their algorithm is an extension to list-scheduling that greedily chooses nodes for each partition attempting to minimize the overall execution time. Lastly, the work by Vasilko and Alt-Boudaoud [315] presents a heuristic partitioning algorithm based on list-scheduling taking into account partial and dynamic reconfiguration.

A very distinct algorithmic approach to this problem has been pursued by other authors. Ouaiss et al. [230] and Kaul and Vemuri [169] formulated temporal partitioning as a 0/1 nonlinear programming, and then into an integer linear programming (ILP) problem. They then use an integer linear programming solver to derive a feasible temporal partitioning solution. Due to the long execution times of the ILP solvers, however, their approach is only practical for small problem instances, relying on heuristics for larger instances [170]. In other work authors have exploited loop fission to split the computations in the body of a loop into distinct loops, thus allowing them to be mapped to the target architecture as each of them now required less resources [171]. Given the typical large number of partitioning options, authors have developed design-space exploration techniques, using search heuristics, to derive good overall solutions. This approach, akin to techniques used in HLS, relies on the description of many implementation variants of each computation and on the aggregation of nodes in the DFG (named tasks), for various resource requirements and performance characteristics. For instance, one task can have an implementation variant using three adders and two multipliers with a specific latency while another variant uses only one adder and one multiplier. Despite its modularity and the ability to generate many combinations of partitions with many degrees of resource sharing, this approach is still time-consuming and lacks a global algorithmic view, preventing it from deriving optimal partitions.

Minimizing the number of temporal partitions is a very desirable goal given the high reconfiguration costs of current reconfigurable architectures. To this effect Pandey and Vemuri [238] describe a *force-directed* list-scheduling algorithm that simultaneously considers resource sharing and temporal partitioning. The algorithm attempts to minimize the overall execution time, exploring a trade-off between the number of partitions and sharing of FUs. The algorithm, however, makes decisions based exclusively on local partition knowledge and thus lacks a global partitioning view. Cardoso [63] describes an enhanced algorithm that combines resource sharing with temporal partitioning. This algorithm derives very good temporal partitioning solutions using a greedy approach, while maintaining a global view of the partitions during the steps of assignment of operations to partitions and resource sharing.

The application of loop transformations poses a set of challenges for temporal partitioning algorithms. Transformations that aim at increasing the overall computation's ILP by the increase in the number of operations associated with each loop iteration lead to direct implementation that exceeds the available hardware resources. To cope with this trend, a compiler can apply two basic loop transformations, respectively, *loop distribution* and *loop dissevering*.

Using *loop distribution*, the compiler partitions a loop into several smaller loops, each of which does not exceed the available hardware resources. Although simple, this transformation may require additional memory to store the values of variables across the execution of the two newly formed loops. Figure 5.11 illustrates this issue where the compiler needs to convert the variable `s` into the array `s_aux` (see scalar expansion in Sect. 4.4.4) to save the various values computed at each iteration of the `i` loop. This loop transformation is thus limited to contexts where the distribution can be applied without violating loop-carried data dependences in the original loop.

Loop dissevering [68] partitions the body of the loop into a set of disjoint configurations, and structures the execution of the loop by executing sequences of these configurations as depicted in Fig. 5.12b. At run-time, each configuration defined by the temporal partitioning of the loop body is activated (e.g., by *context-switching*

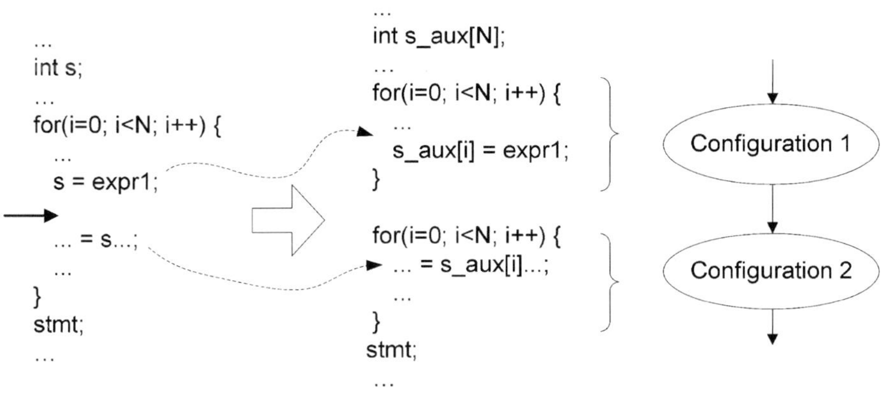

Fig. 5.11 Loop splitting across different temporal partitions using loop distribution (the arrow indicates where the loop is partitioned)

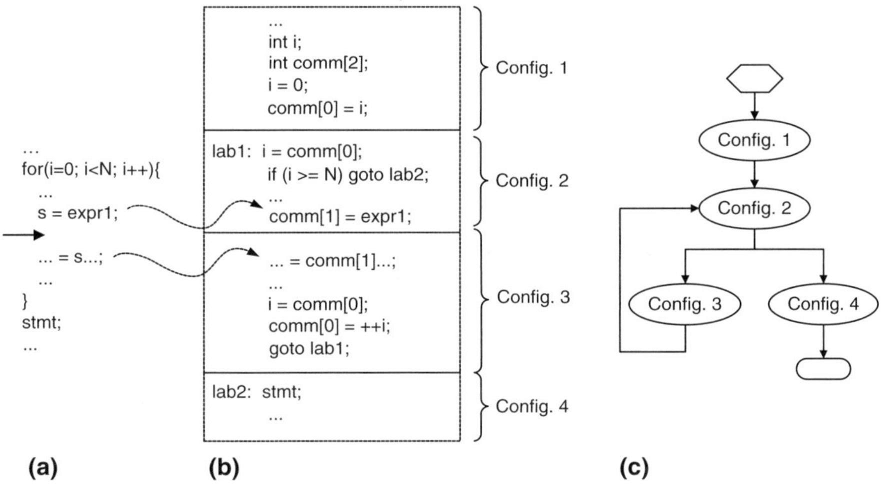

Fig. 5.12 Loop splitting across different temporal partitions using loop dissevering: (**a**) original source code arrows show where the loop is partitioned; (**b**) transformed code with the statements requiring the communication of scalar values between configurations; (**c**) the reconfiguration control-flow graph

between configuration planes or by loading the configuration data from a memory) on demand, and executed using the state of the variables the loop manipulates. The execution is supported by a configuration controller in the architecture [31], and guided by a configuration control graph as illustrated in Fig. 5.12c. As the configurations execute sequentially and respecting the original loop execution order, this transformation can be applied to any loop, even in the presence of arbitrary data dependences.

While reconfiguration times are almost negligible for existing coarse-grained reconfigurable architecture,[5] the application of temporal partitioning techniques that extensively rely on reconfiguration is seriously limited for currently available fine-grained reconfigurable architectures such as FPGAs.[6] To overcome this serious limitation, researchers developed temporal partitioning algorithms aware of the pipelining of reconfiguration and execution of consecutive temporal partitions [119]. Alternatively, the compiler can divide an FPGA into two sections alternating the execution of a temporal partition in one section with the simultaneous reconfiguration of the other section.

5.2.2 Spatial Partitioning

Compilers for reconfigurable architectures use spatial partitioning algorithms when a computation requires more hardware resources than any individual RPU can provide. Spatial partitioning splits a computation into a set of disjoint partitions each of which is then mapped across the RPUs in the target reconfigurable architecture. While spatial partitioning is not constrained by inter-partition dependences as all partitions co-exist in time, it needs, however, to take into account interconnection resource constraints such as inter-device or inter-RPU pins and bus widths.

Partitioning algorithms thus aim at minimizing one fundamental metric, the number of communications between partitions, while maximizing the co-location of data with the computations or operations that manipulate them. The minimization of the communication costs and the maximization of the co-location of data and computations promote the generation of reconfigurable computing implementations with minimal execution time. The minimization of the communication between partitions leads to short interactions and in many instances lower communication buffer requirements. Finally, data and computation co-location avoid long data accesses to remote data promoting fast execution schedules.

The combinatorial nature of spatial partitioning as defined by the constrained partitioning of the computation's DFG has prompted a wide range of algorithmic approaches [266]. Fundamental algorithms rely on graph bi-partitioning [173] and greedy methods [108] or on multiway partitioning extensions [268]. Other approaches are based on generic optimization algorithms such as simulated annealing [176].

Historically, spatial partitioning has been used in early product prototyping phases to split large hardware circuits, typically defined as VLSI gate-level net-lists, to allow them to be mapped on the target prototype systems composed of multiple FPGAs [50, 179, 314]. In the context of mapping of computations to reconfigurable architectures, spatial partitioning was, to the best of our knowledge first reported in

[5] Devices with multiple on-chip contexts exhibit almost negligible reconfiguration times (e.g., one clock cycle) for configurations already loaded on-chip as demonstrated by industrial efforts [113].

[6] A notable exception is the Time-Multiplexed FPGA developed at Xilinx but never commercialized [309].

the literature by Schmit et al. [273] for computations described in VHDL. Also at the algorithmic level, Peterson et al. [244] described an approach targeting multiple FPGAs using simulated annealing whereas Lakshmikanthan et al. [183] present a multi-FPGA partitioning algorithm based on the Fiduccia–Mattheyses recursive graph-partitioning algorithm. Kerkiz [172] uses basic recursive graph partitioning algorithms augmented with heuristics such as topological ordering, to partition an acyclic coarse-grained task graph. The algorithm targets multi-FPGA systems, and attempts to minimize the number of FPGAs used, while considering the constraints on the number of pins, and the number of external and internal memories connected to each FPGA.

The wide range of algorithmic solutions researchers have developed for spatial partitioning underscores the challenging nature of the problem. Specialized algorithmic solutions geared for the specifics of the target architecture at hand will continue to play a role in allowing compilers to effectively exploit the hardware resources at hand. Even with the increasing capacity of FPGA devices, spatial partitioning will very likely continue to be an important mapping technique, not only in the context of multi-FPGA systems, but also when targeting advanced heterogeneous embedded and high-performance reconfigurable computing systems.

5.2.3 Illustrative Example

We now illustrate the application of spatial and temporal partitioning to an example. The target architecture is depicted in Fig. 5.13a and consists of two RPUs, each one with 150 processing elements (PEs) and two local memories. The architecture has a central memory and a crossbar interconnecting the RPUs to the two memories. In this example, we consider the mapping of one application composed by four tasks (`A`, `B`, `C`, and `D`) as depicted by its task-level graph in Fig. 5.13b. This task graph defines the dependences between tasks only allowing tasks `B` and `C` to execute concurrently.

We assume that for each task we have characterizations for two design points corresponding, respectively, to unoptimized and optimized designs considering latency. The unoptimized design has higher latency and uses a minimum number of PEs and is denoted in this table by `NO` (nonoptimized case), whereas the optimized design has minimum latency and is denoted by `OPT` (optimized case). We further assume that there are no routing problems and no resource overhead when mapping each or a combination of tasks to each RPU and that the only resource constraints are the maximum number of PEs for each RPU.

The costs for each design (latency and number of PEs) are depicted in the table in Fig. 5.13b, revealing that for each task, its minimum-latency implementation requires the maximum number of PEs and conversely, its minimum-PE implementation exhibits the maximum latency. As can also be seen in Fig. 5.13b, the maximum latency for the computation considering that all the tasks would fit in the target architecture is 120 and the minimum latency is 70 clock cycles, excluding the configuration time.

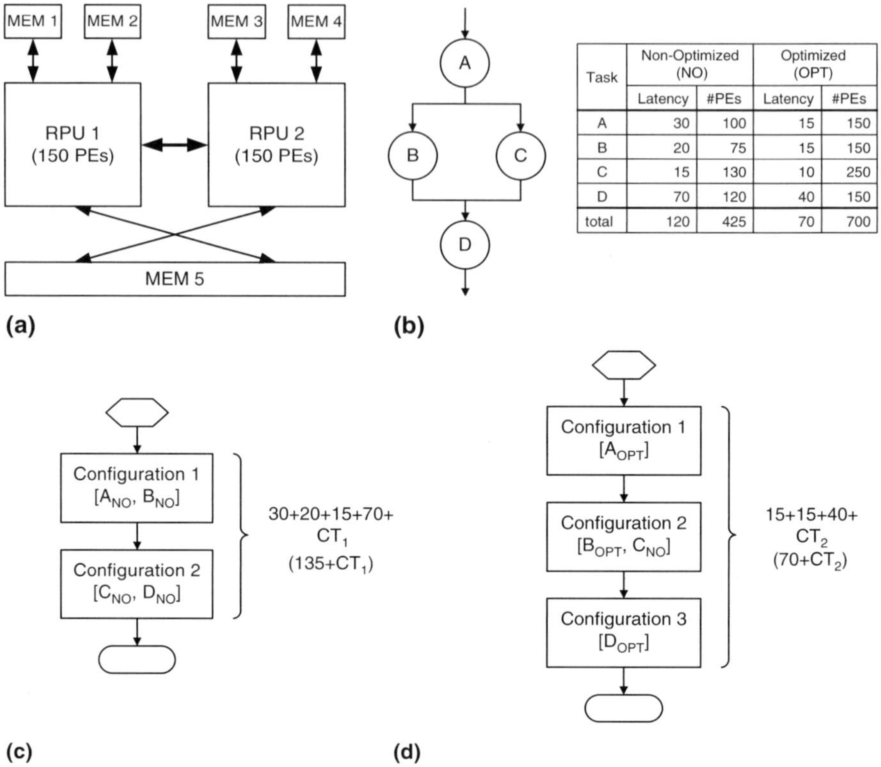

Task	Non-Optimized (NO)		Optimized (OPT)	
	Latency	#PEs	Latency	#PEs
A	30	100	15	150
B	20	75	15	150
C	15	130	10	250
D	70	120	40	150
total	120	425	70	700

Fig. 5.13 Illustrative example of temporal and spatial partitioning: (**a**) target architecture; (**b**) task graph and table of costs; (**c–d**) two possible implementations

Figure 5.13c,d depicts two possible implementations of the example computation after applying temporal and spatial partitioning. In a first implementation, depicted in Fig. 5.13c, all tasks use the minimal number, requiring only two configurations, and thus incurring a single (re)configuration cost. In the first configuration the computation executes the unoptimized tasks A_{NO} and B_{NO} mapped to each of the two RPUs. In a second configuration the computation executes the unoptimized task C_{NO} and D_{NO} resulting in an overall execution time of $135 + CT_1$ clock cycles. Here CT_1 denotes the aggregate reconfiguration cost of this specific partition which may be partially hidden when the architecture supports partial and dynamic reconfiguration.

In a second implementation some tasks have been optimized resulting in three configurations. A first configuration executes the optimized task A_{OPT} entirely occupying one RPU. The second configuration executes the unoptimized task C_{NO} and the optimized task B_{OPT} mapped to distinct RPUs and finally the third configuration executes the task D_{OPT} mapped to either RPUs. The overall execution time of this second implementation is $70 + CT_2$, possibly faster than the first implementation depending on the relative values of their reconfiguration costs CT_1 and CT_2.

As can be seen from this example, tasks in different temporal partitions do not compete for the same hardware resources, allowing the compiler the possibility of using optimized variants of a task. For this particular example, and because of the inter-task dependences, the compiler is able to derive temporal and spatial partitions that, although requiring an additional reconfiguration, may lead to better execution time. To hide, possibly partially, the cost of this extra reconfiguration, the compiler could overlap the execution of one RPU while the second RPU was being loaded with one of the tasks of the second configuration. Data produced by the task in the first configuration could then be readily accessible to the second configuration by using the memory shared between the RPUs.

5.3 Mapping Program Constructs to Resources

We now describe basic techniques for the mapping of high-level programming constructs and operators to the available hardware resources in the target reconfigurable architecture. We begin by describing the assignment of scalar variables to registers followed by the assignment of operations to FUs and the implementation of control-flow constructs. Next we address resource sharing and conclude with the combined mapping of multiple instructions to RPUs.

5.3.1 Mapping Scalar Variables to Registers

As with traditional architectures, the mapping of scalar variables to registers invariably relies on a register assignment and a register allocation algorithm. Compilers must select which of the scalar variables are to be mapped at each point in the execution of the program to the limited number of registers (see, e.g., [52]). Unlike traditional architectures, however, registers in reconfigurable architectures can assume a variety of forms. They can be organized as a traditional centralized or distributed register file, very limited capacity RAMs or even as spatially distributed discrete registers.

Although we focus in this section on the mapping of scalar variables to discrete and spatially distributed registers commonly found in fine-grained reconfigurable architectures, the techniques described here are equally applicable when targeting the coarser storage structures of distributed RAMs. Nevertheless, techniques such as live-range analysis and SSA representation are still the base for the more elaborate mapping techniques used when targeting reconfigurable architectures.

We can classify the strategies a compiler for reconfigurable architecture uses when mapping scalar variables to registers into three broad categories.

A first, and very naive, mapping strategy assigns a distinct register to each scalar variable in the program and includes hardware structures such as multiplexers to allow the values originating from multiple assignments to update the value of the

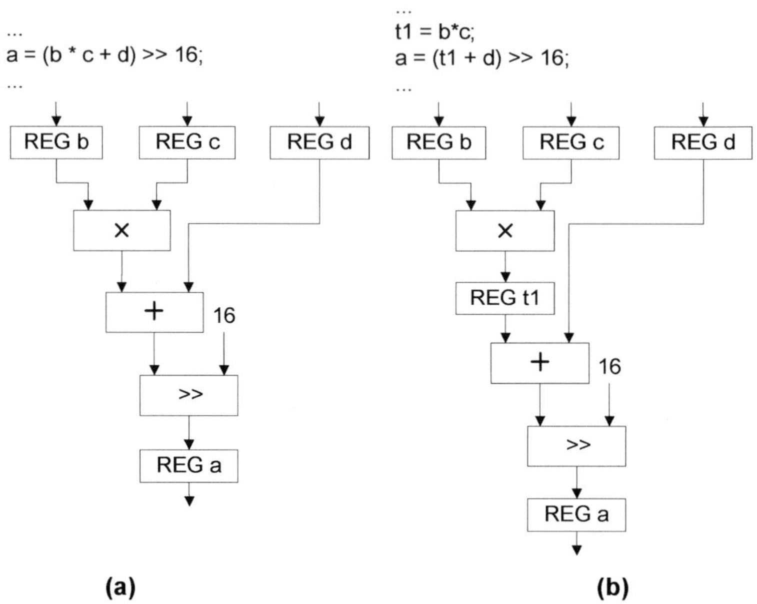

Fig. 5.14 Syntax-oriented hardware compilation with register assignment: (**a**) original source code and its DFG; (**b**) inclusion of an auxiliary variable leading to a new register in the DFG

register. This approach, used in the early hardware compilers, ignores the issue of register allocation entirely. It is extremely wasteful of registers and can, therefore, only be used when registers are plentiful.

A second mapping strategy assigns a distinct register to each assignment in the source code, similar to direct mapping of the data-flows associated with each statement or instruction.[7] In this syntax-oriented approach, assignments to variables define a new clock cycle boundary,[8] allowing the programmer to control these boundaries by decomposing/composing the expressions and statements in the source program. Implicitly these boundaries defined the chaining of operations in each clock cycle. Figure 5.14a depicts an example of the application of this strategy for two statements.

A common transformation when using this mapping strategy consists in the elimination of registers by promotion to wires as depicted by the example in Fig. 5.14. By using liveness analysis [9], the compiler can determine that the variable `t1` is not used in any subsequent instructions in the program. The register used to store the value of `t1` is not needed and the implementation may use wires to communicate its

---

[7] In some assignments such as the initialization of scalar variables to zero, common in loop constructs, the compiler can take advantage of hardware logic *reset* signals of the flip-flops that compose a register holding the variables' values. This optimization is common in fine-grained reconfigurable architectures as without it the hardware implementation would have to include a multiplexer to allow the zero value to be written to the register as a regular value.

[8] This means that expressions in the right side of a statement are directly implemented as operations performed in each clock cycle.

value to the input of the adder operator as depicted in Fig. 5.14b. As this transformation directly impacts the critical path of the hardware located between registers, it is the role of the scheduling phase to remove (or insert) registers to adjust the attained clock rate of the overall hardware implementation.

A third and clearly more systematic approach uses an SSA intermediate representation that exposes the live ranges of each variable and thus the values that must be retained in registers. The compiler can convert the SSA to a DFG representation associating each scalar variable value in the SSA representation to an edge in the DFG. SSA ϕ-functions define join points for the values of variables which are translated to a multiplexer. As with the previous strategy, the compiler can now rely on the insight of the scheduling step to insert registers and thus defining the hardware implementation clock rate.

This SSA representation also allows the compiler to easily capture loop carried dependences via scalar variables as these variables will elicit the inclusion of a ϕ-function in the loop header. Each of these variables is assigned to a register in addition to the other registers used in the hardware implementation of the body of the loop, determined using any of the other mapping techniques described above. In addition to these registers, the compiler may also need to insert additional registers to store the input/output values of operators that share an FU (see Sect. 5.3.4).

As registers are a premium resource, compilers attempt to aggressively reuse them across multiple uses and whenever the live ranges of the variables mapped to them allow. In fine-grained reconfigurable architectures, however, this reuse is seldom justified. To reuse a register in these architectures the hardware implementation must use additional resources such as multiplexers, which typically overwhelm the area used in the transformed hardware implementation. For coarse-grained reconfigurable architectures, where the inputs and output of the FUs are commonly registered and registers are organized as distributed or local register files, sharing might be naturally captured by the data mapping to register files and subsequent register allocation algorithms.

5.3.2 Mapping of Operations to FUs

Operations in the input source program are mapped to an FU that supports its execution either natively, as in the case of coarse-grained architectures, or indirectly by relying on the instantiation of a hardware operator in a fine-grained architecture.

The mapping of operations to FUs is entirely analogous to the mapping of operators found in common high-level synthesis tools as described in Chap. 3. There are, however, some transformations compilers perform during the translation of the high-level input program constructs to their intermediate representation that directly impact this mapping, namely the use of combined-operations and the selection and sharing of operators for operations that use various bit-widths.

Given their prevalence in numerically intensive computations, many architectures directly support the execution of combined arithmetic operations such as multiplication and addition instructions known as `mult-add` or `mult-acc` the latter accumulating in a special register the value of the multiplication. The compiler can therefore reorganize the input computation to expose these operations and exploit the direct target architecture support for these operations (e.g., the XPP [31] architecture). A possible downside of this operation combination, and as it increases the granularity of the computation, is that it reduces the potential for resource sharing among operations (see Sect. 5.3.4).

Many compiler techniques exist for the recognition of basic instruction idioms [9, 245] in particular in the context of automatic program vectorization [332]. A common example consists in the recognition and efficient implementation of a dot-product of two vectors, where the compiler can generate a hardware implementation that accumulates in a `sum` variable the consecutive products of the vectors extensively using the `mult-acc` instructions.

When the operation's bit-width requirements exceed the available bit-width directly supported by the FU, the compiler must decompose the operation into a sequence of canonical/primitive operations. This decomposition can lead to a non-negligible impact in the latency and schedule of the computation thus prompting the compiler to evaluate the cost/benefit of using a wider FU instead, whenever possible.

The complexity of the mapping of operations to FUs can be aggravated when a given operation can be assigned to more than one FU type. This is a common scenario in fine-grained reconfigurable architectures when dealing with different implementations of arithmetic operators with distinct area and latencies. In this context, compilers resort to mapping heuristics in combination with scheduling analyses. One such approach uses the fastest FUs for the operations in the critical paths of the computation and uses FUs with fewer resources, and therefore slower, for operations in the other paths [65].

There are also mapping opportunities when dealing with program constants, as are the classic cases of constant multiplier coefficients common in signal processing applications [328]. Individual constants are folded into and propagated to the implementation of the hardware of the operations that use them. When dealing with large arrays of constants, however, constants are mapped to discrete registers or to discrete logic (e.g., implemented using Look-Up Tables (LUTs) in fine-grained reconfigurable architectures) to increase their availability.

5.3.3 Mapping of Selection Structures

The mapping of data selection constructs either arising directly from control-flow constructs or from the mapping of multiple values in the internal representation of values (e.g., ϕ-functions in SSA) can be implemented in hardware by multiplexers or by sharing lines/buses accessed via tri-state buffers.

The selection of which implementation variant to choose depends on the granularity and multiplexer support in the target architecture. When the architecture includes multiplexer structures of the form N:1 (N inputs to 1 output) can be implemented as a tree of 2:1 multiplexers, or by a single N:1 multiplexer. This use of multiplexers is, nevertheless, only an efficient solution for small number of data sources. For larger numbers, and depending on the input/output ratio of the natively supported multiplexers, the number of multiplexers used can overwhelm the hardware implementation in terms of area and critical path delay. For larger number of inputs, the use of tri-state connections, when efficiently supported, is therefore a better solution.

5.3.4 Sharing Functional Units FUs

When mapping operations to one or more FUs, the compiler will have to negotiate a trade-off between concurrency and FU resource sharing. Although it is possible to share FU resources in both fine-grained and coarse-grained reconfigurable architectures, the techniques and benefits differ slightly.

In coarse-grained architectures that include generic FUs, such as ALUs that support different types of operations, the compiler reuses an FU by time-multiplexing and thus serializing the execution of the operations.

For fine-grained architectures, however, the advantages of FUs sharing are less clear. While sharing the FUs leads to savings in hardware resources, these savings are offset by the need to include additional hardware as depicted in the two sharing scenarios in Fig. 5.15. Figure 5.15a depicts a hardware implementation with three generic operators op1, op2, and op3 and without any resource sharing. Under the assumption that op1 and op2 are identical, the hardware implementation that shares these operators is depicted in Fig. 5.15b. Here, the additional hardware multiplexers are responsible for directing the inputs of each original operations to the shared unit and selecting the corresponding output values (at the appropriate time) from the output of the shared unit. Because of the sharing, the hardware implementation also requires the two output values, labeled u and v to be registered, which incidentally precludes the chaining of the three operators. Finally, Fig. 5.15c depicts a hardware implementation sharing op1 and op3 under the assumption that these operators are identical. As with the previous example, this hardware implementation includes not only multiplexers but also output registers for the u and e values. Lastly, and in addition to the multiplexers and registers, all these hardware designs that share operators require more sophisticated controllers and scheduling to manage more control signals and to orchestrate the flow of data through the shared resource.

Compilers can also exploit operator commutative properties, in particular for arithmetic operators. The compiler can swap the input operands of a shared FU to increase the commonalities between input operands and thus reduce the number of multiplexers needed [121].

In some cases, however, resource sharing does not require the use of additional registers or a more sophisticated controller. As illustrated in Fig. 5.16, when two compatible operations are present in mutually exclusive execution paths arising

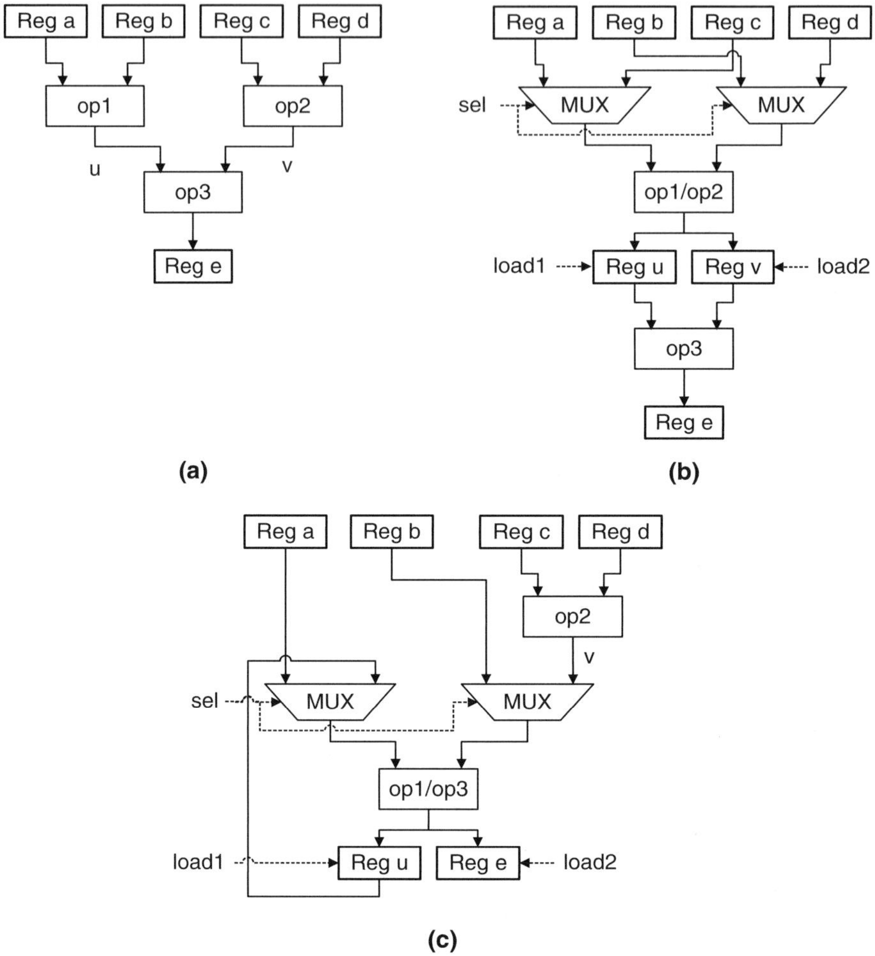

Fig. 5.15 Hardware implementations of two multiplications: (**a**) without FU sharing; (**b**) with FU sharing for `op1/op2`; (**c**) with FU sharing for `op1/op3`

from control-flow constructs, the same FU can be used. Sharing may, nevertheless, degrade the critical path delay as is the case in this example.

5.3.5 Combining Instructions for RFUs

Reconfigurable architectures organized as a general-purpose processor tightly coupled to reconfigurable function units (RFUs) expose compilers to other mapping challenges. For these architectures, compilers aim at identifying sequences of operations which can be mapped to the RFUs as macro-operations, akin to

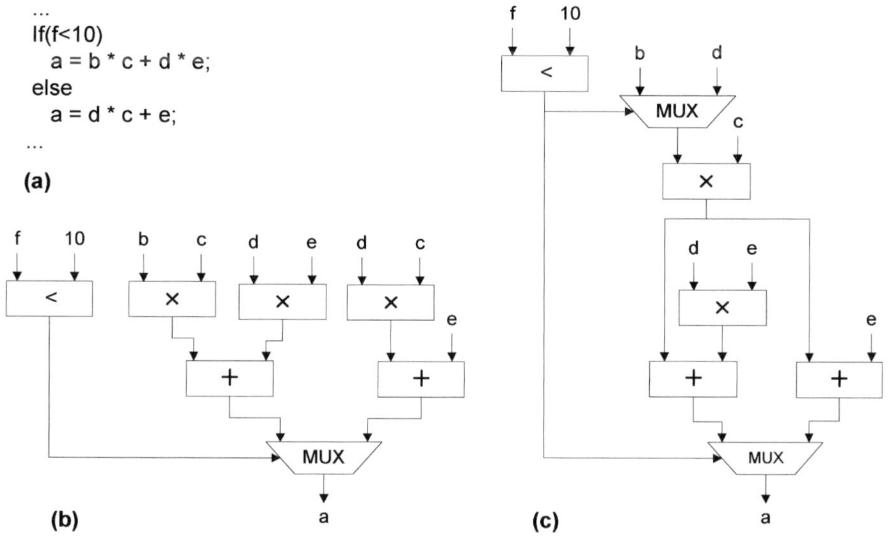

Fig. 5.16 Hardware implementations of a simple example (**a**): (**b**) without FU sharing; (**c**) sharing one multiplier in mutually exclusive execution paths

the compilation techniques used to define instruction-set extensions (ISEs) in Application-Specific Instruction-Set Processors (ASIP) [41].

Generically, the identification of which operations to aggregate depends on the characteristics of the target RFUs. For example, the Chimaera architecture RFU supports operators with up to nine inputs and only one output [152], whereas the Configurable Compute Accelerator (CCA) [80, 156], whose two sample possible architectures are depicted in Fig. 5.17, can accommodate in each specialized instruction up to four inputs and up to two outputs. Further constraints of the mapping of instructions to this particular architecture include a maximum number of predefined level of operations (four in the examples depicted in Fig. 5.17), where even operator levels perform logic operations and odd levels perform logic and simple arithmetic operations, excluding multiplication and division.

When mapping a computation to an RFU in these architectures, the compiler must invariably engage in a matching between the characteristics of the RFUs and the computational patterns in the input program. A simple algorithmic approach consists in the identification of regions of the code, either at the source or intermediate representation levels (e.g., DFG), where the operations can be aggregated with a specific number of inputs and outputs. Two types of regions, illustrated in Fig. 5.18, have been addressed extensively in the literature, respectively, MISO (Multiple-Input, Single-Output) and MIMO (Multiple-Input, Multiple-Output) regions [41, 117, 118, 246]. Given the potential exponential time complexity of generic matching techniques, researchers have developed algorithms that combine greedy techniques and solution-space exploration heuristics [156].

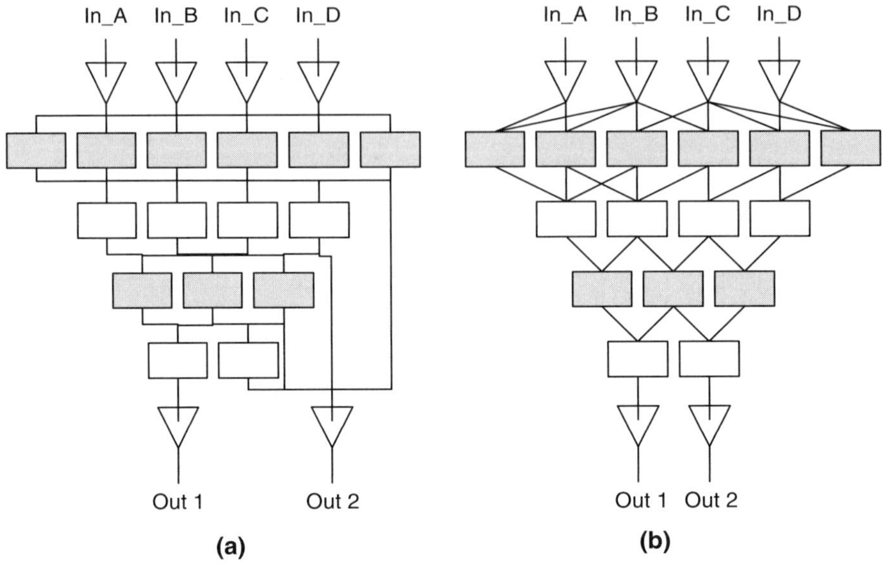

Fig. 5.17 CCA, an example of an RFU: (**a**) with full crossbars between stages (full interconnection); (**b**) with sparse interconnect between stages (sparse interconnection)

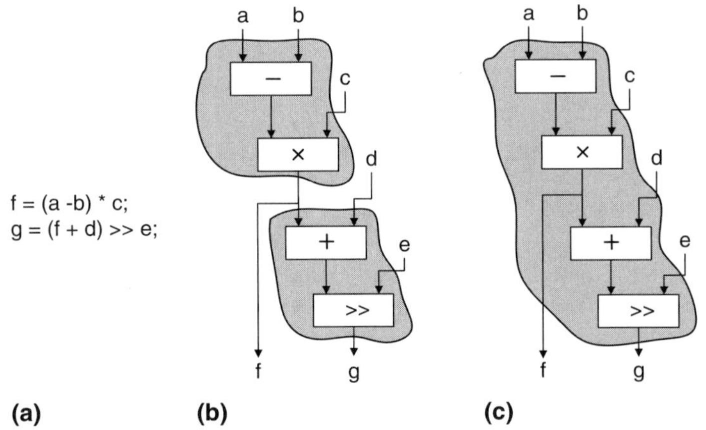

Fig. 5.18 Region examples: (**a**) source code; (**b**) MISO regions; (**c**) MIMO region

5.4 Pipelining

This important execution technique aims at increasing the throughput of a computation by (partially) overlapping the execution of a sequence of operations, subject to data and/or control dependences [154]. This technique can be exploited, even simultaneously, at various levels of operation granularity. When applied to individual instructions, pipelining splits their execution into a sequence of execution steps, or microinstructions (e.g., fetching, decoding, and execution), each of which is executed in a specific clock cycle and by a specific FU. The net result is that at a given point of time, multiple instructions are being executed, and although their individual execution latency is unchanged, the overall execution throughput is substantially increased. For coarse-grained operations, such as the aggregated sequence of instructions in the execution of an iteration of a loop, the concept of pipelined execution allows for the overlapped execution of the instructions corresponding to multiple loop iterations.

Reconfigurable architectures present many opportunities for application-specific pipelining execution via the customization of memories, FUs, and pipeline interstage connectivity. In the context of arithmetic FUs, authors have developed sophisticated pipelined arithmetic operators that can handle multiple, and mixed, data width formats for floating-point representation [95]. Other authors have also used the flexibility of fine-grained reconfigurable architectures to define customs execution pipelines that can implement restricted, yet effective, forms of multithreading, for the pipelined execution of loops [298]. Still, other authors have developed mixed-grained instruction decomposition of high-level constructs which they then heavily pipeline using programmable execution units [55].

In the next sections, we describe various forms of pipelined execution enabled by reconfigurable architectures, for which they are better suited given their ability for resource customization.

5.4.1 Pipelined Functional and Execution Units

Pipelined FUs are organized internally as a sequence of pipeline stages, each of which implements a specific function and when composed carries out a complex operation.

Given the complexity of some arithmetic operations and therefore of the FUs that implement them, these FUs are commonly pipelined. Floating-point arithmetic functional units typically include three pipeline stages. In a first stage the implementation normalizes the exponents of the two input numbers with the corresponding realignment of the mantissa(s). A second stage performs the core operation (e.g., a multiplication or addition of the mantissas) in itself also using pipelined execution techniques. A third and last stage normalizes the result.

A variant of the implementation of pipelined arithmetic FUs can use serial arithmetic [188, 239] or implementation techniques similar to bit-slicing [214] as described recently by Maruyama and Hoshino [202]. In this approach, the compiler decomposes arithmetic operations as micro-operations over sets of k bits to increase pipelining throughput. The slicing also promotes operation chaining as the least significant k bits of the result of an operation can be used by the next operation without waiting for the completion of the computation of the entire result.

An approach that allows compilers to efficiently exploit the pipelined capabilities of FUs relies on the use of pipelined execution models. These execution models

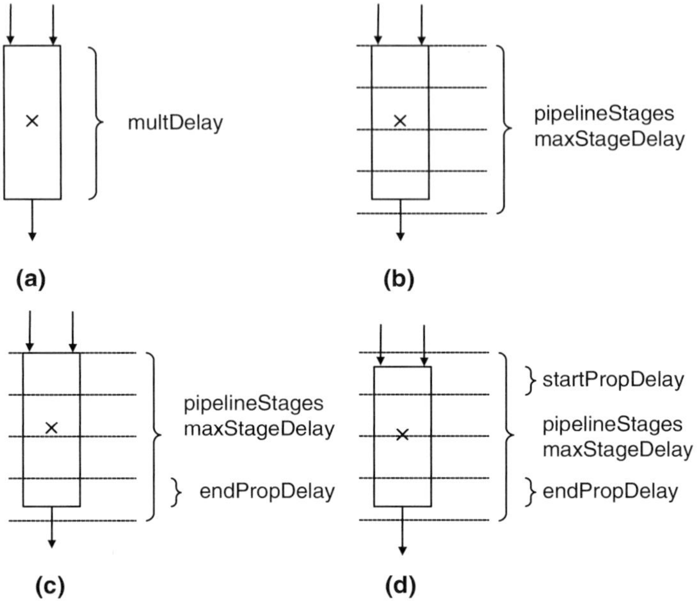

Fig. 5.19 Example of pipelining latency models for a multiplier

focus on the description of time-related execution parameters allowing compilers to perform high-level computation scheduling decisions. Figure 5.19 illustrates a possible set of simple pipelining execution models for a multiplier FU. In a simple nonpipelining model, depicted in Fig. 5.19a, an FU can be characterized by its maximum delay denoted by `multDelay`. Figure 5.19b depicts the simplest pipelining model where each of the `pipelineStages` stage has a maximum stage delay of `maxStageDelay`, thus defining the minimum possible clocking period for the FU to operate correctly. In this model, the overall multiplication execution time is thus given by `pipelineStages` × `maxStageDelay`. This model also assumes that the multiplier uses all its stages and no chaining with other operations is allowed either in the first or in the last execution stage. The models depicted in Figs. 5.19c and d represent the cases where the FU has delay slots at either the start and/or at the end stages, denoted, respectively, by `startPropDelay` and `endPropDelay`. For the model in Fig. 5.19c, the execution time is given by $(\texttt{pipelineStages} - 1) \times \texttt{maxStageDelay} + \texttt{endPropDelay}$.

While the models with delay slots are well suited for fine-grained reconfigurable architectures [285], the model depicted in Fig. 5.19b is commonly used when targeting coarse-grained reconfigurable architectures.

When pipelining the execution of a data-path, a key transformation is the balancing of the execution paths from its inputs to the outputs. The balancing of the paths is performed by the insertion of cascades of registers at selected internal data-path edges such that the latencies from any data-path input of the data-path to any of its outputs are identical. When all the inputs to a data-path are simultaneously

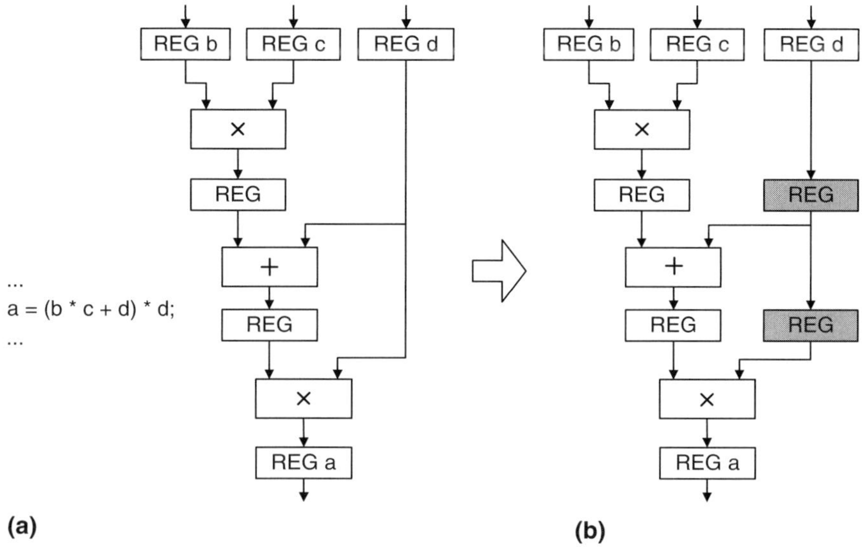

Fig. 5.20 Example of execution path balancing using registers: (**a**) original source code and an implementation with register stages; (**b**) pipelined implementation after execution path balancing

available, path balancing ensures that all the data-path outputs, corresponding to a given set of input values, are available at the same clock cycle. With path balancing, the compiler can schedule the execution of multiple computations over the data-path by submitting a set of input values at each clock cycle, thereby attaining maximum computational throughput. Figure 5.20b illustrates the application of path balancing to the data-path in Fig. 5.20a corresponding to the expression in the statement `a=(b*c+d)*d;`. The balancing of this data-path is accomplished by the two registers (shaded boxes) in the transformed data-path depicted in Fig. 5.20b thus ensuring that the clock cycle latency from the inputs `b`, `c`, and `d` to the output `a` exhibits the same latency of three clock cycles.

Another important base transformation, common in any contemporary logic synthesis tool, for pipelining execution techniques is hardware *retiming* [82]. Retiming aims at balancing pipeline stage delays by moving registers that define stage boundaries either backwards or forwards along the flow of data in the pipeline. In some cases the movement of one register requires the insertion of additional registers as is the case when a register moves backwards across a multiple-input operator. Retiming does not change the latency of the hardware implementation while enabling higher clocking rates and is commonly used by logic synthesis tools to enable the use of pipelining of hard macros (e.g., DSP blocks and embedded multipliers) in current FPGAs. An example of the addition of a cascade of registers in the output of a data-path and the use of backwards retiming is illustrated in Fig. 5.21b for the data-path depicted in Fig. 5.21a.

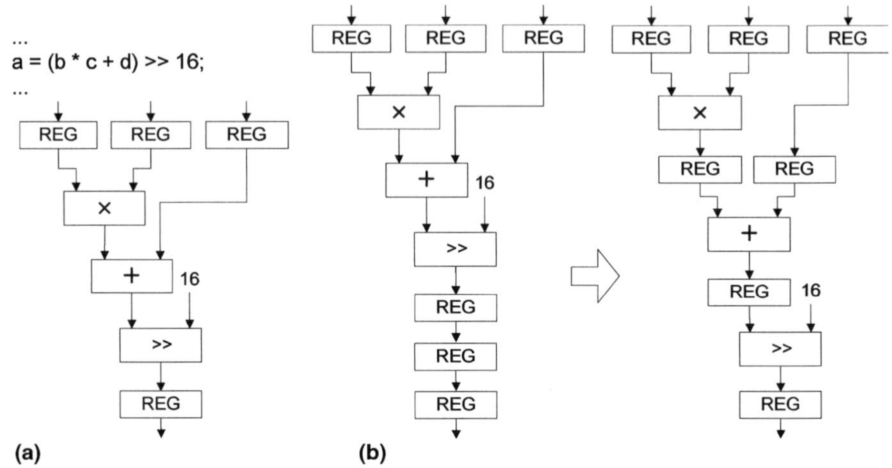

Fig. 5.21 Example illustrating the use of retiming to create pipelining levels: (**a**) original data-path and corresponding source code computation; (**b**) data-path with retiming registers and backward movement of two registers

5.4.2 Pipelining Memory Accesses

When supported by the underlying architecture, pipelining of memory accesses is an important execution technique for reducing the aggregate latency of accessing memory. Reconfigurable architectures are no exception and several commercial reconfigurable computing boards support this memory access mode [19, 166].

The common support for pipelined memory accesses requires the use of custom address generation units and custom interfaces to memory interface units. In this interface, implementations may use registers to stagger the read and write memory operations requests through a FIFO queue, possibly implemented as a RAM or as a tapped-delay line of registers. After an initial access latency, data is retrieved from the memory interface one memory word every k clock cycles. Write operations also rely on registers or write buffers and, in the absence of data dependences or read-after-write hazards, have their latencies totally hidden by the memory interface unit.

In Fig. 5.22, we illustrate a simple example of the use of pipelined memory accesses for a vector external product computation, assuming that memory loads and memory stores require three and two clock cycles, respectively. Figure 5.22b depicts a schedule considering loop pipelining, without pipelining of memory accesses, exhibiting a throughput of three clock cycles per loop iteration. In comparison the schedule of the same loop exploiting the pipelining of memory access reveals a throughput of one clock cycle per loop iteration as depicted in Fig. 5.22(c).

In this context, researchers have developed frameworks exploiting pipelined memory accesses for streaming-data applications [112] and computations that access array variables with very regular access patterns [241]. These frameworks take advantage of the programmability and customization of the address generation units

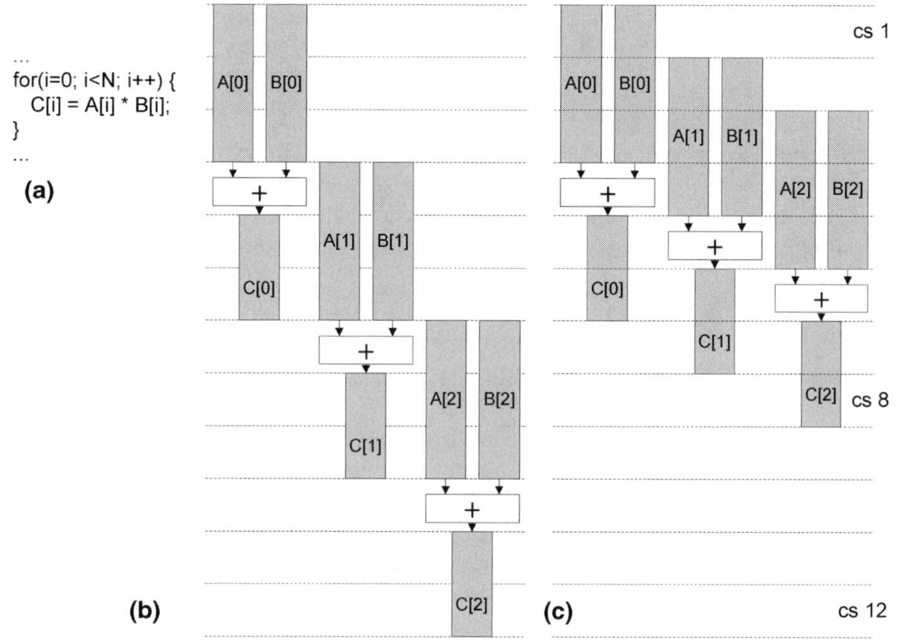

Fig. 5.22 Pipelining memory accesses: (**a**) code; (**b**) scheduling without pipelining memory accesses; (**c**) scheduling with pipelining memory accesses

allowing the controllers to orchestrate the flow of data in and out of the memory interface unit, with seamless integration with the data-path consuming and generating data values.

5.4.3 Loop Pipelining

Loop pipelining is a technique that aims at reducing the execution time of loops by overlapping the computation of consecutive loop iterations. The latency of the iterations of the loop is unchanged, but the rate, or throughput, at which the execution completes loop iterations is greatly increased, thus substantially improving the loop execution performance. As with traditional architectures where *software pipelining* [222] has been extensively used, loop pipelining is also particularly well suited for reconfigurable architectures.

The vast majority of loop pipelining compilation efforts for hardware have focused on the analysis and mapping of "well-structured" loops, i.e., loops that are perfectly or quasi-perfectly nested, have symbolically constant or even compile-time constant loop bounds, and manipulate arrays with affine index access functions. For this class of loops, compilers can rely on powerful analyses to determine the data dependences between statements of the loop and the possible dependence distances (measured in terms of number of iterations of each loop in the nest) across which the dependence occurs. With this information, compilers can be very precise about which statements to pipeline and when and thus control the pipelined hardware implementation for the loop.

In this description, we distinguish between two loop pipelining strategies, namely, pipelining of innermost loops and pipelining of an outer loop of a loop nest. Although both strategies can be exploited when mapping computations to reconfigurable architectures, only recently has the latter strategy been addressed in the literature.

With respect to the mapping of inner loops to hardware using pipelined execution techniques, we can classify the approaches into two broad categories. One category includes approaches based on pipeline vectorization, whereas a second category includes approaches based on software pipelining, of which techniques based on iterative modulo scheduling have been extensively used.

The technique of loop pipelining using pipeline vectorization was originally developed by Weinhardt and Luk [323] for fine-grained reconfigurable architectures and later adapted to a coarse-grained reconfigurable architecture [68]. The basic idea of pipeline vectorization is to build a hardware implementation derived from the computation's data-flow graph (DFG) and then repeatedly execute, in a pipelined fashion, all the iterations of the loop over that hardware implementation. Using this technique, the compiler applies a wide range of loop transformations to expose the adequate amount of ILP in the innermost loop of a nest. It then replaces conditionally executed statements in the loop by predicated statements, merging multiple assignments to variables using selection constructs which will be translated to hardware structures with multiplexers (as described in Sect. 5.3.3). These analyses allow the compiler to derive the DFG of the body of the loop, which is then translated to a hardware representation. To this DFG the compiler next inserts feedback registers to capture loop-carried dependences. Lastly, the compiler generates a hardware implementation for pipelined execution by inserting pipeline registers, and generates a controller that schedules the execution and the various memory accesses. To reduce the number of memory accesses per loop iteration, memory values which are reused in subsequent iterations can be saved in register delay lines [322] (cf. Sect. 4.4.3).

Another approach to inner loop pipelining is based on *software pipelining* techniques [222], also known in the context of high-level synthesis *as loop folding* [114]. The basic idea in software pipelining is to find a core schedule (the kernel) for the execution of the various operations corresponding to overlapped loop iterations. This core schedule depends on the specific hardware resources available and defines the initiation and latency values that characterize the performance of the pipelined execution. In addition to the core schedule, a software pipelining implementation also requires a prologue/epilogue that has to be executed before/after the steady-state execution of the core schedule. A common compiler algorithm for the definition of the core schedule and the prologue/epilogue sections is the Modulo Scheduling algorithm [185].

Figure 5.23 depicts an example of the application of *software pipelining* where we have omitted the derivation of the DFG of the body of this loop and the corresponding hardware implementation. In Figs. 5.23a and b we depict the datapath (FSMD) representation for the execution of the computation without and with software pipelining, respectively. In this example, we consider that arrays `A`, `B`, and `C` are mapped to three distinct memories with 1 clock cycle load/store latency. In this setting, new values of `tmp1` and `tmp2` can be loaded concurrently with the execution of the `tmp1` × `tmp2` multiplication. With software pipelining the

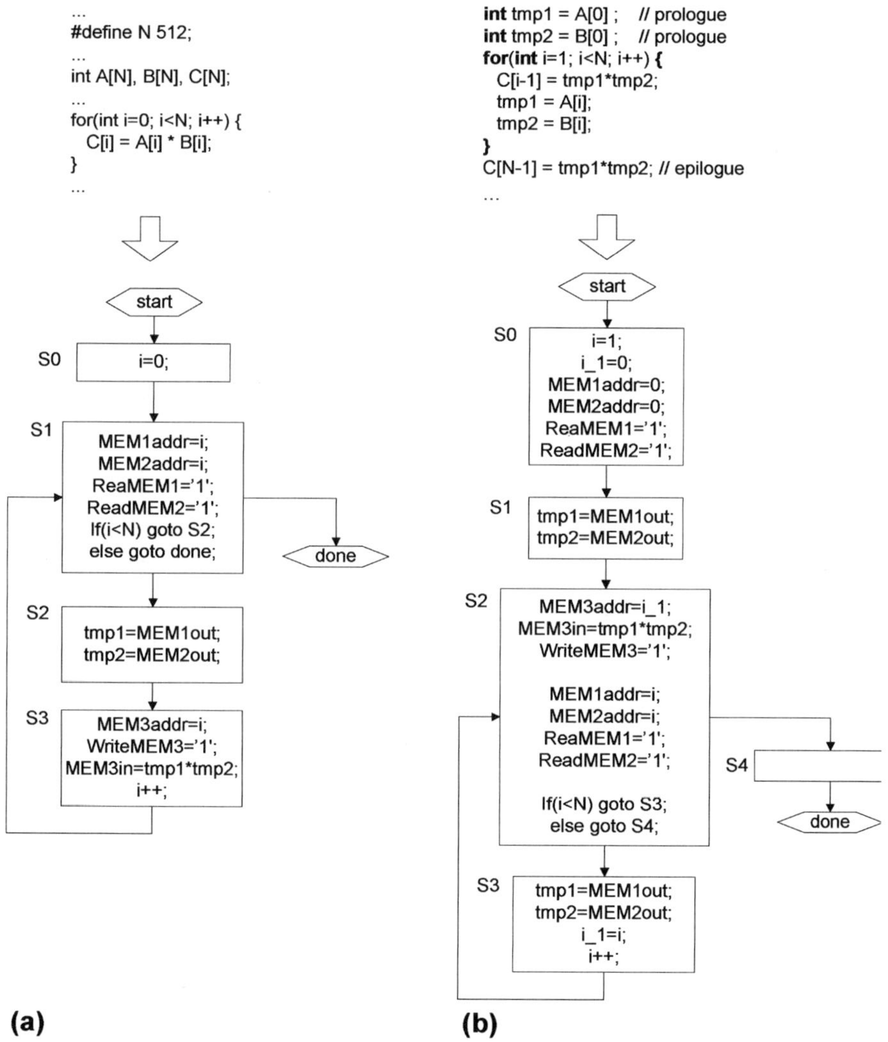

Fig. 5.23 Loop pipelining example: (**a**) original code and possible FSMD representation; (**b**) possible software pipelining and FSMD representation

implementation requires $2 \times \mathtt{N} + 2$ clock cycles to execute the N loop iterations, whereas the nonpipelined implementation requires $3 \times \mathtt{N} + 2$, yielding an asymptotic speedup of 1.5.

When mapping the original code example in Fig. 5.23a to a coarse-grained reconfigurable architecture, in this case the XPP, the compiler can generate the hardware design as the one depicted in Fig. 5.24b, that like the implementation on fine-grained reconfigurable architectures does not include a prologue and an epilogue. Instead, the hardware implementation includes two registers to hold the values of the loop control variable `i` while the hardware performs, for each iteration, the accesses to the input data and samples the multiplication result, in a pipeline vectorization execution scheme. The nonpipelined hardware implementation for this computation

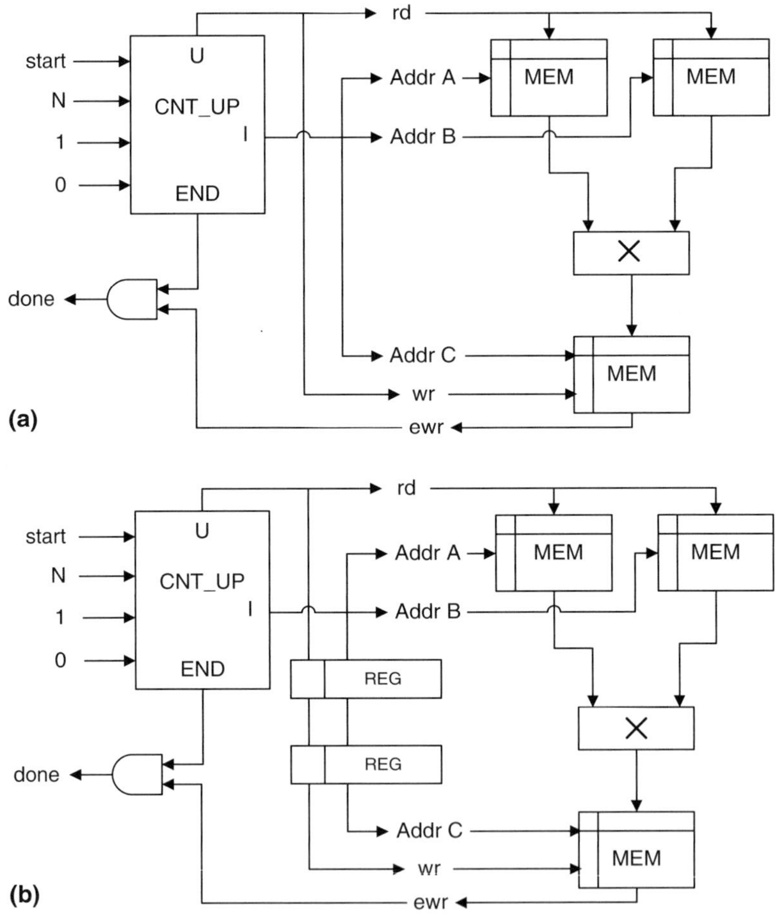

Fig. 5.24 Possible implementations in an architecture similar to the XPP for the example shown in the previous figure: (**a**) without and (**b**) with loop pipelining

does not use delay-line registers, but relies on the hand-shaking of the various signals to stall the counter controlling the execution of the iterations of the loop.[9]

Many compiler implementations of software pipelining rely on the iterative modulo scheduling (IMS) algorithm [255] when targeting reconfigurable architectures such as the *garpcc* [62], the MATCH project [141], the NAPA-C compiler [128], and the compiler described by Snider [285]. The loop pipelining approach used in the MATCH compiler also uses a list-scheduling resource constrained algorithm in order to limit the number of operations active per stage, and the increasing number of resources needed. Snider's approach uses an iterative modulo scheduling version that considers retiming to optimize the pipelining throughput and exploits the insertion of pipeline stages between operations. The *garpcc* [62] targets a reconfigurable architecture with a fixed clock period and pipeline intrinsic stages, and does not require exploitation of the number of stages and retiming optimizations in its scheduling algorithm.

Despite the differences of implementation of the two main approaches to loop pipelining, pipeline vectorization and software pipelining, they share the goal of improving the overall loop execution time. This goal is often, but not always, to maximize the loop pipelining throughout by reduction of the clock period and the latency of the kernel, as depicted in Table 5.1 for a representative sample of state-of-the-art compilers.

When the compiler wishes to exploit concurrency that is beyond what the individual operations or statements of the inner loop provide, it can exploit pipelining at an outer loop. In this pipelining approach, the compiler overlaps consecutive iterations of a loop containing other loops nested within, while maintaining the pipelined execution of the inner loops [267]. In addition to the registers required for the pipelined implementation of the inner loops, the implementation uses memories to save data contexts corresponding to the various pipelined executions of the inner loops [266].

Table 5.1 Comparison of loop pipelining schemes (SPC [323], *garpcc* [60], and Snider's compiler [285])

Compiler	Loop pipelining scheme	Algorithm base	Target architecture characteristics	Goal	Applicability
SPC	Pipeline vectorization	Pipeline vectorization with retiming	Fixed clock period, pipelined FUs with fixed stages	Maximum throughput	well-structured inner FOR-type loops with affine array index functions
garpcc	Software pipelining	IMS (iterative modulo scheduling)	Fixed clock period, native pipeline stages	Maximum throughput	A broad class of inner loops with affine array index functions
Snider's compiler	Software pipelining	IMS (iterative modulo scheduling) with retiming	Pipelined FUs with fixed stages	Exploit throughput versus area (by adding stages)	A broad class of inner loops with affine array index functions

[9] In an architecture that does not have the support for low-level signal hand-shaking, the counter would have to include `k` stall cycles to account for the latency of the computation in each loop iteration.

5.4.4 Coarse-Grained Pipelining

Compilers for reconfigurable architectures can also exploit coarse-grained pipelining execution techniques for computations structured as a sequence of tasks. Of particular interest are computations in the domain of image and signal processing applications, where tasks can be defined as individual loop nests that manipulate array variables.

As with any pipelined execution scheme, the data dependences between tasks limit the exploitable concurrency. If one task reads (consumes) data another task writes (produces) then they cannot execute concurrently as one task must execute completely before the second task begins executing. Despite these data dependences a compiler can use coarse-grained pipelining scheme that interleaves the execution of sequences of tasks. Tasks may overlap part of their execution based on producer/consumer dependences.

Compilers can identify the opportunities for coarse-grained pipelining by analyzing the source program and recognizing producer/consumer relationships between tasks. When tasks consist of loop nests that manipulate array variables, compilers can again rely on a wealth of array data-dependence analyses to determine the data dependences between iterations of the same loop and across distinct loops.

For computations organized as a sequence of tasks inside an outer *control loop* the compiler can explore coarse-grained pipelining in a combination of two strategies. In one strategy, the compiler organizes each loop nest in the control loop as an individual task and uses the dependences across loop nests to pipeline the execution of the tasks. Each task, however, executes sequentially as is depicted in the illustrative example in Fig. 3.12a in Chap. 3. In this approach, the compiler builds a task graph and determines using dependence iteration distances, the sizes of the pipelining inter-stage buffers used to save and retrieve data that is, respectively, produced and consumed by each task. In a second strategy, each task is also executed using the pipelining techniques described in Sect. 5.4.3 as is depicted in the illustrative example in Fig. 3.12c in Chap. 3.

The concept of coarse-grained pipelining for sequences of loops has been recently explored in the mapping of array-based computations to reconfigurable architectures. The work by Ziegler et al. [351,353] uses classic array data-dependence analyses to define the pipeline stages. The synchronization between the execution in the stages is performed via hand-shaking and the communication of data between them relies on FIFO buffers. This work focuses on finding appropriate sized communication buffers, constrained to loops that induce the same producer/consumer order, and thus possibly sacrificing concurrency. The approach described by Rodrigues et al. [263], however, uses a fine-grained, data-driven, synchronization scheme between stages as illustrated in Fig. 5.25. The fine-grained synchronization scheme[10] allows for a larger overlap of the computation in any two stages and consequently to lower execution time. One advantage of this scheme lies in its ability to consider any

[10] Similar in spirit to the empty/full tagged memory scheme used in the context of shared memory multiprocessor architectures [283].

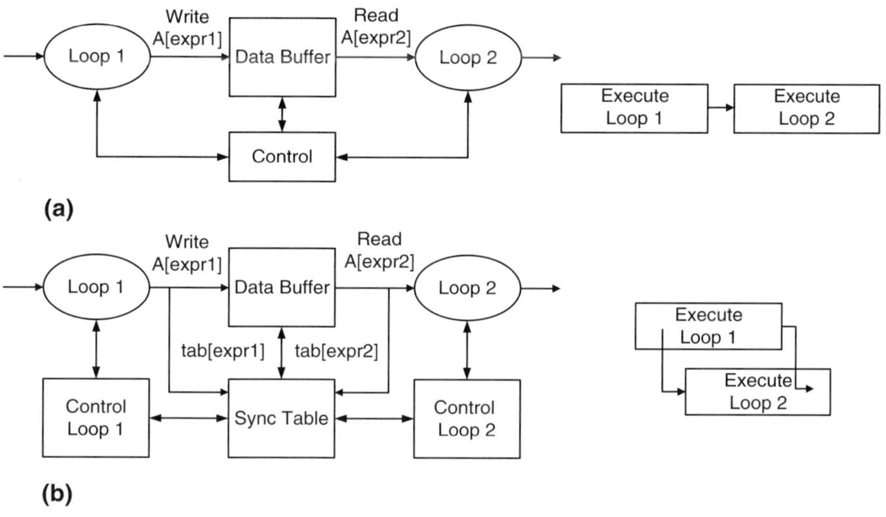

Fig. 5.25 Coarse-grained pipelining: (**a**) original implementation without pipelining; (**b**) implementation with pipelining

irregular (out-of-order) produced/consumed relationship, achieving in many practical computations a performance speedup close to the theoretical speedup limit and still with very small communication buffers.

5.4.5 Pipelining Configuration–Computation Sequences

The steps of loading and configuration of resources on contemporary reconfigurable architectures incur non-negligible latencies.[11] These latencies are bound to increase as devices increase in capacity and therefore in the number of individual configurable points.

To mitigate the costs associated with reconfiguration, compilers rely on two approaches. In a first approach, a compiler can attempt to reduce the number of reconfigurations needed. Recently developed techniques identify and aggregate dependent computations in configurations as to minimize the overall execution configuration time [107].

In a second approach, a compiler can exploit latency-hiding techniques such as prefetching and pipelining. With pipelining and prefetching techniques, the hardware implementation overlaps the execution of an active configuration with the loading and storing in on-chip caches a subsequent configuration. Alternatively, and in architectures without on-chip configuration caches or configuration context

[11] Even when using multicontext devices, the loading of the configuration data onto the inactive planes takes several clock cycles.

planes [195], but with partial reconfiguration support, the reconfiguration latency can be hidden, possibly fully, by using half of the device to run the current configuration and the other half to configure the next one [119].

These latency-hiding techniques, however, can only be used to maximum benefit whenever the configurations can be scheduled in a deterministic fashion. Despite the obvious relationship to compilation techniques, we have not discussed here these aspects of scheduling and management of configurations as they are commonly seen as operating system or run-time system issues.

5.5 Memory Accesses

In the next sections, we describe three basic compiler transformations and mapping techniques that aim at increased data availability and reducing memory access latency. While these transformations are common in the mapping of computations to traditional architectures, the diversity of the hierarchy of memory structures with distinct capacity sizes, access latencies, number of access ports, and data width organizations, found in today's reconfigurable computing platforms, substantially enhances their application in improving the performance of the resulting hardware designs.

5.5.1 Partitioning and Mapping of Arrays to Memory Resources

The significance of data partitioning has long been recognized when compiling for distributed memory multicomputers (see, e.g., [254]) and more recently in the arena of embedded systems [73]. Partitioning and mapping of data to disjoint, and possibly local memories, substantially improves the data availability as Processing Elements (PEs) can access the various data items concurrently without contention in shared intercommunication resources. This data partitioning is particularly important for large data arrays extensively used in many loop-based computationally intensive applications for which parallel execution is essential.

While many of the previously developed techniques for traditional parallel machines, such as data distribution (described in Sect. 4.4.1), are also applicable to reconfigurable architectures, the possibility of customizing the memories and their interconnection substantially increases the complexity of their application. As a result, researchers either adapted existing techniques or developed newer algorithms to deal with this challenging problem of data partitioning and mapping. Of the compiler techniques for the mapping of array data to memories, we focus on memory bank disambiguation and generic array mapping.

In memory bank disambiguation, the compiler uses array data-dependence analyses to determine when a given computation needs to simultaneously access disjoint subsets of the data arrays. These array sections, e.g., odd-indexed and even-indexed array items, are then mapped to distinct memory banks. Memory bank disambiguation can also be profitably combined with loop unrolling in a technique called *modulo unrolling* [30, 291]. Given a specific number of memory banks, the compiler selects the unrolling factor that leads to a data access pattern of the computation where the identified data subsets can be matched to the underlying memory bank structure. In addition to increased data availability and consequently increased performance, bank disambiguation and data partitioning also allow compilers to map to memory arrays that exceed the capacity of the individual memory banks.

Figure 5.26 illustrates the application of memory disambiguation and modulo unrolling for the example code depicted in Fig. 5.26a. The compiler performs memory bank disambiguation identifying six sections of the arrays `a` and `b` in the original code. These sections are transformed to six smaller arrays, respectively, `a0`, `a1`, `a2` and `b0`, `b1`, `b2`, as depicted in Fig. 5.26b. Figure 5.26c illustrates the mapping of these arrays to six distinct memory banks. The transformation allows each iteration of the loop to concurrently access, in the same clock cycle, all the six data elements it requires.

```
...
#define W 3
...
int a[W][W], b[W][W], c[W];
...
for(x=0; x < W; x++) {
  sum = (a[x][0] * b[0][x]);
  sum += (a[x][1] * b[1][x]);
  sum += (a[x][2] * b[2][x]);
  c[x] = sum;
}
```

(a)

```
#define W 3
...
int a0[W], b0[W];
int a1[W], b1[W];
int a2[W], b2[W];
int c[W];
...
for(x=0; x < W; x++) {
  sum = (a0[x] * b0[x]);
  sum += (a1[x] * b1[x]);
  sum += (a2[x] * b2[x]);
  c[x] = sum;
}
...
```

(b)

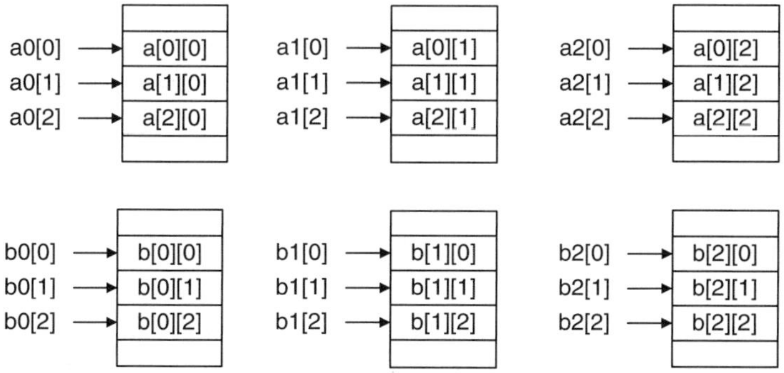

(c)

Fig. 5.26 Loop unrolling and memory bank disambiguation: (**a**) C code after unrolling; (**b**) C code after bank disambiguation; (**c**) arrays mapped to six memories with the mapping of each array element to the original arrays

Fine-grained reconfigurable architectures require more sophisticated data partitioning and array mapping approaches as these architectures expose to a compiler all the low-level execution details. In this context, researchers have developed various techniques, some of which take into account scheduling and latency of the operations in the computations and are thus akin to scheduling and mapping techniques developed for high-level synthesis.

Gokhale and Stone [126] describe an algorithm for the mapping of array variables to memory banks based on partitioning of the computation's precedence graph (a form of data-dependence graph), where each operation in the computation is represented by a node with edges connecting it to the input and output data array nodes. The algorithm then exhaustively attempts various partitions and mappings of the graph to minimize the number of used memories, and subject to their capacity constraints with the overall goal of minimizing execution time. In a similar approach, but targeting embedded systems, researchers in the ATOMIUM [73, 337] compilation and synthesis system proposed an approach for the problem of array data mapping to RAMs, taking into account the dependences of the operations so that all operations can be scheduled in a given cycle budget, while minimizing storage and bandwidth.

Weinhardt and Luk [322] describe an integer linear programming approach for the inference of on-chip memories with the goal of reducing the number of memory accesses for loop pipelining vectorization. Their approach also relies on very simple affinity-based mapping decisions and like the previous work focuses exclusively on a single level of storage hierarchy. Ouaiss and Vemuri [233] describe an approach that targets a reconfigurable memory hierarchy. They use an integer linear programming approach to find an optimal mapping of a set of array data sections to a set of memories. Gong et al. [133] describe an algorithm that partitions the arrays' data in various RAMs based on a loop's iteration space and arrays' data foot-prints with the overall goal of minimizing remote memory accesses. They rely on the notion of the size of data space along specific directions to evaluate the foot-print and integrate a tentative data partitioning to estimate the number and latency of the memory accesses. Lastly, Baradaran and Diniz [27] describe a compiler approach that combines loop transformations such as loop unrolling and scalar replacement with low-level critical path and scheduling information. Their algorithm greedily explores a wide range of loop transformations to map array data to either discrete registers or internal RAMs on an FPGA.

5.5.2 *Improving Memory Accesses*

While data partitioning and mapping techniques aim at increasing the data availability by distributing data among distinct memories, several other techniques can be used to ameliorate the cost of individual memory accesses. We now briefly describe three such techniques, respectively, pipelining of memory accesses, customized address generation units, and data packing/unpacking.

Memory access pipelining offers the simplest form of data access cost reduction. As with other pipelining execution schemes, the initial data access latency is amortized for a large aggregate set of accesses. Typically, the implementation requires the setup of a set of hardware resources (i.e., registers) that define the base address and stride of consecutive memory accesses. Pipelining is particularly suited for streaming data accesses pervasive in program that manipulate array variables using affine index functions.

The customization opportunities offered by reconfigurable architectures allow implementations to greatly simplify memory interface structures, such as memory access controllers, address generation units, and input/output buffers. These simplifications can be substantial for fine-grained reconfigurable architectures such as FPGAs, as they lead to substantial reduction of the amount of programmable resources, i.e., device area, and consequently promote smaller and faster implementations. As a memory controller deals with the specific details of the physical interface (e.g., data pin, timing, or protocol), it can be customized for the specific width and number of memory access paths. Similarly, an address generation unit can be customized for specific physical and virtual address ranges, and stride of accesses. The savings can be substantial as for very limited access ranges the implementation may use very specific address generation logic, replacing, expensive and lengthy, address calculation operations with trivial operations efficiently implemented in hardware.

These opportunities have been extensively explored in the context of HLS for ASICs [275] and more recently when targeting FPGAs. Park and Diniz [241] describe a complete compiler analysis and code generation approach for FPGA custom memory controllers and input buffering. The compiler analysis provides information about the memory access patterns for pipelining of data references corresponding to array references across multiple iterations of nested loops. The compiler also derives information about the relative rate among various array references and embeds that knowledge into the scheduling of memory operations.

Packing and unpacking of data items allows the implementation to reduce the number of memory accesses. When the basic memory transfer unit or block is larger than the individual data items the computation manipulates, the implementation can associate many data items to a single memory word. An individual memory access thus fetches multiple data items, thereby reducing the number of memory accesses when the computation requires all the items need to be fetched. This mapping technique is particularly beneficial for computations that access consecutive array data elements or when the stride is known at compile time, and the compiler customizes the data layout to match the data access patterns of the computation [261, 291].

Figure 5.27 illustrates the application of packing and unpacking for a computation that operates on 5-bit array elements. In Fig. 5.27b the compiler has packed every six consecutive elements of the `a` array into a single 32-bit element of the `a32` array. It then laid out the `a32` array in memory by padding the two most significant bits in each element. For each read access the compiler translates the basic memory access with `mask` and `shift` arithmetic and logic bit-level operations as depicted in Fig. 5.27b, revealing the huge saving as all six individual data items are now accessed by a single memory read operation. Write operations, however, are more

```
int:5 a[N]; // array of 5-bit integers

if((N % 6) == 0) {
  for(i=0; i < N; i += 6) {
    ... = a[i+0];
    ... = a[i+1];
    ... = a[i+2];
    ... = a[i+3];
    ... = a[i+4];
    ... = a[i+5];
  }
}
```

(a)

```
int:32 a[N]; // array of 32-bit integers

if((N % 6) == 0) {
  for(i=0; i < N; i += 6) {
    w = a[i];
    ... = (w & 0x0000001F):5;
    ... = ((w & 0x000003E0) >> 5):5;
    ... = ((w & 0x00007C00) >> 10):5;
    ... = ((w & 0x000F1000) >> 15):5;
    ... = ((w & 0x01F00000) >> 20):5;
    ... = ((w & 0x3E000000) >> 25):5;
  }
}
```

(b)

Fig. 5.27 Packing and unpacking example of 5-bit items into 32-bit words: (**a**) original code; (**b**) code using unpacking to access individual array elements and assuming elements are packed in memory

complicated as the implementation may have to first read the memory word, mask the bits corresponding to the specific data item and them write it back to memory. Despite the memory savings and the reduction of the number of memory accesses (see Fig. 5.27a and b), unpacking operations may impose non-negligible overheads in both latency and hardware resources. In fine-grained reconfigurable architectures, however, the unpacking operations in the loop body of Fig. 5.27b can be performed very efficiently via interconnection resources (wires).

5.6 Back-End Support

The back-end is responsible for the generation of data-path and control unit structures for the specific target reconfigurable architecture. In some architectures, as in the case of FPGAs, the back-end is also responsible for the generation of the configuration data or bit-stream used to program the reconfigurable device. We now briefly describe the main functions and techniques that support these capabilities.

5.6.1 Allocation, Scheduling, and Binding

The three classical steps of allocation, scheduling, and binding[12] have been extensively studied and developed in the context of high-level synthesis [114] and

[12] Ideally these three steps would be fused. The inherent algorithmic complexity of any of these steps, however, has forced implementations to decouple them and imposed a specific execution order (with possible re-execution). While in specific contexts some of the steps are absent, it is common that allocation precedes binding, while binding and scheduling can be arbitrarily ordered.

generically described in Chap. 3. When the compilation flow targets fine-grained reconfigurable architectures and uses traditional high-level synthesis tools as part of its back-end, these mapping steps are transparently applied by the compiler. When using logic synthesis without high-level synthesis tools or when targeting coarse-grained reconfigurable architectures, however, the compiler must engage at some level of the mapping in these three steps.

In the allocation step, the compiler is responsible for assigning each computational element to each type of architectural resource. It assigns each operation to each type of FU, each data unit (scalar or array) to each storage type, and each data transfer operation to each type of interconnection (e.g., buses, wires). This allocation step thus takes into account the specific needs of each computational element and the specific support of the architectural resources in terms of supported instructions, storage capacity, and bandwidth, and typically consists of a straightforward resource matching procedure. After allocation, scheduling is the process of assigning operations to a discrete execution cycle or step, usually a clock cycle, and possibly exploiting resource sharing by scheduling two or more operations at the same FU in distinct time steps. As a by-product of the scheduling step, the compiler generates a State Transition Graph (STG) it uses to derive a control unit, e.g., using a finite-state machine (FSM), that will coordinate data-path execution. Lastly, high-level synthesis flows perform a binding step where they assign each computational element previously bound to a given type of resource to a specific physical instance of that resource. For example, two addition operations can be allocated to the same type of ALU unit, and during binding each operation can be bound to a distinct ALU instance.

When targeting fine-grained reconfigurable architectures, and in the absence of high-level synthesis tools, the compiler relies on the traditional algorithms for scheduling, namely ASAP (As Soon As Possible), ALAP (As Late As Possible), list scheduling, and force-directed list scheduling [114,210]. In this context, researchers have merged basic blocks into *hyperblocks* [200], to enhance the scope and thus the effectiveness of the scheduling steps. For coarse-grained architectures, and in the absence of resource sharing, the scheduling step focuses almost exclusively on supporting memory accesses [148] and on pipelined execution of loops [68].

5.6.2 Module Generation

We now describe module generation techniques for fine-grained and coarse-grained reconfigurable architectures. For coarse-grained architectures, where most of the high-level operations are directly supported by the FUs in each cell, neither a circuit generator nor logic synthesis is usually needed to generate the data-path and control structures. Complex operations, as is the example of the square-root (`sqrt`) operation, can nevertheless rely on circuit generators even for these architectures.

When targeting a fine-grained architecture, compilers resort to techniques for generating the hardware structures of FUs, respectively, logic synthesis tools, or module generators, in some instance combining them synergetically in the same flow, as synthesis tools themselves may rely on module generators.

Module generators allow compilers to quickly generate a description of hardware structure for a specific hardware operator. The generated circuit description can be done at the resource level, natively supported by the target architecture, e.g., LUTs in the case of an FPGA, or at a higher level of abstraction, e.g., at the logic gate level. While the descriptions at both levels still require the use of placement and routing for the generation of the architecture configuration specification (e.g., bit-streams), when specifying a circuit at the logic gate level, the compiler may still need to perform logic synthesis. Mapping is, nevertheless, required. Irrespective of the code generation strategy, however, the use of module generators drastically reduces the synthesis time and in some cases leads to hardware implementations with fewer resources (area) and with shorter execution time (delay) than solutions derived using logic synthesis. In some extreme and very specific cases, module generators can directly generate structures containing preplacement information that can reduce the overall placement and routing time.

In terms of implementation, these module generators are commonly structured as scripts or parameterized language constructs such as the `generate` constructs found in VHDL. These language features have been used in the back-end of several compilers, e.g., the Nenya [65] and the *garpcc* [60] compilers. More sophisticated implementations may even use a domain-specific language and interpreters as is the case of the DIL language and compiler [55].

Other more flexible module generators offer higher-level language interfaces. The JHDL framework [36] allows designers to describe the data-path at RTL in a subset of Java extended by special APIs [328]. Such a description can be independent of the target FPGA architecture and thus require the use of mapping, placement, and routing to generate the configuration data. The Jbits [136] tool generates bit-streams from a Java description integrating placement and routing steps and has been used as the back-end of the Abstract-Machines compiler [287]. This compiler performs some low-level optimizations, at the LUT-level for the Xilinx's Virtex FPGA, namely LUT/register merging, register/LUT merging, and LUT combination.

In other approaches, compilers rely on commercial logic synthesis and placement and routing tools for the generation of the architecture hardware structures. The compiler generates a description of the desired architecture in common HDLs (such as VHDL or Verilog) in structural and/or behavioral RTL forms. Other compilers, however, generate algorithmic HDL descriptions and rely on external HLS tools to generate the RTL description of the architecture. Compilers relying on either of these two approaches invariably use some internal hardware architecture template as is the case of the DEFACTO [47]. While this approach incurs long run-times for the generation of the target device configuration, it offers the benefit of a high-level code generation abstractions and relieves the compiler of the burden of low-level optimizations commonly performed at the lowest levels of hardware implementation.

5.6.3 Mapping, Placement, and Routing

The back-end of the compilation flow includes the three steps of mapping, placement, and routing, to generate the configuration (i.e., a bit-stream) that once loaded into the target reconfigurable device will configure the desired Reconfigurable Processing Unit (RPU) internal structure. We now briefly describe these three steps, well known in the CAD (Computer-Aided Design) community [78] and extensively used in commercial synthesis tools when targeting FPGAs.

The mapping combines or decomposes the computation operations to the specific hardware blocks of the target RPU. When targeting a Xilinx FPGA, for example, mapping combines various logic gates corresponding to the computation to be implemented as the FPGA's Look Up Tables (LUTs). For coarse-grained reconfigurable architectures mapping is used, for example, to assign two or more arithmetic or logic operations to a given Processing Element (PE). After mapping, placement is responsible for assigning each RPU resource, or block, to a specific block in the target RPU (e.g., identified as `x, y` coordinates in a two-dimensional reconfigurable architecture). Lastly, routing assigns physical interconnection resources in the reconfigurable architecture to connections between the blocks, previously placed.

Given the inherent algorithmic complexity of these steps, their implementations are forced to rely on heuristics and generic optimization methods [266], such as simulated annealing techniques [176]. Naturally, the internal structure of the target RPU tremendously influences the complexity of each of these steps. If a PE of a given RPU can only implement a single operation on a specific execution step, a simpler one-to-one mapping is required. The interconnection topology of the RPU drastically impacts the complexity of placement and routing. For fine-grained RPUs such as FPGAs, placement and routing are extremely complex steps, often implemented in a sequential fashion, possibly repeated. For coarse-grained RPUs, however, these steps tend to be very simplified given the simplicity of the net-lists involved and the coarser granularity of the underlying PE structures. When targeting a simple VLIW-based RPU, placement is reduced to assigning the mapped operations to the PE able to execute the operations. There are no routing issues, as routing is emulated by load/store of data from/to a global register file. Similarly, when targeting a network-on-a-chip architecture (NoC) where routers can dynamically define the data communication paths, no static routing is required.

5.7 Summary

In this chapter we presented an overview of mapping and execution techniques for reconfigurable architectures. While many of these techniques have been developed for traditional architectures, the spatial nature of reconfigurable architectures substantially increases the complexity of their application.

We have described opportunities for reconfigurable architectures to exploit advanced execution techniques and the very challenging problems of temporal and

Table 5.2 Qualitative comparison of the applicability of some mapping techniques in reconfigurable architectures and general-purpose processors

Technique	Target	
	General purpose architectures	Reconfigurable computing architectures
Temporal partitioning		✓
Spatial partitioning		✓
Loop pipelining	✓	✓
Memory accesses reduction by Rotating-/shift-register	✓	✓
Memory accesses reduction by packing	✓	✓

spatial partitioning. We also described the basic resource and operator mapping techniques and loop pipelining, a very important execution technique that exploits the spatial computing resources and custom control structures for high-throughput. Lastly, we have described techniques that ameliorate the cost of memory accesses, and highlighted the mapping techniques in the back-end phases of a compilation and synthesis flow for reconfigurable architectures.

In Table 5.2, we summarize the applicability of some of the most significant mapping techniques when targeting reconfigurable architectures, qualitatively comparing their applicability to general-purpose processors. For the techniques in this table, we note that all but spatial and temporal partitioning are applicable to reconfigurable architectures and general-purpose processors. The application of these common mapping techniques, however, exhibits very distinct potential impact in the two architecture classes.

Chapter 6
Compilers for Reconfigurable Architectures

This chapter describes the most prominent academic efforts on compilation and synthesis of application codes written in high-level programming languages to reconfigurable architectures. The maturity of some of the compilation and mapping techniques described in Chaps. 4 and 5, and the stability of the underlying reconfigurable technologies, have enabled the emergence of commercial compilation solutions, such as the MAP compiler from SRC Computers [292] and the High-Level Compiler from Nallatech [223], both of which support the mapping of programs written in a subset of the C programming language to FPGAs.

In this chapter, we distinguish between compilation efforts that target fine-grained commercially available reconfigurable devices, such as well-known FPGAs, and efforts that target architectures with proprietary reconfigurable devices, typically coarse-grained devices. Despite their granularity distinction, and thus the different mapping techniques used, these efforts exhibit many commonalities. We begin with a brief historical perspective on early compilation efforts, which naturally focused on fine-grained architectures. We then describe various representative compilation efforts, highlighting their use of the transformations and mapping techniques described in the previous two chapters. We conclude by summarizing and highlighting the differences between the described compilation efforts.

6.1 Early Compilation Efforts

The early compilation efforts were naturally constrained by the inherent resource limitations of early fine-grained reconfigurable devices, such as FPGAs and PLDs and the low-level abstractions offered to program them. Consequently, the first compilation efforts provided relatively simple, yet powerful, translation schemes of limited scope. The basic approach focused on straightforward one-to-one mapping schemes which translated high-level programming language operators and simple syntactic constructs directly to hardware structures (see, e.g., [326]). In this approach, each assignment statement is translated into a data-path element controlled

DOI 10.1007/978-0-387-09671-1_6,

directly by a specific state in a finite state machine (FSM) controller. The compiler aggregates multiple data-path elements to form a large data-path and corresponding controller responsible for the hardware execution of the entire computation.

Several early compilation efforts to FPGAs reflected this simple translation approach. The work by Page and Luk [236] mapped occam programs [165] directly into hardware. The Transmogrifier C compiler [116] and the compiler developed by Wo and Forward [330] considered the mapping to an FPGA of a subset of the C programming language. A similar translation approach was used by the Handel-C compiler [235] exploiting the explicit concurrency of language constructs to aggregate multiple assignment statements in a single FSM controller state.

While early compilers targeted a fine-grained standalone reconfigurable architecture, the PRISM I [21] and PRISM II [7] compilers increased the reach of target architectures by compiling C programs to a system consisting of a GPP and an RPU [20]. The compilation to the RPU focused on low-level optimizations, at the gate or logic levels, still with limited scope and not supporting advanced data structure access constructs.

Spatial partitioning was also a key technique used in early compilers and tools. They addressed the issues raised by the very limited amount of hardware resources in each FPGA in important applications such as rapid prototyping and the emulation of hardware, by partitioning large circuits to circuit boards with multiple FPGAs. While most of spatial partitioning efforts focused on fairly low-level partitioning using as input specifications of circuit net-lists, the work by Schmit et al. [273] exploited spatial partitioning at the behavioral and structural levels. An example of a compiler including spatial partitioning of C programs targeting multi-FPGA platforms is described in [244].

With the increasing capacity of reconfigurable devices, compiler techniques and tools reflected the need to raise the level of abstraction offered to programmers. In this context, various efforts led to prototype compilers that interacted with high-level synthesis (HLS) tools and could therefore leverage all the techniques developed by the HLS research community. As an example, the work by Doncev et al. [97] used a commercial HLS tool to synthesize specific architectures targeting FPGA substrates from a behavioral algorithmic-level VHDL description.

After the earlier and arguably more timid efforts, we have witnessed a growing interest in academia for compilation of high-level languages to FPGAs. Rather than forcing programmers to code in hardware-oriented programming languages, many research efforts took the pragmatic approach of directly compiling to hardware high-level languages such as C or Java. Most of these efforts produce behavioral RTL-HDL descriptions used by RTL/logic synthesis tools. While many of these efforts originated in academia (e.g., [224,323]), the increase in FPGA capacity and popularity stimulated a growing interest by industry in this area, leading to various industry compilation efforts (e.g., Forge compiler [339], Nios II C-to-Hardware Acceleration Compiler (C2H) [187], Impulse-C [243]) explicitly targeting FPGAs.

Largely for economic reasons, early compilation efforts to reconfigurable architectures focused mostly on fine-grained architectures. Compilation efforts targeting recently available coarse-grained reconfigurable architectures have their roots in the translation approaches for Systolic, VLSI, and Wavefront arrays [178, 181] of which the Xputer compiler [34, 148] is considered one of the first. The suitability of coarse-grained reconfigurable architectures for computationally intensive algorithms, requiring common arithmetic precision while exhibiting very desirable power and energy characteristics, made them the target of recent research efforts in academia and industry. For these architectures, spatial and temporal partitioning alongside instruction scheduling and placement and routing are very important mapping techniques. Compilation efforts for these architectures could leverage, at least, from a conceptual stand-point, experiences and insights of the same techniques developed for finer-grained reconfigurable architectures.

6.2 Compilers for FPGA-Based Systems

We now describe compilation efforts that exclusively target FPGA-based systems through a wide variety of approaches and for distinct input programming languages and computational models. We begin with a description of compilation efforts for C programs and then describe efforts considering other languages (e.g., MATLAB or Java). In terms of hardware implementation generation, these efforts rely on one of two, not completely orthogonal approaches. One approach leverages the use of component libraries and thus directly maps high-level programming constructs to these systems. A second approach relies on external HLS tools and uses algorithmic VHDL specifications as an intermediate compilation step.

6.2.1 The SPC Compiler

The SUIF Pipeline Compiler (SPC) focuses on automatic vectorization techniques [323] for synthesizing custom hardware pipelines for loops in C programs. The compiler directly generates RTL-VHDL descriptions for the corresponding hardware implementations and relies on RTL/logic synthesis and placement and routing tools to generate an FPGA bit-stream. SPC has its roots in the early research efforts by Weinhardt [321].

The SPC analyzes all program loops, focusing on innermost loops with no data dependences or with regular loop-carried dependences. SPC generates pipelined implementations of those loops aggressively exploiting instruction-level parallelism opportunities for hardware execution. The compiler synthesizes address generators for accesses to multidimensional arrays, and generates hardware implementations that extensively use shift-registers for input data reuse, thus eliminating redundant memory read operations. Pipeline vectorization takes advantage of several loop transformations to meet hardware resource constraints, while maximizing available parallelism. The compiler also uses simple array memory allocation strategies to increase data availability and array access transformations to reduce the cost, and even eliminate memory operations [322].

6.2.2 A C to Fine-Grained Pipelining Compiler

Maruyama and Hoshino [202] developed a prototype compiler that maps loop computations expressed in C programs to fine-grained custom pipelined hardware solutions implemented on FPGA devices. As with other similar early efforts, this compiler also generates an FPGA device bit-stream from an RTL-VHDL hardware description using RTL/logic synthesis and placement and routing tools.

The compiler aggressively splits arithmetic operations into cascading 8-bit wide operations, a transformation known as decomposition, and uses speculative execution techniques between loop iterations for higher pipelining throughput. In the presence of memory bank dependences, the pipeline is stalled and the accesses serialized. Feedback dependences, either through scalar or array variables, cause speculative operations in the pipeline to be cancelled. These speculative operations are then restarted after the operations in the previous loop iterations have completed their updates to memory, thus guaranteeing the correctness of subsequent operations. The compiler also supports the mapping of limited recursive function calls by converting them to iterative constructs. In addition, the compiler front-end supports a limited set of concurrency annotations that allow the compiler to take advantage of coarse-grained parallelism.

6.2.3 The DeepC Silicon Compiler

The DeepC silicon compiler [23, 24] maps C or Fortran programs to a two dimensional mesh of tiles where each tile consists of reconfigurable logic connected to local memories and an inter-tile communication channel.

Internally, each generated tile design consists of a data-path and the definition of the various communication channels along with an FSM-based control unit. The compiler back-end generates technology independent behavioral RTL Verilog models and relies on commercial RTL/logic synthesis and placement and routing tools to generate complete hardware implementations for each tile. The compiler uses state-of-the-art static pointer analysis in the SUIF framework [30, 189] for bank disambiguation and partitioning of array data across memories to collocate data to the title that manipulates it. It also performs bit-width analysis [296] and supports the translation of floating-point data types and operations to sequences of integer bit-level micro-operations.

6.2.4 The COBRA-ABS Tool

The COBRA-ABS tool [99, 100] synthesizes custom architectures for digital signal processing algorithms written in a subset of the C programming language. The target architecture consists of a multi-FPGA system with various arithmetic ASICs and global and local memories.

The tool uses commercially available synthesis tools to generate the various FPGA bit-stream configurations. It uses a high-level synthesis approach developed for ASICs to create a target architecture based on a VLIW style with a large register file and centralized control unit. Internally, the tool performs spatial partitioning, scheduling, mapping and allocation using simulated annealing techniques.

6.2.5 The DEFACTO Compiler

The DEFACTO (Design Environment For Adaptive Computing TechnOlogy) compiler [47] maps computations, expressed in high-level languages such as C and Fortran to FPGA-based computing platforms such as the Annapolis WildStar board [19]. It partitions the input program into a component that executes on a GPP and a component that is translated to behavioral algorithmic VHDL to execute on one or more FPGAs.

DEFACTO combines parallelizing compiler technology with commercially available high-level VHDL synthesis tools. DEFACTO uses the SUIF framework and performs several traditional parallelizing compiler analyses and transformations such as loop unrolling, loop tiling, data and computation partitioning. It also generates customized memory interfaces and maps data to internal storage structures. In particular, it uses data reuse analysis coupled with balance metrics to guide the application of high-level loop transformations [290]. When performing hardware/software partitioning, the compiler is responsible for generating the data management (copying to and from the memory associated with each FPGA) and synchronizing the execution of every FPGA in a distributed memory parallel computing style of execution.

6.2.6 The Streams-C Compiler

The Streams-C compiler [127] relies on a Communicating Sequential Processes (CSP) parallel programming model [155]. The programmer uses annotations to explicitly declare and manage processes, streams, and signals. Streams-C processes are independently executing objects with their bodies specified by a C routine and using signals to synchronize their execution. Programmer is also responsible for the definition of the data streams and associated input/output ports for each process, explicitly controlling the execution of read and write operations with primitives functions.

Internally, the compiler builds a process graph decorated with the corresponding data stream information. It then maps the computation on each process to an FPGA and uses the Malleable Architecture Generator (MARGE) tool [121] to generate the specific data-path VHDL code (structural RTL model) from C routine of each process. It inserts synchronization and input/output operations by converting the annotations in the source C to library function calls. The MARGE tool is also responsible for scheduling the execution of loops in each process body in a pipelined fashion [112].

6.2.7 The Cameron Compiler

The Cameron compiler [44, 45] maps programs written in a C-based single-assignment language called SA-C onto an architecture composed of a GPP and an FPGA. The compiler translates SA-C programs into data-flow graphs (DFGs) and then onto synthesizable VHDL designs [260] relying on predefined and parameterized library templates. A back-end pass uses commercially available synthesis tools, such as Synplicity's Synplify [301] and placement and routing tools to generate the target FPGA bit-streams.

The SA-C language includes constructs that relax the execution order of computations, such as arithmetic reduction operators, windowing primitives over one- and two-dimensional arrays, and variable bit-width specification. The SA-C compiler exploits the semantics of these constructs alongside information extracted from source-level *pragmas*, regarding array and loop bound definition, for the selection of loop unrolling, loop tiling transformations as well as fixed-precision arithmetic operators. Efforts on the SA-C compiler [318] also included the compilation to Morphosys [283], a coarse-grained reconfigurable architecture.

6.2.8 The MATCH Compiler

The MATCH compiler [25,224] translates MATLAB programs [307] to behavioral RTL-VHDL descriptions [142] which are subsequently mapped to FPGAs using commercial RTL/logic synthesis and placement and routing tools. A novel aspect of the compiler is the integration of intellectual property (IP) cores in its compilation flow using an IP core repository with EDIF/HDL, performance, area and interface descriptions.

The compiler leverages MATLAB's library of predefined operators. To improve the quality of the generated hardware implementations, and in addition to user directives, the compiler performs static array shape and dimension analyses of vector/matrix operations. Vector and matrix operations are translated into loop nests and subject to various loop-based transformations for concurrent execution on multiple FPGAs. The compiler performs arithmetic precision, bit-width inference analysis, and converts floating-point data types to fixed point. Lastly, it also performs pipelining and scheduling of loop-level computations using modulo scheduling. For pipelined loops the compiler schedules the memory accesses based on the number of ports, the available memories, and on the delays of each IP core used.

6.2.9 The Galadriel and Nenya Compilers

The Galadriel compiler translates Java bytecodes [193] to an architectural synthesis tool (Nenya) specific for FPGAs [65, 67]. The compilers target architectures based on a single commercial FPGA connected to one or more memories. The Galadriel compiler acts as a front-end and exposes parallelism at different levels of granularity, namely, operation, basic block, and functional, for each Java method being compiled [66].

The Nenya compiler relies on a fine-grained scheduler to orchestrate the operations in each method, which considers different macrocell alternatives for a given FU. This scheduler also takes into account the bit-width of each operand and the area/delay estimation of each component in a hardware library, modeled using curve fitting for each target device. Nenya uses temporal partitioning techniques for designs that exceed the target FPGA capacity. It generates, for each temporal partition, a control unit and a data-path unit with the corresponding memory interfaces. The control unit is output in behavioral RTL-VHDL and the data-path in structural RTL-VHDL, both ready for commercial RTL/logic synthesis. Lastly, FPGA bit-streams are generated using vendor-specific placement and routing tools. Early versions of Nenya relied on circuit generators to target the Xilinx XC6200 FPGA [341].

6.2.10 The Sea Cucumber Compiler

The Sea Cucumber (SC) compiler [310] is a Java to FPGA compiler that takes a pragmatic approach to the problem of concurrency extraction. It uses the Java thread model to recognize task-level or coarse-grained parallelism. The communication between the Java threads is defined by the CSP model and is based on one-way, non-buffered, self-synchronized channels. The programmer is responsible for avoiding deadlocks.

The compiler extracts fine-grained concurrency using conventional control-flow and data-flow analyses at the statement level and across multiple statements in each task. Internally, it uses a hyperblock representation to increase the amount of fine-grained parallelism and uses *if-conversion* to facilitate mapping in space. A scheduler is responsible for generating a data-path and control unit for each hyperblock. The back-end generates hardware specifications in EDIF (Electronic Design Interchange Format) using JHDL [36], which are then translated to FPGA bit-streams using a placement and routing tool.

6.2.11 The Abstract-Machines Compiler

This compiler leverages the abstraction of objected-oriented programming in defining the set of predefined execution methods for objects of every class that extends a Machine [287] object. Classes define the machine-specific *input*, *output* and *step* methods the compiler uses to define the interfaces to each hardware object that instantiates the software object counterpart. The programmer naturally defines coarse-grained concurrency as each object is mapped to a distinct hardware component. The compiler then explores the execution methods in each class to extract and match to hardware ILP opportunities.

Internally, the compiler uses the hyperblock and the SSA intermediate representations. To expose more ILP it unrolls loops, maps array variables to RAMs, and uses predicated execution. It uses traditional source-level transformations, such as dead-code elimination and constant propagation, and performs bit-width narrowing. It also limits the use of multiplexers in the implementation of nested conditional constructs. In the middle-level of the compilation flow, the compiler uses retiming, micropipelining, and digital serial arithmetic for higher pipelined throughputs. In the back-end, the compiler performs Virtex-specific transformations to decrease the number of slices used relying on the JBits tool [136] to generate the FPGA bit-streams.

6.2.12 The CHAMPION Software Design Environment

The CHAMPION software design environment [229] maps applications specified in the Cantata [349] graphical programming environment to a board of FPGAs with local memories. Cantata allows programmers to graphically describe their applications by interconnecting, in an acyclic fashion, icons, representing functions, named *glyphs*. Each *glyph* is mapped to a given hardware component, whose behavior is described in C code. Each *glyph* hardware component is synthesized, and placed and routed beforehand, thus providing the compiler, during mapping, with accurate information about its size and delay. The VHDL code (behavioral RTL) of each component is generated using a commercial high-level synthesis tool that accepts as input C code using fixed-point data types. To generate the FPGA bit-streams the compiler relies on commercial logic synthesis and placement and routing tools.

CHAMPION focuses mainly on three design aspects. First, it uses a task-level graph to explicitly represent the control and data dependences between the various computations. This representation facilitates the spatial partitioning and simple forms of temporal partitioning of the tasks when the hardware resources to implement a set of nodes in the graph exceeds the FPGA's capacity. Second, and given a data-driven execution model, it facilitates the design of synchronization and communication primitives between components. Lastly, by using the attributes of each *glyph* the compiler can match and adjust (by padding or truncating) port bit-widths between components.

6.2.13 The SPARCS Tool

The SPARCS (Synthesis and Partitioning for Adaptive Reconfigurable Computing Systems) tool [230] partitions and synthesizes designs for reconfigurable architectures with multiple FPGA devices. The tool accepts as input a task graph where each task is specified in behavioral algorithmic-level VHDL. It then applies temporal and spatial partitioning techniques to map the individual tasks to the target FPGAs.

Internally, it uses the unified specification model (USM) [231] as an intermediate representation and relies on high-level synthesis, RTL/logic synthesis, and placement and routing tools to generate FPGA configurations. The authors formalize a joint temporal and spatial partitioning problems taking into account the additional storage required to save intermediate data given a temporal partitioning of a task. The tool uses integer-linear programming techniques to find a feasible temporal partitioning of the tasks and a genetic algorithmic approach perform spatial partitioning. The tool suffers from long run-times as it is dominated by design-space exploration. This exploration relies on area and resource estimation provided by commercial logic synthesis and placement and routing tools.

6.2.14 The ROCCC Compiler

The Riverside Optimizing Compiler for Configurable Computing (ROCCC) is a C to hardware compiler that targets FPGA-based acceleration of frequently executed code segments, most notably loop nests [137].

ROCCC uses a variation of the SUIF2 and MachSUIF [284] compilation infrastructure, called CIRRF (Compiler Intermediate Representation for Reconfigurable Computing) [138]. In addition to common loop-based transformations such as loop-unrolling and strip-mining, this compiler uncovers and exploits input data reuse in windowing operations by analysis of array subscripts in perfectly nested loops [137]. Using predefined hardware buffering primitives and library modules, the compiler generates dedicated structures to hold the data and schedules external memory operations. It generates RTL-VHDL hardware specifications and relies on commercial RTL/logic synthesis and placement and routing tools to generate FPGA bit-streams.

6.2.15 The DWARV Compiler

The Delft Workbench Automated Reconfigurable VHDL (DWARV) Generator [346] translates *pragma*-identified C functions to VHDL designs targeting the Molen architecture [316].

Internally, the compiler is organized as two modules: the DFG Builder and the VHDL Generator. The DFG Builder constructs a hierarchical data-flow graph (HDFG) from the SUIF2 intermediate representation [10]. It then performs scalar replacement, *if-conversion*, and transformation to SSA form, in addition to standard source-level optimizations. The VHDL Generator schedules the operations in the HDFG, taking into account memory and register file characteristics (e.g., access times) specified in a configuration file. The Generator outputs a behavioral RTL-VHDL FSM-based design using the Molen architecture generation interface [182]. Existing commercial tools are then used to synthesize, place and route, and generate the final FPGA bit-stream which is then merged with the remainder Molen architecture design.

6.3 Compilers for Coarse-Grained Reconfigurable Architectures

Other research and commercial projects took the alternative route of considering specific reconfigurable architectures and developed their own translation and mapping tools. Examples of such efforts include the compilers for the PipeRench [132], RaPiD [101], Xputer [149], and the XPP [31] architectures.

6.3.1 The DIL Compiler

The PipeRench compiler [55] maps computations described in an intermediate single assignment language, called Data-flow Intermediate Language (DIL) [129], into the PipeRench architecture [132]. The DIL language allows the description of unidirectional pipelined circuits using a C-like syntax with operators using fixed-point type variables with arbitrary bit-widths. The compiler performs bit-width inference for all but input and output variables [56] as one of the 30 analyses passes before generating hardware stripe configurations.

Internally, the compiler expands the input program using function and module inlining techniques, as well as loop unrolling, generating a large straight-line single assignment program representation. It then constructs a global hierarchical acyclic DFG with nodes representing operations, I/O ports, and delay-registers and where each operator node can be a DFG itself. After the generation of the global DFG, the compiler performs a variety of common transformations (e.g., common subexpression elimination, algebraic simplifications, and dead code elimination). It then uses module generators to expand the arithmetic operators and applying hardware retiming techniques and interconnection simplifications. To generate the virtual hardware stripes, the compiler performs a placement and routing phase over the DFG using a deterministic linear-time greedy algorithm based on list scheduling [58].

6.3.2 The RaPiD-C Compiler

The RaPiD-C compiler [84] relies on RaPiD-C, a C-like, architecture-specific concurrent programming language, to facilitate the mapping of high-level computation descriptions to the RaPiD architecture [101]. RaPiD-C allows programmers to specify parallelism, data movement, and data partitioning across the multiple elements of the RaPiD array. In particular, RaPiD-C introduces the notion of space-loop, or *Sloop*. The compiler unrolls all the iterations of a *Sloop* and maps them onto the architecture. The designer, however, is responsible for permuting and tiling a loop to fit onto the architecture and for introducing and managing the communication and synchronization in the unrolled versions of the loops. Specifically, the programmer must assign variables to memories and ensure the correct data is written to the RAM modules using the language-provided synchronization primitives, *Wait* and *Signal*.

Internally, the RaPiD-C compiler extracts from each loop a control tree per each concurrent task [84] defined by a *Par* statement in the language. Each task control tree has as interior nodes sequential statements defined by *Seq* constructs and *For* loop statements. At the leaves the control tree the compiler inserts synchronization dependences between the *Wait* and *Signal* nodes. During compilation, the RaPiD-C compiler inserts registers for scalar variables and ALUs for arithmetic operations, in effect creating a DFG for the entire computation to be mapped to a stage in the architecture. The compiler then extracts address and instructions generators that are used to control the transfer of values between stages. The RaPiD-C compiler uses two control techniques, called *multiplexer merging* and *FU merging*, respectively. In the multiplexer merging the compiler aggregates several multiplexers into a single larger multiplexer and modifies the control predicates for each of the inputs taking into account the net-list of multiplexers created as a result of the implementation of conditional statements. The FU merging exploits the fact that ALUs can be merged if their inputs are mutually exclusive in time and the union of their inputs does not exceed a fixed bit-width value.

The compiler represents in its control tree, scenarios in which the control is data dependent, i.e., by defining the dependency as an event with a condition evaluated at run-time, directly translated into hardware. For example, the first iteration of a loop can be represented by the *i.first* condition being true only at the first iteration of a `For` loop, and the carry of an ALU operation is accessed by the *alu.carry* signal. The compiler aggregates these predicates into instructions and generates the corresponding decoding that drives each of the available control lines of the architecture, so that the control signals can be present at the corresponding stage during execution.

6.3.3 The CoDe-X Compiler

The CoDe-X [34] compiler maps C applications to a system consisting of a general-purpose processor (GPP) and Xputers [146]. The compiler maps selected segments of C code to the rDPA applying a number of loop parallelization transformations such as loop distribution and strip-mining to expose and leverage task-level concurrency. It also performs loop unrolling, vectorization, and parallelization of loops when they operate on different array sections.

Internally, the compiler identifies the tasks to be mapped to the coarse-grained rPDA array, generating for each task a description of its computations using ALE-X, a language to represent arithmetic and logic expressions. Each ALE-X description is then synthesized to an rDPA using a data-path synthesis (DPSS) tool [148]. The DPSS tool generates the configurations for the rDPA and the controller of the various task configurations. As the rDPA only executes data-flow computations, the compiler uses the *if-conversion* technique.

The DPSS tool is also responsible for scheduling, using a dynamic list-scheduling algorithm [148], the operations to be mapped to the array, with the constraint of a single I/O operation per each step (the Xputer uses only one bus to stream I/O data). The final step uses a mapper, based on simulated annealing, that performs the placement and routing of each task's data-path onto the rDPA array and generates the various array configurations and corresponding controllers.

6.3.4 The XPP-VC Compiler

The XPP-VC compiler [68,69] maps C programs to the XPP [31], a coarse-grained, reconfigurable architecture. XPP-VC uses the SUIF intermediate representation and generates a structural description resembling functional elements of the XPP in NML, the native mapping language of the XPP. These NML descriptions are then input to a placement and routing tool for generating the XPP configuration bit-streams. A stylized C form is accepted by the compiler to embed previously optimized NML modules in C programs [70]. The compiler aggressively exploits loop pipelining using the pipeline vectorization technique developed in the context of mapping computations to FPGAs [323] and adapted for targeting the XPP.

The compiler relies on input source code annotations to control loop unrolling and to specify the binding of array variables to internal or external memories. The compiler also includes temporal partitioning techniques to split computations unable to be mapped in a single configuration, i.e., when requiring more hardware resources than the available in the target XPP. Finally, and as the XPP architecture directly implements a data-flow, data-driven execution scheme, with a ready/acknowledge synchronization protocol, the compiler needs to be aware of the implicit synchronization based on data availability between architecture components such as FUs and/or interconnect resources.

6.3.5 The DRESC Compiler

The DRESC (Dynamically Reconfigurable Embedded System Compiler) [207] maps C programs to the ADRES architecture [206,208,299]. The compiler relies on execution profiling for identifying the computationally intensive loops (kernels) in the input programs which are mapped to the two dimensional coarse-grained reconfigurable array mode (also known as view) whereas other portions of the code are executed using the VLIW mode. In this compilation flow, source-level transformations (e.g., loop transformations) are considered and applied manually to improve implementations in the ADRES architecture.

Internally, the compiler uses the *Lcode* intermediate representation output by the IMPACT compiler infrastructure [76, 159] to perform scheduling and other optimizations. It also generates code for communication between the VLIW and the reconfigurable array views alongside their schedulers. The compiler uses a novel modulo scheduling algorithm which combines scheduling, placement and routing to map pipelined loop kernels onto the reconfigurable array. A novel aspect of the compilation flow is the possibility to target a family of ADRES architectures by modification of an architectural description. Examples of this flexibility have been shown for different routing topologies among the PEs of the architecture, as well as for heterogeneous FUs [206].

6.4 Compilers for Hybrid Reconfigurable Architectures

We now describe illustrative examples of compilers that target hybrid architectures, that include in the same VLSI chip traditional processors and reconfigurable elements.

6.4.1 The Chimaera-C Compiler

The Chimaera-C compiler [347] maps C programs to Chimaera [152], a hybrid RISC/RFU (Reconfigurable Function Unit) architecture where both components, the RISC and the RFU, are tightly coupled via a register file. The compiler uses the GNU's C compiler (*gcc*) framework to identify suitable multiple-input single-output sequences of instructions that it then translates into RFU customized instructions.

This compiler focuses on two key instruction-level transformations. First, it uses *control localization* whereby it combines several basic blocks into a larger basic block. This merging of instructions increases the likelihood of finding good candidate sequences for RFU custom instructions. The second transformation is akin to multimedia ISA extensions whereby registers are split into disjoint fields operated on by instructions on a field-by-field fashion as in an SIMD style. Given the opportunities exposed by these analyses, the compiler then identifies the instructions and generates the RFU operations. The code generation and instruction scheduling is simplified under the assumption that RFU custom instructions execute in a single clock cycle. Loading of a configuration for a selected set of RFU instructions is performed via special registers [152].

6.4.2 The Garp and the Nimble C Compilers

The Garp reconfigurable architecture C compiler, called *garpcc*, maps C programs to the Garp reconfigurable architecture [60]. The Garp architecture exports a GPP/RPU coprocessor model whereby communication of data between the GPP and the RPU (a fine-grained reconfigurable array) is accomplished via memory-mapped registers. The loading of the RPU configuration is controlled by the GPP and is performed via the data memory bus.

Internally, the compiler uses the SUIF compiler framework [325] and identifies hyperblock regions of instructions, mostly in loops, that are suitable for implementation in the RPU. The compiler also integrates software pipelining techniques [62] and predicated execution in hardware. The compiler uses predefined module generators to generate the configurations for the RPU which are mapped to the architecture using dynamic programming strategies by the Gama tool [59]. Gama also generates from the DFG a specific array configuration for the RPU by integrating a specific placement and routing phase.

The basic concepts of the *garpcc* compiler were incorporated in the Synopsys Nimble compiler [192]. The Nimble compiler, however, targets a tightly coupled CPU/RPU system. It uses profiling information to identify inner loops for implementation on a specific data-path in the FPGA-based RPU. Based on the profiling data, Nimble partitions the input code between the CPU and the RPU. The hardware component is mapped to the RPU by the ADAPT data-path compiler. The ADAPT compiler uses module descriptions for creating the data-path and generates a sequencer for scheduling possible conflicts resulting from memory accesses and for orchestration of loops. The compiler also considers floor-planning and placement during this phase. Placement information of each data-path is fed to the placement and routing FPGA vendor tool to generate the bit-streams. As with other efforts, the software component of the input code is compiled using the CPU native C-compiler.

6.4.3 The NAPA-C Compiler

The NAPA-C compiler [121, 125] maps C programs to a coupled CPU/RFU reconfigurable architecture exposing a coprocessor execution model where the CPU and the RPU (an FPGA) share the same memory space. The compiler relies on source-code extensions that specify concurrency and bit-widths of integer types [125] and on programmer annotations (or *pragmas*) to define the input code sections that are to be mapped to the RPU. Among its key mapping techniques is the automatic mapping of array variables to memory banks taking into account the operator precedence between instructions of the code's data-flow graph [126]. The NAPA-C compiler has been retargeted for distinct hybrid architectures, namely the National Semiconductor's CLAy FPGA [121] and the NAPA (RISC+FPGA) device [125, 264]. The NAPA-C compiler has been recently augmented with a Stream-C language [127] front-end to support stream-based computation abstractions.

Internally, the compiler uses the MARGE (Malleable Architecture Generator) tool to generate a custom-specific instruction for each basic block of instructions to be implemented in the RPU [121]. MARGE uses as input intermediate representation a three-address code annotated with operand bit-widths. Each custom instruction consists of a data-path leveraging a library of parameterized macros/modules such as ALUs, counters, encoders, SRAMs, and register banks. Some of the library elements are preplaced and prerouted, drastically reducing the total compilation time [121]. Macros are generated using the `Modgen` tool whereby the logic structure (defined as a function of the bit-width of the operands, geometric shape) of each macro can be described in a C-like language. The output of MARGE is an RTL description containing `Modgen` components. FUs are shared by operations whenever possible, e.g., whenever they have similar bit-widths, offer the same functionality, and are not being used on a given schedule cycle. MARGE also generates the controllers that orchestrate the execution of the generated designs.

6.5 Compilation Efforts Summary

The previous sections introduced some of the most representative research efforts regarding the compilation to reconfigurable architectures. Table 6.1 presents a characterization of these efforts, grouped according to the supported programming model (either sequential or concurrent) and the abstraction level provided to programmers

Table 6.1 Characterization of a representative number of compilation efforts

			Target architectures			**Domain specialization**	
			Commercial FPGAs	**Microprocessor coupled with reconfigurable processing units (RPUs)**	**Coarse-grained RPUs**	**Architecture-Specific**	**Application-Specific**
Programming model	**Sequential**	**Low level**	Transmogrifier-C				
		High-level	PRISM, DEFACTO, ROCCC, SPC, Trident-C, MATCH, SA-C, DeepC, Galadriel & Nenya, XPP-VC, DWARV	DRESC, Code-X, *garpcc*, Chimaera-C, DWARV	DRESC, Code-X, DIL, XPP-VC	DIL	
	Concurrent (e.g., CSP)	**Low level**	SPARCS				
		High-level	Handel-C, Stream-C, Sea Cucumber, Abstract-Machines		RaPiD-C	RaPiD-C	Stream-C

(either high or low). Also represented in the table are the types of reconfigurable architectures they target, respectively, commercial FPGAs, GPPs coupled with RPUs, or coarse-grained reconfigurable architectures. Also noteworthy is the domain specialization as architecture-specific or application-specific. Not surprisingly, most compilers use a high-level sequential programming model and target commercial FPGAs, given the wide acceptance of imperative programming languages.

Tables 6.2 through 6.8 summarize various characteristics for most of the compilers described here, namely, the Transmogrifier-C [116], PRISM [21], Handel-C [235], Galadriel & Nenya [65], SPARCS [230], COBRA-ABS [99], DEFACTO [47], SPC [323], DeepC [24], C to Fine-Grained Pipeline [202], MATCH [25], CHAMPION [229], Cameron [44], NAPA-C [125], Stream-C [127], *garpcc* [60], Nimble [192], Chimaera-C [347], Abstract-Machines [287], ROCCC [137], DWARV [346], DIL [55], RaPiD-C [84], CoDe-X [34], and the XPP-VC [68].

A separation mark in each table splits the compilers targeting fine-grained architectures from those targeting coarse-grained architectures. Each table indicates, for each compiler, the most relevant information and compilation techniques (✓ symbols identify supported techniques and x symbols identify unsupported or nonapplicable techniques). Table 6.2 presents for each compiler the year of the first known scholarly publication, the location where the compiler has been implemented, the input language accepted, the granularity of the description, and the programming model used. Table 6.3 indicates for each compiler the front-end used, the data types supported, the intermediate representations used, and the level of parallelism exploited. Table 6.4 indicates for each compiler the support of loops, array variables, floating-point operations, pointers, recursive functions, and sharing of FUs.

Table 6.5 indicates for each compiler the support of bit-width narrowing, bit optimizations, the approach used when mapping the existent arrays onto the target architecture memories, the support of loop pipelining, the use of shift-registers, and packing to reduce the number of memory accesses. Table 6.6 indicates the support for array, temporal, spatial, and hardware/software partitioning. Table 6.7 indicates the representation model used for the output, the tool used to generate the hardware structure, and the tool used to generate the configuration data. Finally, Table 6.8 indicates for each compiler the target platform corresponding to published experimental results.

In addition to the compilation efforts described in this chapter, there have been continuing research efforts. The Trident C-to-FPGA compiler [311] is one of those examples. Trident has been specifically developed for mapping scientific applications described in C to FPGAs. The compiler addresses floating-point computations (both using standard and user-defined formats) and uses analyses and code transformations to identify and expose high levels of ILP and generate pipelined hardware implementations.

A number of research compilers have been adopted by companies as the basis for their internal research and development, or even in product lines. As an example, techniques used in the MATCH compiler [25, 224] were transferred to AccelChip, Inc. [3]. The early work on hardware compilation from Handel-C performed at Oxford University [235] in the second half of the 1990s ultimately led to

Table 6.2 Main characteristics of some of the considered compilers: General Information

Compiler	Year (1st pub.)	Affiliation	Input programming language	Granularity of description	Model Used
Transmogrifier-C	1995	Univ. of Toronto, Canada	C-subset	Operation	Software, imperative
PRISM-I, II	1992	Brown Univ., USA	C-subset	Operation	Software, imperative
Handel-C	1996	Oxford Univ., Celoxica, UK	Concurrency + channels + memories (C-based)	Operation	Delay, CSP model, each assignment in one cycle
Galadriel & Nenya	1998	INESC-ID, Univ. of Algarve, Portugal	Any language compiled to Java bytecodes (subset)	Operation	Software, imperative
SPARCS	1998	Univ. of Cincinnati, USA	VHDL tasks	Operation	VHDL and tasks
COBRA-ABS	1997	Univ. of Aberdeen, UK	C-like (subset)	Operation	Software, imperative
DEFACTO	1999	Univ. of South. California/Information Sciences Institute, USA	C-subset	Operation	Software, imperative
SPC	1996	Univ. Karlsruhe, Germany, London Imperial College, UK	C, Fortran: (subsets)	Operation	Software, imperative
DeepC	1999	MIT, USA	C, Fortran: (subsets)	Operation	Software, imperative
C to Fine-Grained Pipeline	2000	Univ. of Tsukuba, Japan	C-subset	Operation	Software, imperative
MATCH	1999	Northwestern Univ., USA	Matlab	Operation and/or functional blocks	Software, imperative
CHAMPION	1999	Univ. of Tennessee, USA	Khoros/Cantanta – Glyphs in fixed-point C	functional blocks (modules/glyphs)	Data-driven
Cameron	1998	Colorado State Univ., USA	SA-C	Operation	Software, functional
NAPA-C	1997	Sarnoff Corporation, USA	C-subset extended	Operation	Software, imperative added with concurrency
Stream-C	2000	Los Alamos National Laboratory, Sarnoff Corporation, Adaptive Silicon, Inc., USA	C-subset extended	Operation	Software, stream-based, processes
garpcc	1998	Univ. of California at Berkely, USA	C	Operation	Software, imperative
Nimble	2000	Synopys, USA	C	Operation	Software, imperative
Chimaera-C	2000	Northwestern University, USA	C	Operation	Software, imperative
Abstract-Machine	2001	Hewlett-Packard Laboratories, USA	C++ (subset) extended to specify Machines	Operation	Machines (process/thread) Notion of update per cycle
ROCCC	2003	University of California at Riverside, USA	C-subset	Operation	Software, imperative
DWARV	2007	Delft University of Technologies, The Netherlands	C-subset	Operation	Software, imperative
DIL	1998	Carnegie Mellon Univ., USA	DIL	Operation	Imperative with Delay annotations
RaPiD-C	1997	Univ. of Washington, USA	RaPiD-C	Operation	Specific to RaPiD, par, wait, signal, and pipeline statements
CoDe-X	1995	Univ. of Kaiserlautern, Germany	C-subset, ALE-X	Operation	Software, imperative
XPP-VC	2002	PACT XPP Technologies, Inc., Munich, Germany	C-subset (extended)	Operation	Software, imperative

Table 6.3 Main characteristics of some of the considered compilers (cont.): Front-End Analysis

Compiler	High-level mapping to hardware	Front-end	Data types	Intermediate representations	Parallelism
Transmogrifier-C	Integrated	Custom	Bit-level	AST	Operation
PRISM-I, II	Integrated	Lcc	Primitive	Operator Network (DFG)	Operation
Handel-C	Integrated	Custom	Bit-Level	AST ?	Operation
Galadriel & Nenya	Integrated	Custom: GALADRIEL	Primitive	HPDG + global DFG	Operation, inter basic block, inter-loop
SPARCS	Integrated HLS	Custom	Bit-level	USM	Operation, task-level
COBRA-ABS	Integrated HLS	Custom?	?	?	Operation
DEFACTO	Commercial HLS	SUIF	Primitive	AST	Operation
SPC	Integrated	SUIF	Primitive	DFG	Operation
DeepC	Commercial RTL synthesis	SUIF	Primitive	SSA	Operation
C to Fine-Grained Pipeline	Integrated	Custom	Primitive	DDGs (data dependence graphs)	Operation
MATCH	Commercial RTL synthesis	Custom	Primitive	AST, DFG for pipelining	Operation
CHAMPION	Commercial C-to-VHDL compiler + LS	Custom	Primitive, fixed-point	SFG (signal flow graph)	Functional (Glyphs/modules)
Cameron	Commercial LS	Custom	Bit-Level	Hierarchical DDCF (Data Dependence and Control Flow) + DFG + AHA graph	Operation
NAPA-C	Integrated	SUIF	Pragmas (bit-level)	AST	Operation
Stream-C	Integrated	SUIF	Pragmas (bit-level)	AST	Operation
garpcc	Integrated	SUIF	Primitive	Hyperblock + DFG	Operation, inter basic blocks
Nimble	Integrated	SUIF	Primitive	Hyperblock + DFGs	Operation, inter basic blocks
Chimaera-C	Integrated	GCC	Primitive	DFG	Operation
Abstract-Machines	Integrated	Custom	Bit-level	Hypergraph + DFG	Operation, machines
ROCCC	Integrated	SUIF2	Primitive	CIRRF	Operation
DWARV	Integrated	SUIF2	Primitive	SUIF2 IR + HDFG	Operation
DIL	Integrated	Custom	Bit-level (fixed-point)	Hierarchical and acyclic DFG	Operation
RaPiD-C	Integrated	Custom	Primitive + pipe + RAM	Control Trees	Functional, operation
CoDe-X	Integrated	Custom	Primitive	DAG	Operation, loops
XPP-VC	Integrated	SUIF	Primitive	HTG+, CDFG	Operation, inter basic block, inter-loop

the creation of Celoxica Ltd. [75]. The research work on the Streams-C hardware compiler [127] was licensed by Impulse Accelerated Technologies, Inc. [160, 243], and the work on the *garpcc* compiler [60] was used by Synopsys in the Nimble compiler [192].

Table 6.4 Main characteristics of some of the considered compilers (cont.): Supported Features

Compiler	Loops	Array variables	Floating-point operations	Pointers	Recursive functions	Sharing of functional units (FUs)
Transmogrifier-C	✓	×	×	×	×	×
PRISM-I, II	✓	×	×	×	×	×
Handel-C	✓	×	×	×	×	×
Galadriel & Nenya	✓	✓	×	×	×	(only on distinct conditional paths)
SPARCS	✓	✓	×	×	×	✓
COBRA-ABS	✓	✓	×	×	×	✓
DEFACTO	✓	✓	×	×	×	✓
SPC	✓ (inner)	✓	×	×	×	×
DeepC	✓	✓	✓	✓	×	✓
C to Fine-Grained Pipeline	✓	✓	×	×	limited	×
MATCH	✓	✓	Converted to fixed-point	×	×	×
CHAMPION	✓	✓	×	×	×	×
Cameron	✓	✓	×	×	×	×
NAPA-C	✓	✓	×	×	×	✓
Stream-C	✓	✓	×	×	×	✓
garpcc	✓ (inner)	✓	Software	✓	Software	×
Nimble	✓	✓	Software	Software	Software	×
Chimaera-C	×	×	Software	Software	software	×
Abstract-Machine	× (unrollable)	✓	×	×	×	✓
ROCCC	✓	✓	×	×	×	×
DWARV	✓	✓	On-going	✓	×	×
DIL	× (unrollable)	× (arrays are used to specify interconnections)	×	×	×	×
RaPiD-C	✓	✓ (used to access I/O data)	×	×	×	✓
CoDe-X	✓	✓	×	×	×	×
XPP-VC	✓	✓	×	×	×	×

Table 6.5 Main characteristics of some of the considered compilers (cont.): Optimizations

Compiler	Bit-width narrowing	Bit-optimizations	Arrays-to-multiple-memories mapping	Loop pipelining	Memory accesses reduction by shift-Register	Memory accesses reduction by packing
Transmogrifier-C	×	✓	×	×	×	×
PRISM-I, II	×	✓	×	×	×	×
Handel-C	×	×	Explicit use of memories	Manual	Manual	Manual
Galadriel & Nenya	✓	✓	(exhaustive or manual)	×	×	×
SPARCS	×	✓	✓	?	?	×
COBRA-ABS	×	×	×	?	?	×
DEFACTO	×	×	×	✓	✓	✓
SPC	×	×	✓ (ILP)	✓	✓	×
DeepC	✓	×	✓	×	×	×
C to Fine-Grained Pipeline	×	×	×	✓	×	×
MATCH	✓	✓	×	✓	×	✓
CHAMPION	×	✓	×	×	×	×
Cameron	×	×	×	✓	✓	×
NAPA-C	×	×	✓ (implicit enumeration)	✓	×	×
Stream-C	×	×	✓ (implicit enumeration)	✓	×	×
garpcc	×	×	×	✓	×	× (queues are used to grap a cache line at a time)
Nimble	×	×	×	✓	×	×
Chimaera-C	×	×	×	×	×	×
Abstract-Machine	✓	✓	×	✓	×	×
ROCCC	×	×	?	?	✓	?
DWARV	×	×	Relies on RAM inference of the synthesis tools for the local arrays	×	×	×
DIL	✓	✓	×	✓	×	×
RaPiD-C	×	×	Explicit use of memories	✓	×	×
CoDe-X	×	×	×	✓	×	✓
XPP-VC	×	×	✓ (one array per internal memory)	✓	✓	×

Table 6.6 Main characteristics of some of the considered compilers (cont.): Forms of Partitioning

Compiler	Array partitioning	Temporal partitioning	Spatial partitioning	Hardware/software partitioning
Transmogrifier-C	×	×	×	×
PRISM-I, II	×	×	×	×
Handel-C	×	×	×	×
Galadriel & Nenya	×	✓	×	×
SPARCS	×	✓	✓	×
COBRA-ABS	×	×	✓	×
DEFACTO	×	×	×	✓
SPC	×	×	×	×
DeepC	✓	×	×	×
C to Fine-Grained Pipeline	×	×	×	×
MATCH	×	×	✓	✓
CHAMPION	×	✓	✓	×
Cameron	×	×	×	×
NAPA-C	×	×	×	× (annotations)
Stream-C	×	×	×	×
garpcc	×	×	×	✓
Nimble	×	×	×	✓
Chimaera-C	×	×	×	✓
Abstract-Machine	×	×	×	×
ROCCC	×	×	×	×
DWARV	×	×	×	×
DIL	×	× (the architecture is automatically virtualized)	×	×
RaPiD-C	×	×	×	×
CoDe-X	×	×	×	✓
XPP-VC	×	✓ (includes loop dissevering)	×	×

Table 6.7 Main characteristics of some of the considered compilers (cont.): Back-End Support

Compiler	Output of the compiler: (1) : RTL-HDL (2) : algorithmic-HDL (3) : bit–streams	Generation of the hardware structure: VLS: Vendor Logic Synthesis CG: Circuit Generators OO: one-to-one mapping	Back-end (bit–stream generation): CPR: commercial place and route tools
Transmogrifier-C	?	CG	CPR
PRISM-I, II	?	CG	CPR
Handel-C	(1)	CG	CPR
Galadriel & Nenya	(1)	Data-path: CG Control unit: VLS	CPR
SPARCS	(1)	VLS	CPR
COBRA-ABS	(1)	VLS	CPR
DEFACTO	(2)	VLS	CPR
SPC	(1)	CG	CPR
DeepC	(1)	VLS	CPR
C to Fine-Grained Pipeline	(1)	VLS	CPR
MATCH	(1)	VLS	CPR
CHAMPION	(1)	VLS	CPR
Cameron	(1)	VLS	CPR
NAPA-C	(1)	CG	CPR
Stream-C	(1)	CG	CPR
garpcc	(3)	CG	Proprietary: Gama
Nimble	(1)	CG	CPR
Chimaera-C	?	Manually ?	-
Abstact-Machine	(3)	CG	Proprietary + Jbits
ROCCC	(1)	VLS	CPR
DWARV	(1)	VLS	CPR
DIL	(3)	CG	Proprietary
RaPiD-C	(3)	OO	Proprietary
CoDe-X	(3)	OO	Proprietary
XPP-VC	(3)	OO	Proprietary: xmap

Table 6.8 Main characteristics of considered compilers (cont.): Target Platform

Compiler	Target platform
Transmogrifier-C	1 FPGA
PRISM-I, II	1 FPGA
Handel-C	1 FPGA
Galadriel & Nenya	1 FPGA connected to multiple memories
SPARCS	Multi-FPGA, Multiple Memories
COBRA-ABS	1 global memory bus-connected with multiple FPGAs (Motorola MPA-1000): each one with 1 local memory or custom/ASIC arithmetic resource
DEFACTO	Multi-FPGA, multiple memories
SPC	1 FPGA connected to multiple memories ?
DeepC	A mesh of tiles each one with 1 FPGA connected to 1 memory
C to Fine-Grained Pipeline	1 FPGA connected to multiple memories
MATCH	Multi-FPGAs, each one connected to one memory
CHAMPION	Multi-FPGAs, each one with local memory
Cameron	1 FPGA connected to multiple memories
NAPA-C	1 FPGA connected to multiple memories
Stream-C	1 FPGA connected to multiple memories
Garpcc	μP (Garp) connected to a proprietary RPU
Nimble-C	Garp, ACE2 Card (a uSPARC CPU and Xilinx 4085 FPGAs), ACEV (ACE Card and a Xilinx XCV 1000 FPGA)
Chimaera-C	μP (SimpleScalar) connected to an RFU
Abstract-Machine	1 FPGA connected to memories
ROCCC	1 FPGA
DWARV	1 FPGA
DIL	PipeRench RPU
RaPiD-C	RaPiD RPU
CoDe-X	Multi-KressArrays connected to a host system
XPP-VC	1 XPP connect to memories

Chapter 7
Perspectives on Programming Reconfigurable Computing Platforms

Despite tremendous progress in the development and integration of compilation and synthesis techniques, the challenging nature of the compilation and synthesis for reconfigurable architectures has defied the establishment of a de facto standard methodology. In this chapter, we begin by providing an overall perspective of what we believe is missing to make reconfigurable computing an ever increasing reality. We then outline several outstanding issues suggesting a set of research directions in compilation techniques for these architectures. In this context, we have focused on compilation techniques and have deliberately omitted system-level aspects of reconfigurable architectures such as dynamic reconfiguration and operating system-level services. We then describe a vision, albeit speculative, of a compilation flow augmented by the synergetic integration of language description and transformation specification techniques as well as the notion of resource virtualization. Finally, we discuss how reconfigurable technologies can play an important role in future VLSI devices where unreliability is an important issue [57, 130]. In this context, we highlight how compilation techniques for reconfigurable architectures can also play a role in emerging nanotechnology systems.

7.1 How to Make Reconfigurable Computing a Reality?

The last 15 years have witnessed a great enthusiasm for reconfigurable computing as a new and broad computing paradigm with great computational flexibility and performance potential [83,90,122]. Despite many research efforts, first in academia and more recently in industry, reconfigurable computing has not been widely adopted as the dominant computing paradigm. We believe there are several key factors that contribute to this, as addressed in the next sections.

J.M.P. Cardoso, P.C. Diniz, *Compilation Techniques for Reconfigurable Architectures*,
DOI 10.1007/978-0-387-09671-1_7,

7.1.1 Easy of Programming

To make reconfigurable computing approachable to the average programmer, programming tools must offer a set of high-level programming abstractions programmers can easily grasp, and execution models they can easily reason about. As with early compilers for traditional architectures, compilers for reconfigurable architectures must hide the complexity of the low-level programming details while exploiting a wide range of mapping choices in the pursuit of effective computing solutions.

In this context, researchers have proposed various high-level programming language approaches. While imperative languages such as MATLAB offer the clear benefits of sequential semantics, uncovering the underlying concurrency is an extremely complex problem. Some approaches relaxed the sequential semantics of some of its constructs to facilitate the extraction of concurrency from a sequential program (e.g., SA-C [44]), while other efforts have focused on explicitly concurrent languages inspired by the CSP programming model that better matches the spatial nature of reconfigurable architectures [127].

While there is no obvious path that offers the best of both worlds, we envision three main, and possibly complementary, approaches that can ameliorate the programming challenges for reconfigurable architectures, namely:

- Augmenting Imperative Languages: In this approach, programmers would use concepts based on aspect-oriented programming [109, 174] to augment an application where information compilers are (currently) unable to derive. For example, aspects can allow the programmer to specify execution modes for specific regions of the code, to indicate data properties such as streaming data rates from input devices, or to add complementary information about an algorithm, not present in the programming model used. The programmer would retain the benefits of an imperative programming language while relying on the richness of aspects to aid the compiler in the mapping of the application to the underlying architecture.
- Transactional-Based Languages: In this approach the language allows the programmer to explicitly define regions of the code that execute sequentially, *transactions* [198], but whose execution order can be arbitrary, provided they execute atomically. Transactions offer a programming model that is concurrent in nature, but isolate the programmer from having to explicitly manage concurrency and data orchestration throughout the execution [247, 336]. In combination with emerging productivity-oriented parallel programming languages (e.g., X10 [77]) that provide mechanisms for high-level synchronization and assignment of data to locus of computations, these approaches might represent promising avenues for programming reconfigurable architectures.
- Domain-Specific Languages: In this, nongeneric programming approach, the language would include domain-specific constructs and/or knowledge about the specific target architecture (such as with the DIL [55] and the RaPiD-C [84] languages). Features such as the partitioning among hardware resources with

different execution models, and the direct indication of which computation to assign to which kind of resources, would help the compiler in its mapping. The use of a programming language with a limited scope would allow programmers to better understand the impact of compiler mapping techniques and code transformations.

While there is no obvious single generic programming solution, the approaches outlined above could coexist synergetically. The ability to exploit architecture-specific aspects in a language with transactional-based abstractions would allow compilers to exploit the knowledge about the underlying architecture. The compiler would select which of the aspects were relevant to the specific architecture at hand and ignore others that describe features of the computations, or of the architecture, that are either nonapplicable or lead to clearly unprofitable implementations.

It is even possible to envision the concept of virtual abstract machines whereby an external mechanism, the programmer targets a set of abstract machines with distinct instruction-set architectures (ISA), execution models, and configuration parameters. In addition to the virtual machine description that would reflect the underlying architecture, a separate programming mechanism would define an execution model, exposing notions akin to tasks, processes, or transactions. The programmer would still define an application in terms of these computing abstractions, relying on the compiler to map them to a concrete abstract machine that better matches, or facilitates, the mapping to the specific reconfigurable architecture.

7.1.2 Program Portability and Legacy Code Migration

This is a very important economic issue given the huge industry investment in their code basis and is very likely the key to enable reconfigurable computing to become mainstream. While a disruptive programming evolution approach would likely be the most expeditious process for the emergence of a common programming language, the economics of such an approach makes this scenario extremely unlikely. Furthermore, the variety of programming approaches proposed in recent years reinforces the difficulty of a consensus ever being reached.

An incremental, nondisruptive approach is likely to be the only economically feasible option. In this context, it is possible to envision a series of evolution stages relying on the techniques described in the previous section.

In a first stage, programmers would augment their C-based application codes with specific algorithm-related and target architecture-related aspects. This would allow them to immediately rip the benefits of reconfigurable architectures while retaining the integrity of their codes. Specific code patterns could be recognized and implemented as domain-specific *softcores* creating an intermediate layer between the program and the fine-grained structures of some reconfigurable fabrics.

In a second stage, selected portions of the application would be translated to either domain-specific languages and/or use transaction-based techniques to improve the performance of specific subcomputations. This translation effort would be related to the desired increase in application performance. Still, in this scenario, the programmer would retain an application code that could be easily translated to a sequential programming language.

7.1.3 Performance Portability

The diversity of architectures, reconfigurable devices can emulate, leads to a wide variety of possible implementations for the same functionality, and hence many mapping and scheduling decisions. Some of these decisions are fairly sensitive to variations of the underlying architecture, in particular for coarse-grained reconfigurable architectures. For example, the use of a long interconnection in an ALU-based reconfigurable architecture might imply the use of additional clock cycles and data buffering along the routing path. The variety of an application implementation scenarios makes it very hard for a compiler to establish a very robust performance basis. The potential heterogeneity of RPUs and the porting of specific mapping and scheduling strategies to an architecture with distinct underlying mechanisms further exacerbate this issue.

We can envision two basic approaches that can address this problem of performance portability. A first and less satisfactory approach would rely on the compiler to be conservative in its mapping and scheduling phases, not pushing to the limit the device capacities.[1] The spare device capacity would allow compilers to make mapping decisions that would be less sensitive to device features. When moving to a new architecture with similar features, the compiler could reuse the same application mapping decision and rely on a low-level emulation of device features to effectively recast the computation on the new architecture.

A second more satisfying approach would leverage the notion of resource virtualization. Here, the compiler could rely on the notion of emulation of abstract machines, possibly, with specific execution and control models, to facilitate the mapping, and more importantly the portability, of applications across architectures. For a selected combination of execution models and architectures, some of these abstract models could be supported natively by the underlying architecture, thus exploiting the architecture's full potential. When these abstract models could not be directly supported, the compiler would attempt to recast them to other directly supported abstract models.

[1] With the increase in device capacity, device occupancy is bound to be an increasingly less important concern, as occurred in the 1990s with traditional processors with respect to the quality of compiled code.

7.2 Research Directions in Compilation for Reconfigurable Architectures

We now outline several open issues for compilers for reconfigurable architectures that naturally reflect the broad issues discussed in the previous section. In this description, we focus on aspects related to the compilation process and less on the overall concepts of program and performance portability.

7.2.1 Programming Language Design

Most approaches on compilation to reconfigurable architectures have addressed imperative programming languages (e.g., [44, 125, 323]), possibly augmented with *annotations* or *pragmas*, due to their wide acceptance, and consequently their large codes basis in generic and embedded computing domains. Given the many challenges this approach imposes, many researchers have advocated the use of alternative programming models. For instance, there have been substantial research efforts on hardware compilation for declarative languages (e.g., Ruby [197]), and functional languages (e.g., Lava [42], SAFL [278]) as well as on hardware compilation of synchronous programming languages such as Esterel (e.g., [102]). Although significant, these efforts have been limited by the confined acceptance and adoption of these languages.

Domain-specific languages can also play an important role in mitigating some of the complexity issues plaguing the compilation for reconfigurable architectures. Given their focus, domain-specific languages could allow programmers and/or library designers to describe a wide range of programmable hardware resources, possibly exposing the programmer to the issues of unreliability and alternative implementations. These features, possible beyond the reach of the average programmer, would allow the compiler to internally explore alternative architectures and run-time adaptive strategies, thus promoting the generation of flexible hardware solutions.

7.2.2 Intermediate Representation

A common goal of an intermediate representation is to explicitly represent the concurrency in the input computation to match the available parallelism in the target reconfigurable architecture. The common approach has consisted in augmenting an existing compilation infrastructure, such as the popular SUIF compilation framework [325], with a graph-based representation derived by the knowledge gained from analysis of the input program. Furthermore, a robust front-end in the framework can easily accommodate other programming languages, with the added benefit of allowing a simple migration path for the components of the application that are mapped in a reconfigurable computing system to traditional processors.

As a result of the many cost benefits of using an existing framework, there has been very little research in this area. A novel intermediate representation is usually tied to a new programming language, where the semantic gap between the language and the internal representation is not wide. The easiest development path for an intermediate representation with explicit concurrency seems to be the development of a concurrent programming language. Although many such languages exist, none has emerged as the dominant paradigm that offers substantial benefits over the approach of automatic derivation of concurrency from imperative high-level programming languages.

7.2.3 Mapping to Multiple Computing Engines

The mapping of computations to multiple computing engines is becoming an increasingly important issue. While this mapping can be viewed as a generalization of the hardware/software partitioning problem found in today's reconfigurable platforms, the complexity of the problem is compounded in the presence of multiple, and possibly, heterogeneous architecture components. These multiple components may include general-purpose processors (GPPs), application-specific instruction-set processors (ASIPs), heterogeneous hardware templates (possibly different coarse-grained reconfigurable arrays). These components might be hardwired or even implemented as *soft-macros* defined over fine-grained reconfigurable units.

Although hardware/software partitioning has been extensively researched in the context of hardware/software codesign [213], in that domain the hardware components of the architecture have mostly been considered nonprogrammable and thus also nonreconfigurable. Techniques developed in this context can, nevertheless, be adapted for mapping computations to multiple computing engines in reconfigurable architectures.

To effectively address the complexity of the problem of partitioning and mapping of computations to reconfigurable architectures, tools will undoubtedly have to rely on accurate resource and execution time modeling/estimation techniques [242] with which they can quickly assess a key issue in partitioning: profitability. In addition, researchers will have to develop generalized spatial and temporal partitioning algorithms capable of coping with the ability of the reconfigurable resources to implement, in a time-multiplexed fashion, diverse hardware templates throughout the execution of the application.

7.2.4 Code Transformations

Low-level and instruction-level transformations have been intensively explored in hardware high-level synthesis (see, e.g., [210]). Transformations for high-level constructs, in particular functions and loops, however, have only recently been addressed (see, e.g., [139]).

Existing efforts on compilation to hardware have leveraged the encapsulation provided by functions to effectively define, in many instances, the scope of the mapping process. Support for recursive functions is nevertheless commonly ignored. This is particularly important in the context of functional descriptions where algorithmic solutions, naturally, have recursive formulations. A subset of recursive functions known as tail-recursive functions[2] can be easily transformed to iterative formulations. Other more general recursive functions still require new code transformation and implementation techniques to be efficiently implemented in reconfigurable architectures.

Loop constructs have also provided a fruitful domain for code transformations, in particular `for` loop constructs with compile-time known bounds that manipulate array variables using affine index functions [186]. These constructs exhibit very regular behavior for which a wealth of transformations and analyses from the arena of parallelizing compilation can be applied [12]. As described in Chap. 4, however, the application of these transformations, when targeting reconfigurable architectures, is far from trivial. Their indiscriminate application can quickly lead to a shortage of hardware resources and thus infeasible implementations. In this context it is thus important to develop high-level models of the application of transformations, possibly combined with estimation, to effectively predict the characteristics of the corresponding hardware implementations.

7.2.5 Design-Space Exploration and Compilation Time

To be practical, compilers for reconfigurable computing architectures need to provide programmers with feasible compilation times, possibly comparable to compilation times experienced when targeting traditional architectures. This is a challenge, as compilers for reconfigurable architectures require substantially more sophisticated mapping and transformations processes, in particular during its optimization and back-end phases.

Of particular significance is the complexity raised by the diversity of architecture characteristics and the large number of mapping and transformation choices, leading to huge implementation spaces [2]. Exploring these spaces and generating an implementation for each possible design-space point are clearly infeasible, typically leaving designers with two very unsatisfying options: either wait for an exploration of several design points which leads to a global extremely long compilation and synthesis time, possibly days or weeks or settle for a suboptimal or even low-performing design.

Three key techniques have been pursued to ameliorate or mitigate the design-space exploration issues compilers face for reconfigurable architectures. These techniques focus on the most demanding phases of a compilation and synthesis flow,

[2] In tail-recursive functions, the recursive call is the last operation of the function, i.e., there are no pending operations at each recursive call.

respectively, the selection of which mapping and code transformations to apply and the actual generation of the bit-streams to configure the target architecture:

- **Estimation:** The use of estimation and modeling [180,290] has been shown to be a very effective technique to reduce design exploration time. A key issue for this promising approach, however, and in particular for fine-grained reconfigurable architectures, is the ability of deriving accurate estimates [43,49,180] in feasible time, while still allowing the compiler to make correct mapping decisions.
- **Module Generation:** The use of module generators integrated with the DFG (data-flow graph) representing the overall program enables the specialization of each module instance without incurring in long code generation times. The use of preplaced and prerouted soft-macros is a key technique in this setting. The key issue, in particular for coarse-grained reconfigurable architectures, lies in the ability not to excessively fragment the overall hardware implementation. In addition, module generators can also interact synergetically with estimation models for providing accurate estimates for the various parameter settings they are designed for.
- **Placement and Routing:** Compared to traditional placement approaches commonly based on simulated annealing [266], strategies based on faster algorithms, such as force-directed approaches [219] or approaches combining clustering and hierarchical simulated annealing [269], have yielded very short execution times with acceptable results. The development of alternative placement and routing algorithms, possibly customized for specific architectures, is a very desirable and promising approach that must be validated for arbitrary input computations in terms of mapping time and quality of the resulting mapping.

Although some preliminary evidence exists to suggest that these approaches are very effective in reducing the compilation and synthesis time for reconfigurable architectures (see, e.g., estimation [288]), they need to be generalized in the presence of changing application requirements and evolving architecture characteristics.

7.2.6 Pipelined Execution

Pipelining is an extremely effective execution technique when mapping loop constructs to reconfigurable architectures. Common loop pipelining schemes rely exclusively on static scheduling knowledge to derive the definition of the pipeline stages. They often assume specific latencies for PEs or FUs that compose their stages thus leading to suboptimal implementations.

In practice the application of loop pipelining techniques is limited to normalized, well-behaved loops with statically determined loop carried dependences. Aggressive loop pipelining techniques are required to deal with a wider spectrum of loops, possibly using dynamic analyses and data-dependence analyses techniques, so that compilers are not unnecessarily constrained in the mapping to the reconfigurable architectures of many real-life applications.

While there has been plenty of techniques developed for loop pipelining, these efforts have mostly focused on the pipelining of innermost loops in a nest. Exploiting coarse-grained forms of pipelining (e.g., at task level) [263,353] at an outer most loop level [46] has only recently been addressed and the combination of both forms of pipelining for more general computation cases is still an open area of research.

7.2.7 Memory Mapping Optimizations

The diversity and the number of distributed memory resources in advanced reconfigurable architectures create an exceedingly complex data partitioning, mapping, and management problem. As with traditional architectures, the local registers (usually in a very limited number) have extremely low access time and off-chip memory with much higher capacity. Internal memories represent a compromise between access time and capacity, but need to be managed explicitly. This problem is exacerbated by the possibility of memory customization and nonuniformity of data access time even within the same storage category. This is for example the case when mapping data to block RAMs in FPGAs which can be located fairly close to an FU or fairly distant, thus possibly requiring additional clock cycles to access.

A key to address the complexity of this mapping and management problem lies, very likely, on the development of sophisticated algorithms (e.g., [27]) that can cope with the diversity of the target storage structures. As with the application of other transformations, modeling and estimation of data access times for each mapping/allocation should guide the search to quickly find an efficient memory structure design and corresponding data mapping process.

7.2.8 Application-Specific Compilers and Cores

Specific applications and domains can clearly justify the development of compilers with powerful optimizations that explore specific domain knowledge or specific target architecture characteristics. For example, instances of particular digital filters (e.g., Finite Impulse Response filters) with particular coefficient values can be efficiently mapped to reconfigurable architectures with very specific mapping and transformation algorithms. This approach can also be complemented by the inclusion in the target architectures of application-specific cores, organized as *softcores* or hard-macros, possibly defining an architectural layer with parameterized libraries of cores or building blocks.

These domain/architecture-specific compilers will very likely include simplified variants of the steps of the compilation and synthesis flows described in Chap. 3. Still, and given the many design choices, they will undoubtedly have to internally engage in a selected form of design-space exploration to generate optimized reconfigurable computing implementations. A very desirable goal in the construction of such domain-specific compilation tools is the development of compiler design methodologies that would allow compiler designers to build, and more importantly maintain and adapt, the compilation flows to evolving target reconfigurable architectures.

7.2.9 Resource Virtualization

Resource and execution model virtualization are elegant ways to deal with the diversity and the limitations of hardware resources in reconfigurable architectures. Virtualization, albeit at a possible loss of peak performance, can provide the key to application and programmer portability.

Using virtualization, a programmer, or a library designer, would define abstract virtual machines and virtual resources whereby a model of execution, or abstract resource operations, is specified through primitive data movement and execution operations. Basic pipelining, VLIW, parallel execution, and synchronization would be specified at an abstract level and mapped to specific execution models, supported by the underlying architecture, using an intermediate mapping tool. The closer these abstract operations are to the modes and the instruction natively supported by the architecture, the more efficient the final hardware implementation is.

7.2.10 Dynamic and Incremental Compilation

Current compilation flows are too rigid as programmers must endure long compilation cycles, for the definition of a suitable reconfigurable computing implementation. A possible avenue for mitigating the issues related to long compilation cycles would include the use of dynamic Just-In-Time (JIT) and incremental compilation techniques. A first, quick translation to possible not very efficient mappings, using only the regions of the input code exercised, would allow the execution to proceed as quickly as possible. As the execution would progress, a run-time system would trigger a recompilation of the more frequently exercised structures for recompilation, this time with the benefit of the knowledge of key specific program values. A similar approach was explored by Schmit et al. [274] for dynamic translation to hardware of traditional binary instructions. Additionally, JIT compilation can be an enabling technology to allow portability among different reconfigurable computing platforms.

While appealing, this notion of JIT compilation and incremental refinement of an implementation presents its challenges. For instance, if placement and routing is already complex as an off-line process, using a dynamic approach seems a daunting prospect. While the abundance of hardware resources in current target architectures (in particular for fine-grained architectures) might not make the loss of device occupancy an issue, the loss of performance of the resulting designs might be a concern.

7.3 Tackling the Compilation Challenge for Reconfigurable Architectures

We now outline a conceptual compilation flow that aims at mitigating many of the issues arising when compiling high-level programming languages to reconfigurable architectures. The proposed flow, depicted in Fig. 7.1, would augment, in a synergetical way, a traditional compilation flow with three key techniques, namely, Aspect-Oriented programming [103, 174], History-based and Learning-based techniques, and Resource Virtualization techniques. In addition, the flow would rely on an intermediate domain-specific language, LARA, a LAnguage for

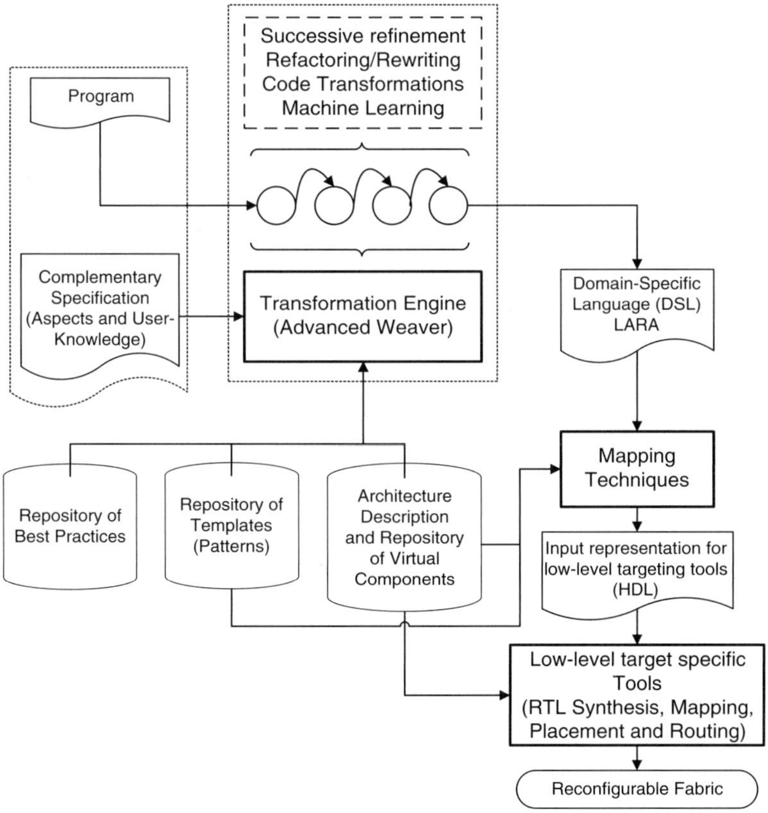

Fig. 7.1 Envisioned compilation flow

Reconfigurable Architectures, and the corresponding transformation engine to leverage the information provided by the other techniques to explore a wide range of reconfigurable computing implementations.

As input to this hypothetical flow is an application code, specified using a traditional imperative programming language, augmented with complementary aspect specifications using Aspect-Oriented programming techniques, aspects would allow programmers to expose domain-specific or algorithm-specific knowledge to the compiler nonintrusively and without compromising the semantics of the original specification. Aspects may ensure the application specifications last longer than its current implementations by not obscuring their description with details used in today's architectures, which might be obsolete in tomorrow's architectures.

The knowledge conveyed by the aspects specification, such as data rate and timing, absent in the input source languages, would be used by the compiler and the architectural synthesis tools towards the implementation of highly specialized implementations. Aspects would also provide a handle into an extremely important and often neglected issue when compiling to reconfigurable architectures: test generation and verification.

The middle-end of the flow includes the core of the transformation engine responsible for the derivation of the overall hardware implementation. The transformation engine would map the input program description to a set of virtual hardware resources and virtual execution modes in the search for a design that is both feasible and meets the input performance specifications. The compiler would match the input program to the target virtual resources by using a set of transformations techniques, such as successive refinement, refactoring and term-rewriting, guided by learning-based techniques using history-based and best-practices knowledge. By understanding which sets of transformations and corresponding parameters lead to the best designs for codes with specific input aspects, these repositories will substantially reduce the size of the design-search-space the compiler would need to cover in the pursuit of efficient, and correct, designs.

These knowledge repositories can be built either with the help of designers for specific hardware/software virtual resource patterns or using machine-learning pattern extraction and pattern matching techniques [6, 74]. For a new architecture or a new set of resource patterns, the approach might be slow in deriving good designs and thus populating the space of best practices. With time, and with the use on many additional codes, the system would use the knowledge of previous design mappings and deliver designs increasingly faster and of increasingly higher quality.

Once the middle-end derives a feasible design, the back-end of the flow would generate a hardware implementation description by translating the selected virtual resources into architecture specific data-path and control structures. The flow would generate this target architecture description using a domain-specific mapping language, LARA, which is envisaged to include explicit elements for reconfiguration and hardware-oriented directives such as data mapping and streaming information. Lastly, the flow would translate this hardware specification into behavioral RTL-HDL using either parameterized hardware patterns or programmable hardware templates for increased efficiency.

7.4 Reconfigurable Architectures and Nanotechnology

Emerging computational substrates as is the case with nanostructures [262] share several characteristics with today's and future silicon-based reconfigurable devices.

First, and like fine-grained reconfigurable architectures, nanoscale computing systems are spatially organized at the architecture level with diverse mechanisms for creating, processing, and preserving state. The notion of state might, however, be distributed in space and time. Second, and unlike today's reconfigurable devices, nanostructures are inherently unreliable [93, 262]. As a result, the prevailing computing paradigm must explore postfabrication defect avoidance techniques, computation and data replication, to attain high levels of assurance.

The unreliability of nanostructures makes the establishment of a well-accepted execution model and programming paradigm for nanostructures even more problematic than for reconfigurable architectures. Nevertheless, reconfiguration and the abundance of resources in nanostructures might prove to be effective techniques to cope with this unreliability.

As with reconfigurable technologies, the key for nanotechnologies to make it as a mainstream computing paradigm lies in their ability to support a well-established programming paradigm. This is a major challenge for which the development of programming languages and compilation techniques for reconfigurable architectures will, we believe, play a key role.

7.5 Summary

In this chapter we have provided a perspective on programming reconfigurable computing platforms and what we believe are the key major issues to make this promising computing paradigm a reality. In this context, we have outlined the most relevant and challenging topics related to compilation to these architectures. We described a vision for a compilation system that aims at mitigating many of the problems that plague today's compilation approaches. This vision relies on several techniques already shown to be effective in other domains, but which have not yet been combined in the context of compiling to reconfigurable architectures. Lastly, we have briefly highlighted the similarities between current reconfigurable computing devices and emerging nanoscale computing systems, pointing out that the techniques currently developed for reconfigurable computing might prove to be a key enabling factor for these technologies.

Chapter 8
Final Remarks

Despite the tremendous progress made over the last decade, efficient automatic compilation from high-level programming languages to reconfigurable architectures, widely believed to be the key to make this promising technology the dominant computing paradigm, still remains an elusive goal.

Several aspects of the compilation process conspire to this effect. First, and foremost, compiler must bridge a widening semantic gap between the high-level imperative programming languages pervasive in existing software basis and the hardware-oriented programming languages required to define the underlying computing architecture. Second, the lack of an accepted high-level programming paradigm, particularly suited for reconfigurable architectures, further exacerbates the complexity of the compilation process. This fact hampers the establishment of a stable, widely available compilation framework, as well as the definition of benchmark codes for qualitative and quantitative compiler and architecture performance analysis. Third, to reach acceptable performance, compilers must apply a plethora of code transformations and mapping techniques at the software and hardware levels. These transformation and mapping processes are extremely bridle as transformations often interfere, forcing the compiler to explore a wide range of transformation combinations and to negotiate a trade-off between compilation time and the quality of final hardware implementations. Lastly, compilers may have to include hardware synthesis steps in their flows, often by the integration of commercial synthesis tools. Despite the maturity of the techniques used by these tools, the inherent algorithmic complexity of synthesis-related steps leads to extremely long, and unacceptable, compilation times for the average programmer. The relentless increase in device capacity and the rapid evolution of reconfigurable architectures further exacerbate this problem.

These compilation challenges are, we believe, not insurmountable, prompting many research opportunities for the development of alternative compilation techniques at various levels. Two areas are of particular interest. The first area includes the definition of newer high-level programming languages and translation approaches from binary code directly to reconfigurable hardware, thus promoting programmer and program portability. The second area includes the modeling of the

J.M.P. Cardoso, P.C. Diniz, *Compilation Techniques for Reconfigurable Architectures*,
DOI 10.1007/978-0-387-09671-1_8,

impact of code transformations and mapping techniques on resources and execution time. This modeling, when coupled with history-based and/or learning techniques, will lead to the reduction of compilation and synthesis times. This reduction, in turn, will ultimately allow compilers to explore a wide range of design choices in the search for efficient reconfigurable computing implementations, thereby promoting performance portability.

Compilation for reconfigurable architectures will very likely also play an important role in emerging computational paradigms. This is the case with nanoscale computing, where high defect rates of nanostructures may require these architectures to strongly rely on cell replication and cell reconfiguration. In addition to low-level programming abstractions that capture and cope with the unreliability of such computing environments, compilers will be instrumental in isolating the programmer from the peculiar low-level characteristics of these architectures, while offering a familiar stable computing paradigm.

We believe compilation techniques for reconfigurable computing platforms offer many exciting research and development opportunities. We hope this book, to our knowledge the first book completely dedicated to the topic of compilation for reconfigurable architectures, will motivate further research efforts in this domain and serve as a base for a deeper understanding of the overall compilation and synthesis problems, current solutions, and open issues.

References

1. Aamodt, T., Chow, P.: Embedded ISA Support for Enhanced Floating-Point to Fixed-Point ANSI-C Compilation. In: Proc. of the 2000 Intl. Conf. on Compilers, Architecture, and Synthesis for Embedded Systems (CASES'00), pp. 128–137. ACM Press, New York, NY, USA (2000)
2. Abraham, S., Rau, B., Schreiber, R.: Fast Design Space Exploration Through Validity and Quality Filtering of Subsystem Designs. Tech. Rep. HPL-2000/98. Hewlett-Packard Corp., Palo Alto, CA, USA (2000)
3. AccelChip, Inc.: URL http://www.accelchip.com
4. ACE, Corp.: DSP-C Specification (2001). URL http://www.dsp-c.org
5. Actel, Corp.: Reconfigurable Programmable Interconnect Architecture. US Patent 5,187,393 (1969)
6. Agakov, F., Bonilla, E., Cavazos, J., Franke, B., Fursin, G., OB́oyle, M., Thomson, J., Toussaint, M., Williams, C.: Using Machine Learning to Focus Iterative Optimization. In: Proc. of the 2006 Intl. Symp. on Code Generation and Optimization (CGO'06), pp. 295–305. IEEE Computer Society Press, Los Alamitos, CA, USA (2006)
7. Agarwal, L., Wazlowski, M., Ghosh, S.: An Asynchronous Approach to Efficient Execution of Programs on Adaptive Architectures Utilizing FPGAs. In: Proc. of 2nd IEEE Workshop on Field-Programmable Custom Computing Machines (FCCM'94), pp. 101–110. IEEE Computer Society Press, Los Alamitos, CA, USA (1994)
8. Agesen, O., Hölzle, U.: Type Feedback vs. Concrete Type Inference: A Comparison of Optimization Techniques for Object-Oriented Languages. In: Proc. of the 10th ACM Conf. on Object-Oriented Programming Systems, Languages, and Applications (OOPSLA'95), pp. 91–107. ACM Press, New York, NY, USA (1995)
9. Aho, A., Lam, M., Sethi, R., Ullman, J.: Compilers: Principles, Techniques and Tools. Addison Wesley, 2 edition, August 31 (2006)
10. Aigner, G., Diwan, A., Heine, D., Lam, M., Moore, D., Murphy, B., Sapuntzakis, C.: An Overview of the SUIF2 Compiler Infrastructure. Tech. Rep. Stanford University, Palo Alto, CA, USA (2000)
11. Allen, J., Kennedy, K., Porterfield, C., Warren, J.: Conversion of Control Dependence to Data Dependence. In: Proc. of the 10th ACM Symp. on Principles of Programming Languages (POPL'83), pp. 177–189. ACM Press, New York, NY, USA (1983)
12. Allen, R., Kennedy, K.: Optimizing Compilers for Modern Architectures: A Dependence-Based Approach. Morgan Kaufmann Pub., Inc., San Francisco, CA, USA (2001)
13. Altera, Corp.: URL http://www.altera.com
14. Altera, Corp.: Programmable Logic Array Device Using EPROM Technology. US Patent 4,774,421 (1989)
15. Altera, Corp.: Stratix™ Programmable Logic Device Family Data Sheet 1.0 (2002). URL http://www.altera.com

16. Altera, Corp.: Nios II® Processor Reference Handbook (2007). URL http://www.altera.com
17. Amerson, R., Carter, R., Culbertson, W., Kuekes, P., Snider, G.: Teramac-Configurable Custom Computing. In: Proc. of the 3rd IEEE Workshop on FPGA's for Custom Computing Machines (FCCM'95), pp. 32–38. IEEE Computer Society Press, Los Alamitos, CA, USA (1995)
18. Anderson, J., Amarasinghe, S., Lam, M.: Data and Computation Transformations for Multiprocessors. In: Proc. of the 1995 ACM Conf. on Programming Language Design and Implementation (PLDI'95), pp. 166–178. ACM Press, New York, NY, USA (1995)
19. Annapolis Microsystems, Inc.: Wildstar™ Reconfigurable Computing Engines. User's Manual R3.3 (1999)
20. Athanas, P.: An Adaptive Machine Architecture and Compiler for Dynamic Processor Reconfiguration. Ph.D. thesis, Brown University, Providence, Rhode_Island, USA (1992)
21. Athanas, P., Silverman, H.: Processor Reconfiguration Through Instruction-Set Metamorphosis: Architecture and Compiler. IEEE Computer **26**(3), 11–18 (1993)
22. August, D., Sias, J., Puiatti, J.M., Mahlke, S., Connors, D., Crozier, K., Hwu, W.: The Program Decision Logic Approach to Predicated Execution. In: Proc. of the 26th Annual Intl. Symp. on Computer Architecture (ISCA'99), pp. 208–219. ACM Press, New York, NY, USA (1999)
23. Babb, J.: High-Level Compilation For Reconfigurable Architectures. Ph.D. thesis, Massachusetts Institute of Technology (MIT), Boston, MA, USA (2000)
24. Babb, J., Rinard, M., Moritz, C., Lee, W., Frank, M., Barua, R., Amarasinghe, S.: Parallelizing Applications into Silicon. In: Proc. of the 7th IEEE Symp. on Field-Programmable Custom Computing Machines (FCCM'99), pp. 70–80. IEEE Computer Society Press, Los Alamitos, CA, USA (1999)
25. Banerjee, P., Shenoy, N., Choudhary, A., Hauck, S., Bachmann, C., Haldar, M., Joisha, P., Jones, A., Kanhare, A., Nayak, A., Periyacheri, S., Walkden, M., Zaretsky, D.: A Matlab Compiler for Distributed, Heterogeneous, Reconfigurable Computing Systems. In: Proc. of the 8th IEEE Symp. on Field-Programmable Custom Computing Machines (FCCM'00), pp. 39–48. IEEE Computer Society Press, Los Alamitos, CA, USA (2000)
26. Banerjee, U., Eigenmann, R., Nicolau, A., Padua, D.: Automatic Program Parallelization. Proc. of the IEEE **81**(2), 211–243 (1993)
27. Baradaran, N., Diniz, P.: Memory Parallelism Using Custom Array Mapping to Heterogeneous Storage Structures. In: Proc. of the Intl. Conf. on Field Programmable Logic (FPL'06), pp. 383–388. Madrid, Spain, August 28–30 (2006)
28. Baradaran, N., Diniz, P., Park, J.: Extending the Applicability of Scalar Replacement to Multiple Induction Variables. In: Proc. of the 17th Workshop on Languages and Compilers for Parallel Computing (LCPC'04), *Lecture Notes on Computer Science (LNCS)*, vol. 3602, pp. 455–469. Springer-Verlag (2004)
29. Baradaran, N., Park, J., Diniz, P.: Compiler Reuse Analysis for the Mapping of Data in FPGAs with RAM Blocks. In: Proc. of the IEEE Intl. Conf. on Field-Programmable Technology (FPT'04), pp. 145–152, Brisbane, Australia, December 6–8 (2004)
30. Barua, R., Lee, W., Amarasinghe, S., Agarwal, A.: Compiler Support for Scalable and Efficient Memory Systems. IEEE Trans. Computers **50**(11), 1234–1247 (2001)
31. Baumgarte, V., Ehlers, G., May, F., Nückel, A., Vorbach, M., Weinhardt, M.: PACT XPP® – A Self-Reconfigurable Data Processing Architecture. J. Supercomputing **26**(2), 167–184 (2003)
32. Beck, G., Yen, D., Anderson, T.: The Cydra 5 Minisupercomputer: Architecture and Implementation. J. Supercomputing **7**(1–2), 143–180 (1993)
33. Becker, J., Glesner, M.: A Parallel Dynamically Reconfigurable Architecture Designed for Flexible Application-Tailored Hardware/Software Systems in Future Mobile Communication. J. Supercomputing **19**(1), 105–127 (2001)
34. Becker, J., Hartenstein, R., Herz, M., Nageldinger, U.: Parallelization in Co-Compilation for Configurable Accelerators. In: Proc. of the 1998 Asia South Pacific Design Automation Conference (ASP-DAC'98), pp. 23–33, Yokohama, Japan, February 10–13 (1998)

35. Becker, J., Vorbach, M.: Architecture, Memory and Interface Technology Integration of an Industrial/Academic Configurable System-on-Chip (CSoC). In: Proc. of the 2003 IEEE Symp. on VLSI (ISVLSI'03), p. 107. IEEE Computer Society Press, Los Alamitos, CA, USA (2003)
36. Bellows, P., Hutchings, B.: JHDL–An HDL for Reconfigurable Systems. In: Proc. of the 6th IEEE Symp. on FPGA for Custom Computing Machines (FCCM'00), pp. 175–184. IEEE Computer Society Press, Los Alamitos, CA, USA (1998)
37. Benini, L., Micheli, G.D.: Networks on Chips: A New SoC Paradigm. IEEE Computer **35**, 70–78 (2002)
38. Bernstein, R.: Multiplication by Integer Constants. Software Practice Experience **16**(7), 641–652 (1986)
39. Betz, V., Rose, J.: VPR: A New Packing, Placement and Routing Tool for FPGA Research. In: Proc. of the 1997 Intl. Workshop on Field Programmable Logic and Applications (FPL'97), pp. 213–222, London, UK, September 1–3, 1997. *Lecture Notes in Computer Science (LNCS)*, vol. 1304, Springer (1997)
40. Bilavarn, S., Gogniat, G., Philippe, J.L.: An Estimation and Exploration Methodology from System-Level Specifications. In: Proc. of the 11th ACM Intl. Symp. on Field-Programmable Gate Arrays (FPGA'03), p. 239. ACM Press, New York, NY, USA (2003)
41. Biswas, P., Banerjee, S., Dutt, N., Pozzi, L., Ienne, P.: ISEGEN: An Iterative Improvement-Based ISE Generation Technique for Fast Customization of Processors. IEEE Trans. Very Large Scale Integration (VLSI) Systems **14**(7), 754–762 (2006)
42. Bjesse, P., Claessen, K., Sheeran, M., Singh, S.: Lava: Hardware Design in Haskell. In: Proc. of the 3rd ACM Intl. Conf. on Functional programming (ICFP'98), pp. 174–184. ACM Press, New York, NY, USA (1998)
43. Bjuréus, P., Millberg, M., Jantsch, A.: FPGA Resource and Timing Estimation from Matlab Execution Traces. In: Proc. of the 10th Intl. Symp. on Hardware/Software Codesign (CODES'02), pp. 31–36. ACM Press, New York, NY, USA (2002)
44. Böhm, W., Draper, B., Najjar, W., Hammes, J., Rinker, R., Chawathe, M., Ross, C.: One-Step Compilation of Image Processing Applications to FPGAs. In: Proc. of the the 9th IEEE Symp. on Field-Programmable Custom Computing Machines (FCCM'01), pp. 209–218. IEEE Computer Society Press, Los Alamitos, CA, USA (2001)
45. Böhm, W., Hammes, J., Draper, B., Chawathe, M., Ross, C., Rinker, R., Najjar, W.: Mapping a Single Assignment Programming Language to Reconfigurable Systems. J. Supercomputing **21**(2), 117–130 (2002)
46. Bondalapati, K.: Parallelizing of DSP Nested Loops on Reconfigurable Architectures Using Data Context Switching. In: Proc. of the 38th ACM/IEEE Design Automation Conference (DAC'01), pp. 273–276. ACM Press, New York, NY, USA (2001)
47. Bondalapati, K., Diniz, P., Duncan, P., Granacki, J., Hall, M., Jain, R., Ziegler, H.: DEFACTO: A Design Environment for Adaptive Computing Technology. In: Proc. of the 6th Reconfigurable Architectures Workshop (RAW'98), *Lecture Notes on Computer Science (LNCS)*, vol. 1388, pp. 570–578. Springer-Verlag (1999)
48. Bondalapati, K., Prasanna, V.: Dynamic Precision Management for Loop Computations on Reconfigurable Architectures. In: Proc. of the 7th IEEE Symp. on Field-Programmable Custom Computing Machines (FCCM'99), pp. 249–258. IEEE Computer Society Press, Los Alamitos, CA, USA (1999)
49. Brandolese, C., Fornaciari, W., Salice, F.: An Area Estimation Methodology for FPGA Based Designs at SystemC-level. In: Proc. of the 41st ACM/IEEE Design Automation Conference (DAC'04), pp. 129–132. ACM Press, New York, NY, USA (2004)
50. Brasen, D., Saucier, G.: Using Cone Structures for Circuit Partitioning into FPGA Packages. IEEE Trans. Computer-Aided Design Integrated Circuits Sys. **17**(7), 592–600 (1998)
51. Brayton, R., Angiovanni-Vincentelli, A., Murgai, R.: Logic Synthesis for Field-Programmable Gate Arrays. Kluwer Academic, Inc. (1995)
52. Briggs, P., Cooper, K., Torczon, L.: Improvements to Graph Coloring Register Allocation. ACM Trans. Program. Lang. Syst. **16**(3), 428–455 (1994)

53. Brooks, D., Martonosi, M.: Dynamically Exploiting Narrow Width Operands to Improve Processor Power and Performance. In: Proc. of the 5th Intl. Symp. on High Performance Computer Architecture (HPCA'99), pp. 13–22. IEEE Computer Society, Washington, DC, USA (1999)
54. Brown, S., Rose, J.: FPGA and CPLD Architectures: A Tutorial. IEEE Design Test Computers **13**(2), 42–57 (1996)
55. Budiu, M., Goldstein, S.: Fast Compilation for Pipelined Reconfigurable Fabrics. In: Proc. of the 7th ACM Intl. Symp. on Field Programmable Gate Arrays (FPGA'99), pp. 195–205. ACM Press, New York, NY, USA (1999)
56. Budiu, M., Goldstein, S., Sakr, M., Walker, K.: Bitvalue Inference: Detecting and Exploiting Narrow Bit-width Computations. In: Proc. of the 6th Intl. European Conf. on Parallel Computing (EuroPar'00), *Lecture Notes on Computer Science (LNCS)*, vol. 1900, pp. 969–979. Springer-Verlag (2000)
57. Butts, M., DeHon, A., Goldstein, S.: Molecular Electronics: Devices, Systems and Tools for Gigagate, Gigabit Chips. In: Proc. of the 2002 IEEE/ACM Intl. Conf. on Computer-Aided Design (ICCAD'02), pp. 433–440. IEEE Computer Society Press, Los Alamitos, CA, USA (2002)
58. Cadambi, S., Goldstein, S.: Efficient Place and Route for Pipeline Reconfigurable Architectures (2000). In: Proc. of the IEEE International Conference on Computer Design: VLSI in Computers & Processors (ICCD'00), Austin, Texas, USA, 2000, IEEE Computer Society, Washington, DC, USA, pp. 423–429
59. Callahan, T., Chong, P., DeHon, A., Wawrzynek, J.: Fast Module Mapping and Placement for Datapaths in FPGAs. In: Proc. of the 6th ACM Symp. on Field Programmable Gate Arrays (FPGA'98), pp. 123–132. ACM Press, New York, NY, USA (1998)
60. Callahan, T., Hauser, J., Wawrzynek, J.: The Garp Architecture and C Compiler. Computer **33**(4), 62–69 (2000)
61. Callahan, T., Wawrzynek, J.: Instruction Level Parallelism for Reconfigurable Computing. In: Proc. of the 8th Intl. Workshop on Field-Programmable Logic and Applications (FPL'98), *Lecture Notes on Computer Science (LNCS)*, vol. 1482, pp. 248–257. Springer-Verlag (1998)
62. Callahan, T., Wawrzynek, J.: Adapting Software Pipelining for Reconfigurable Computing. In: Proc. of the 2000 Intl. Conf. on Compilers, Architecture, and Synthesis for Embedded Systems (CASES'00), pp. 57–64. ACM Press, New York, NY, USA (2000)
63. Cardoso, J.: On Combining Temporal Partitioning and Sharing of Functional Units in Compilation for Reconfigurable Architectures. IEEE Trans. Computers **52**(10), 1362–1375 (2003)
64. Cardoso, J., Neto, H.: An Enhanced Static-List Scheduling Algorithm for Temporal Partitioning onto RPUs. In: Proc. of the IFIP X Intl. Conf. on Very Large Scale Integration (VLSI'99), pp. 485–496. Kluwer Academic Publ. (1999)
65. Cardoso, J., Neto, H.: Macro-Based Hardware Compilation of Java™ Bytecodes into a Dynamic Reconfigurable Computing System. In: Proc. of the 7th IEEE Symp. on Field-Programmable Custom Computing Machines (FCCM'99), pp. 2–11. IEEE Computer Society, Los Alamitos, CA, USA (1999)
66. Cardoso, J., Neto, H.: Compilation Increasing the Scheduling Scope for Multi-Memory-FPGA-Based Custom Computing Machines. In: Proc. of the 11th Intl. Conf. on Field Programmable Logic and Applications (FPL'01), *Lecture Notes on Computer Science (LNCS)*, vol. 2147, pp. 523–533. Springer-Verlag (2001)
67. Cardoso, J., Neto, H.: Compilation for FPGA-Based Reconfigurable Hardware. IEEE Design Test Computers **20**(2), 65–75 (2003)
68. Cardoso, J., Weinhardt, M.: XPP-VC: A C Compiler with Temporal Partitioning for the PACT-XPP Architecture. In: Proc. of the 12th Intl. Workshop on Field Programmable Logic and Applications (FPL'02), *Lecture Notes on Computer Science (LNCS)*, vol. 975, pp. 864–874. Springer-Verlag (2002)
69. Cardoso, J., Weinhardt, M.: From C Programs to the Configure-Execute Model. In: Proc. of the Conf. on Design, Automation and Test in Europe (DATE'03), pp. 576–581. IEEE Press, Piscataway, NJ, USA (2003)

70. Cardoso, J., Weinhardt, M.: Compilation and Temporal Partitioning for a Coarse-Grain Reconfigurable Architecture. In: New Algorithms, Architectures, and Applications for Reconfigurable Computing, Chap. 9, pp. 105–115. Springer (2005)
71. Caspi, E.: Empirical Study of Opportunities for Bit-Level Specialization in Word-Based Programs (2000) M.Sc. Thesis, University of California Berkeley, Berkeley, CA, USA
72. Caspi, E., Chu, M., Huang, R., Yeh, J., Wawrzynek, J., DeHon, A.: Stream Computations Organized for Reconfigurable Execution (SCORE). In: Proc. of the The Roadmap to Reconfigurable Computing, 10th Intl. Workshop on Field-Programmable Logic and Applications (FPL'00), *Lecture Notes in Computer Science (LNCS)*, vol. 1896, pp. 605–614. Springer-Verlag (2000)
73. Catthoor, F., Danckaert, K., Kulkarni, K., Brockmeyer, E., Kjeldsberg, P., van Achteren, T., Omnes, T.: Data Access and Storage Management for Embedded Programmable Processors. Kluwer Academic Publ. (2002)
74. Cavazos, J., Dubach, C., Agakov, F., Bonilla, E., O'Boyle, M., Fursin, G., Temam, O.: Automatic Performance Model Construction for the Fast Software Exploration of New Hardware Designs. In: Proc. of the 2006 Intl. Conf. on Compilers, Architecture and Synthesis for Embedded Systems (CASES'06), pp. 24–34. ACM Press, New York, NY, USA (2006)
75. Celoxica, Ltd.: URL http://www.celoxica.com
76. Chang, P., Mahlke, S., Chen, W., Warter, N., Hwu, W.M.: IMPACT: An Architectural Framework for Multiple-Instruction-Issue Processors. SIGARCH Comput. Archit. News **19**(3), 266–275 (1991)
77. Charles, P., Grothoff, C., Saraswat, V., Donawa, C., Kielstra, A., Ebcioglu, K., Praun, C., Sarkar, V.: X10: An Object-Oriented Approach to Non-Uniform Cluster Computing. In: Proc. of the 2005 ACM Intl. Conf. on Object-Oriented Programming, Systems, Languages, and Applications (OOPSLA'05), San Diego, CA, USA, October 16–20, 2005, pp. 519–538. ACM Press (2005)
78. Chen, D., Cong, J., Pan, P.: FPGA Design Automation: A Survey. Found. Trends Electron. Des. Autom. **1**(3), 139–169 (2006)
79. Chu, M., Weaver, N., Sulimma, K., DeHon, A., Wawrzynek, J.: Object Oriented Circuit-Generators in Java. In: Proc. of the 6th IEEE Symp. on FPGAs for Custom Computing Machines (FCCM'98), pp. 158–166. IEEE Computer Society Press, Los Alamitos, CA, USA (1998)
80. Clark, N., Kudlur, M., Park, H., Mahlke, S., Flautner, K.: Application-Specific Processing on a General-Purpose Core via Transparent Instruction Set Customization. In: Proc. of the 37th IEEE/ACM Intl. Symp. on Microarchitecture (MICRO), pp. 30–40. IEEE Computer Society Press, Los Alamitos, CA, USA (2004)
81. Compton, K., Hauck, S.: Reconfigurable Computing: A Survey of Systems and Software. ACM Comput. Surv. **34**(2), 171–210 (2002)
82. Cormen, T., Leiserson, C., Rivest, R., Stein, C.: Introduction to Algorithms, 2nd edn. McGraw-Hill Publ. (2002)
83. Craven, S., Athanas, P.: Examining the Viability of FPGA Supercomputing. EURASIP J. Embedded Systems **2007**(1), 8 pages (2007)
84. Cronquist, D., Franklin, P., Berg, S., Ebeling, C.: Specifying and Compiling Applications for RaPiD. In: Proc. of the 6th IEEE Symp. on FPGAs for Custom Computing Machines (FCCM'98), pp. 116–125. IEEE Computer Society Press, Los Alamitos, CA, USA (1998)
85. Cytron, R., Ferrante, J., Rosen, B., Wegman, M., Zadeck, F.: Efficiently Computing Static Single Assignment Form and the Control Dependence Graph. ACM Trans. Program. Lang. Syst. **13**(4), 451–490 (1991)
86. Dehnert, J., Hsu, P., Bratt, J.: Overlapped Loop Support in the Cydra 5. In: Proc. of the 3rd Intl. Conf. on Architectural Support for Programming Languages and Operating Systems (ASPLOS-III), pp. 26–38. ACM Press, New York, NY, USA (1989)
87. DeHon, A.: Reconfigurable Architectures for General-Purpose Computing. Ph.D. thesis, Massachusetts Institute of Technology, Cambridge, MA, USA (1996)
88. DeHon, A.: The Density Advantage of Configurable Computing. Computer **33**(4), 41–49 (2000)

89. DeHon, A.: Nanowire-Based Programmable Architectures. ACM J. Emerging Technologies Comput. Systems (JETC) **1**(2), 109–162 (2005)
90. DeHon, A., Hauck, S. (ed.): Reconfigurable Computing: The Theory and Practice of FPGA-Based Computations. Elsevier (2007)
91. DeHon, A., Huang, R., Wawrzynek, J.: Hardware-Assisted Fast Routing. In: Proc. of the 10th IEEE Symp. on Field-Programmable Custom Computing Machines (FCCM'02), p. 205. IEEE Computer Society Press, Los Alamitos, CA, USA (2002)
92. DeHon, A., Markovsky, Y., Caspi, E., Chua, M., Huang, R. Pozzi, S.P., Yeh, L., Wawrzynek, J.: Stream Computations Organized for Reconfigurable Execution. Microprocessors and Microsystems **30**(6), 334–354 (2006)
93. DeHon, A., Naeimi, H.: Seven Strategies for Tolerating Highly Defective Fabrication. IEEE Design Test Computers **22**(4), 306–315 (2005)
94. Diniz, P.: Evaluation of Code Generation Strategies for Scalar Replaced Codes in Fine-Grain Configurable Architectures. In: Proc. of the 13th IEEE Symp. on FPGA for Custom Computing Machines (FCCM'05), pp. 73–82. IEEE Computer Society Press, Los Alamitos, CA, USA (2005)
95. Diniz, P., Govindu, G.: Design of a Field-Programmable Dual-Precision Floating-Point Arithmetic Unit. In: Proc. of the 2006 Inl. Conf. on Field Programmable Logic and Applications (FPL'06), pp. 1–4. Madrid, Spain (2006)
96. Diniz, P., Hall, M., Park, J., So, B., Ziegler, H.: Automatic Mapping of C to FPGAs with the DEFACTO Compilation and Synthesis System. Microprocessors and Microsystems **29**(2–3), 51–62 (2005)
97. Doncev, G., Leeser, M., Tarafdar, S.: High Level Synthesis for Designing Custom Computing Hardware. In: Proc. of 6th IEEE Symp. on Field-Programmable Custom Computing Machines (FCCM'98), pp. 326–327. IEEE Computer Society Press, Los Alamitos, CA, USA (1998)
98. Doshi, G., Krishnaiyer, R., Muthukumar, K.: Optimizing Software Data Prefetches with Rotating Registers. In: Proc. of the 2001 Intl. Conf. on Parallel Architectures and Compilation Techniques (PACT'01), pp. 257–267. IEEE Computer Society, Washington, DC, USA (2001)
99. Duncan, A., Hendry, D., Cray, P.: An Overview of the COBRA-ABS High Level Synthesis System for Multi-FPGA Systems. In: Proc. of 6th IEEE Symp. on Field-Programmable Custom Computing Machines (FCCM'98), pp. 106–115. IEEE Computer Society Press, Los Alamitos, CA, USA (1998)
100. Duncan, A., Hendry, D., Cray, P.: The COBRA-ABS High Level Synthesis System for Multi-FPGA Custom Computing Machines. IEEE Trans. Very Large Scale Integration (VLSI) Systems **9**(1), 218–223 (2001)
101. Ebeling, C., Cronquist, D., Franklin, P.: RaPiD – Reconfigurable Pipelined Data-path. In: Proc. of the Intl. Workshop on Field Programmable Logic and Applications (FPL'95), pp. 126–135. *Lecture Notes in Computer Science (LNCS)*, vol. 1142, Springer-Verlag (1995)
102. Edwards, S.: High-Level Synthesis from the Synchronous Language Esterel. In: Proc. of the Intl. Workshop on Logic and Synthesis (IWLS02) (2002). New Orleans, Louisiana, USA, June 4–7, 2002, pp. 401–406
103. Elrad, T., Filman, R., Bader, A.: Aspect-Oriented Programming: Introduction. Communications of the ACM **44**(10), pp. 29–32 (2001)
104. Estrin, G.: Organization of Computer Systems – The Fixed Plus Variable Structure Computer. In: Proc. of the Western Joint Computer Conference, New York, USA, pp. 33–40 (1960)
105. Estrin, G., Bussell, B., Turn, R., Bibb, J.: Parallel Processing in a Restructurable Computer System. IEEE Trans. Computers **12**(6), 747–755 (1963)
106. Estrin, G., Turn, R.: Automatic Assignment of Computations in a Variable Structure Computer System. IEEE Trans. Computers **12**(6), 755–773 (1963)
107. Fekete, S., Kohler, E., Teich, J.: Optimal FPGA Module Placement with Temporal Precedence Constraints. In: Proc. of the Conf. on Design Automation and Test in Europe (DATE'01), pp. 658–665. IEEE Press, Piscataway, NJ, USA (2001)

108. Fiduccia, C., Mattheyses, R.: A Linear-Time Heuristic for Improving Network Partitions. In: Proc. of the 19th ACM/IEEE Design Automation Conference (DAC'82), pp. 175–181. ACM Press, New York, NY, USA (1982)
109. Filman, R., Elrad, T., Clarke, S., Akşit, M. (eds.): Aspect-Oriented Software Development. Addison-Wesley Publ., Boston, MA, USA (2005)
110. Fisher, J., Faraboschi, P., Young, C.: Embedded Computing: A VLIW Approach to Architecture, Compilers and Tools, 1st edn. Morgan Kaufmann, Inc. (2004)
111. Freeman, R.: Configurable Electrical Circuit Having Configurable Logic Elements and Configurable Interconnects. US Patent 4,870,302 (1989)
112. Frigo, J., Gokhale, M., Lavenier, D.: Evaluation of the Streams-C C-to-FPGA Compiler: An Applications Perspective. In: Proc. of the 9th ACM Intl. Symp. on Field-Programmable Gate Arrays (FPGA'01), pp. 134–140. ACM Press, New York, NY, USA (2001)
113. Fujii, T., Furuta, K., Motomura, M., Nomura, M., Mizuno, M., Anjo, K., Wakabayashi, K., Hirota, Y., Nakazawa, Y., Ito, H., Yamashina, M.: A Dynamically Reconfigurable Logic Engine with a Multi-Context/Multi-Mode Unified-Cell Architecture. In: Proc. of the IEEE Intl. Solid State Circuits Conf. (ISSCC'99), San Francisco, CA, USA, February 15–17, pp. 364–365 (1999)
114. Gajski, D., Dutt, N., Wu, A., Lin, S.: High-Level Synthesis, Introduction to Chip and System Design. Kluwer Academic Pub. (1992)
115. Gajski, D., Vahid, F., Narayan, S., Gong, J.: Specification and Design of Embedded Systems. Prentice-Hall, Inc., Upper Saddle River, NJ, USA (1994)
116. Galloway, D.: The Transmogrifier C Hardware Description Language and Compiler for FPGAs. In: Proc. of the 3rd IEEE Workshop on FPGA for Custom Computing Machines (FCCM'95), pp. 136–144. IEEE Computer Society Press, Los Alamitos, CA, USA (1995)
117. Galuzzi, C., Bertels, K., Vassiliadis, S.: A Linear Complexity Algorithm for the Automatic Generation of Convex Multiple Input Multiple Output Instructions. In: Proc. of the 3rd Intl. Workshop on Applied Reconfigurable Computing (ARC'07), *Lecture Notes on Computer Science (LNCS)*, vol. 4419, pp. 130–141. Springer (2007)
118. Galuzzi, C., Panainte, E., Yankova, Y., Bertels, K., Vassiliadis, S.: Automatic Selection of Application-Specific Instruction-Set Extensions. In: Proc. of the 4th Intl. Conf. on Hardware/Software Codesign and System Synthesis (CODES'06/ISSS'06), pp. 160–165 (2006)
119. Ganesan, S., Vemuri, R.: An Integrated Temporal Partitioning and Partial Reconfiguration Technique for Design Latency Improvement. In: Proc. of the Conf. on Design, Automation and Test in Europe (DATE'00), pp. 320–325. IEEE Press, Piscataway, NJ, USA (2000)
120. Girkar, M., Polychronopoulos, C.: Automatic Extraction of Functional Parallelism from Ordinary Programs. IEEE Trans. Parallel Distributed Systems **3**(2), 166–178 (1992)
121. Gokhale, M., Gomersall, E.: High-Level Compilation for Fine Grained FPGAs. In: Proc. of the 5th IEEE Symp. on FPGA for Custom Computing Machines (FCCM'97), pp. 165–173. IEEE Computer Society Press, Los Alamitos, CA, USA (1997)
122. Gokhale, M., Graham, P.: Reconfigurable Computing: Accelerating Computation with Field-Programmable Gate Arrays, 1st edn. Springer (2006)
123. Gokhale, M., Holmes, W., Kopser, A., D. Kunze, D.L., Lucas, S., Minnich, R., Olsen, P.: SPLASH: A Reconfigurable Linear Logic Array. In: Proc. of the 1990 Intl. Conf. on Parallel Processing (ICPP'90), Urbana-Champaign, IL, USA, August, pp. 526–532 (1990)
124. Gokhale, M., Marks, A.: Automatic Synthesis of Parallel Programs Targeted to Dynamically Reconfigurable Logic Array. In: Proc. of the 5th Intl. Workshop on Field Programmable Logic and Applications (FPL'95), *Lecture Notes on Computer Science (LNCS)*, vol. 975, pp. 399–408. Springer-Verlag (1995)
125. Gokhale, M., Stone, J.: NAPA C: Compiling for a Hybrid RISC/FPGA Architecture. In: Proc. of the 6th IEEE Symp. on FPGAs for Custom Computing Machines (FCCM'98), pp. 126–135. IEEE Computer Society, Washington, DC, USA (1998)
126. Gokhale, M., Stone, J.: Automatic Allocation of Arrays to Memories in FPGA Processors with Multiple Memory Banks. In: Proc. of 7th IEEE Symp. on Field-Programmable Custom Computing Machines (FCCM'99), pp. 63–69. IEEE Computer Society Press, Los Alamitos, CA, USA (1999)

127. Gokhale, M., Stone, J., Arnold, J., Kalinowski, M.: Stream-Oriented FPGA Computing in the Streams-C High Level Language. In: Proc. of the 8th IEEE Symp. on Field-Programmable Custom Computing Machines (FCCM'00), pp. 49–56. IEEE Computer Society Press, Los Alamitos, CA, USA (2000)
128. Gokhale, M., Stone, J., Gomersall, E.: Co-synthesis to a Hybrid RISC/FPGA Architecture. J. VLSI Signal Processing Systems Signal Image Video Technol. **24**(2), 165–180 (2000)
129. Goldstein, S., Budiu, M.: The DIL Programming Language. Tech. Rep., Carnegie-Mellon University, Pittsburgh, PA, USA (1999)
130. Goldstein, S., Budiu, M., Mishra, M., Venkataramani, G.: Reconfigurable Computing and Electronic Nanotechnology. In: Proc. of the IEEE 14th Intl. Conf. on Application-Specific Systems, Architectures and Processors (ASAP 2003), pp. 132–143. The Hague, Netherlands (2003)
131. Goldstein, S., Schmit, H., Budiu, M., Cadambi, S., Moe, M., Taylor, R.: PipeRench: A Reconfigurable Architecture and Compiler. Computer **33**(4), 70–77 (2000)
132. Goldstein, S., Schmit, H., Moe, M., Budiu, M., Cadambi, S., Taylor, R., Laufer, R.: PipeRench: a Co/Processor for Streaming Multimedia Acceleration. In: Proc. of the 26th Annual Intl. Symp. on Computer Architecture (ISCA'99), pp. 28–39. ACM Press, New York, NY, USA (1999)
133. Gong, W., Wang, G., Kastner, R.: Storage Assignment During High-Level Synthesis for Configurable Architectures. In: Proc. of the 2005 IEEE/ACM Intl. Conf. on Computer-Aided Design (ICCAD'05). pp. 3–6, IEEE Computer Society Press, Los Alamitos, CA, USA (2005)
134. Gonzalez, R.: Xtensa™ – A configurable and Extensible Processor. IEEE Micro **20**(2), 60–70 (2000)
135. Gray, J., Kean, T.: Configurable Hardware: A New Paradigm for Computation. In: Proc. of the Decennial Caltech Conf. on VLSI on Advanced Research in VLSI, pp. 279–295. MIT Press, Cambridge, MA, USA (1989)
136. Guccione, S., Levi, D., Sundararajan, P.: Jbits: Java Based Interface for Reconfigurable Computing. In: Proc. of the Military and Aerospace Applications of Programmable Devices and Technologies Conference (MAPLD'0099), pp. 1–9, Laurel, Maryland, USA, September 28–30 (1999)
137. Guo, Z., Buyukkurt, B., Najjar, W.: Input Data Reuse in Compiling Window Operations onto Reconfigurable Hardware. In: Proc. 2004 ACM Symp. on Languages, Compilers and Tools for Embedded Systems (LCTES'04), pp. 249–256. ACM Press, New York, NY, USA (2004)
138. Guo, Z., Najjar, W.: A Compiler Intermediate Representation for Reconfigurable Fabrics. In: Proc. of the 16th Intl. Conf. on Field Programmable Logic and Applications (FPL'2006), pp. 741–744. IEEE Computer Society Press (2006)
139. Gupta, S., Kam, T., Kishinevsky, M., Rotem, S., Savoiu, N., Dutt, N., Gupta, R., Nicolau, A.: Coordinated Transformations for High-Level Synthesis of High Performance Microprocessor Blocks. In: Proc. of the 39th ACM/IEEE Design Automation Conference (DAC'02), p. 898. ACM Press, New York, NY, USA (2002)
140. Gupta, S., Savoiu, N., Kim, S., Dutt, N., Gupta, R., Nicolau, A.: Speculation Techniques for High Level Synthesis of Control Intensive Designs. In: Proc. of the 38th ACM/IEEE Design Automation Conference (DAC'01), pp. 269–272. ACM Press, New York, NY, USA (2001)
141. Haldar, M., Nayak, A., Choudhary, A., Banerjee, P.: A System for Synthesizing Optimized FPGA Hardware from Matlab. In: Proc. of the 2001 IEEE/ACM Intl. Conf. on Computer-Aided Design (ICCAD'01), pp. 314–319. IEEE Computer Society Press, Los Alamitos, CA, USA (2001)
142. Haldar, M., Nayak, A., Choudhary, A., Banerjee, P., Shenoy, N.: FPGA Hardware Synthesis From Matlab. In: Proc. of the 14th Intl. Conf. on VLSI Design (VLSID '01), pp. 299–304. IEEE Computer Society Press, Los Alamitos, CA, USA (2001)
143. Harrison, W.: Compiler Analysis of the Value Ranges for Variables. IEEE Trans. Software Eng. **3**(3), 243–250 (1977)
144. Hartenstein, R.: The Microprocessor is No More General Purpose: Why Future Reconfigurable Platforms Will Win. In: Proc of the Intl. Conf. on Innovative Systems in Silicon (ISIS'97), Austin, Texas, USA, October 8–10 (1997)

145. Hartenstein, R.: A Decade of Reconfigurable Computing: A Visionary Retrospective. In: Proc. of the Conf. on Design, Automation and Test in Europe (DATE'01), pp. 642–649. IEEE Press, Piscataway, NJ, USA (2001)
146. Hartenstein, R., Becker, J., Kress, R., Reinig, H.: High-Performance Computing Using a Reconfigurable Accelerator. Concurrency: Practice and Experience **8**, 429–443 (1996)
147. Hartenstein, R., Herz, M., Hoffmann, T., Nageldinger, U.: Generation of Design Suggestions for Coarse-Grain Reconfigurable Architectures. In: Proc. of the 10th Intl. Workshop on Field-Programmable Logic and Applications (FPL'00), *Lecture Notes on Computer Science (LNCS)*, vol. 1896, pp. 389–399. Springer-Verlag, London, UK (2000)
148. Hartenstein, R., Kress, R.: A Datapath Synthesis System for the Reconfigurable Datapath Architecture. In: Proc. of the 1995 Asia Pacific Design Automation Conference (ASP-DAC'95), Chiba, Japan, Aug. 29 – Sept. 1, pp. 479–484 (1995)
149. Hartenstein, R., Kress, R., Reinig, H.: A New FPGA Architecture for Word-Oriented Datapaths. In: Proc. of the 4th Intl. Workshop on Field-Programmable Logic and Applications (FPL'04), pp. 144–155. Springer-Verlag, London, UK (1994)
150. Hartley, R.: Optimization of Canonic Signed Digit Multipliers for Filter Design, IEEE International Symposium on Circuits and Systems, Singapore, June 11–14, 1991, pp. 1992–1995 (1991)
151. Hauck, S.: The Roles of FPGAs in Reprogrammable Systems. Proc. of the IEEE **86**(4), April 1998, 615–638 (1998)
152. S.Hauck, Fry, T., Hosler, M., Kao, J.: The Chimaera Reconfigurable Functional Unit. IEEE Trans. Very Large Scale Integr. Syst. **12**(2), 206–217 (2004)
153. Hauser, J., Wawrzynek, J.: Garp: A MIPS Processor with a Reconfigurable Coprocessor. In: Proc. of the 5th IEEE Symp. on FPGAs for Custom Computing Machines (FCCM'97), pp. 12–21. IEEE Computer Society Press, Los Alamitos, CA, USA (1997)
154. Hennesy, J., Patterson, D.: Computer Architecture: A Quantitative Approach, 3rd edn. Morgan Kaufmann Pub., Inc., San Francisco, CA, USA (2003)
155. Hoare, C.A.R.: Communicating Sequential Processes. Prentice-Hall, Inc. (1985)
156. Hormati, A., Clark, N., Mahlke, S.: Exploiting Narrow Accelerators with Data-Centric Subgraph Mapping. In: Proc. of the Intl. Symp. on Code Generation and Optimization (CGO'07), pp. 341–353. IEEE Computer Society Press, Los Alamitos, CA, USA (2007)
157. Huang, R., Wawrzynek, J., DeHon, A.: Stochastic, Spatial Routing for Hypergraphs, Trees, and Meshes. In: Proc. of the 11th ACM Intl. Symp. on Field-Programmable Gate Arrays (FPGA'03), pp. 78–87. ACM Press, New York, NY, USA (2003)
158. IEEE Computer Society: IEEE 754 Standard for Binary Floating-Point Arithmetic (1985)
159. The impact research group. URL http://www.crhc.uiuc.edu/Impact/
160. Impulse Accelerated Technologies, I.: URL http://www.impulsec.com
161. Inoue, A., Tomiyama, H., Okuma, H., nd, H.K., Yasuura, H.: Language and Compiler for Optimizing Data-path Widths of Embedded Systems. IEICE Trans. Fundamentals **E81-A**(12), 2595–2604 (1998)
162. Institute of Electrical and Electronics Engineers (IEEE): 1076-2000 IEEE Standard VHDL Language Reference Manual (2000)
163. Institute of Electrical and Electronics Engineers (IEEE): 1364-2001 IEEE Standard Verilog Hardware Description Language (2001)
164. Iseli, C., Sanchez, E.: Spyder: A Reconfigurable VLIW Processor using FPGAs. In: Proc. of the IEEE Workshop. on FPGAs for Custom Computing Machines (FCCM'93), pp. 17–24. IEEE Computer Society Press, Los Alamitos, CA,USA (1993)
165. Jones, G., Goldsmith, M.: Programming in OCCAM®2. Prentice Hall, Englewood Cliffs, NJ, USA (1989)
166. Jones, M., Scharf, L., Scott, J., Twaddle, C., Yaconis, M., Yao, K., Athanas, P., Schott, B.: Implementing an API for Distributed Adaptive Computing Systems. In: Proc. of the 7th IEEE Symp. on FPGA for Custom Computing Machines (FCCM'00), pp. 222–230. IEEE Computer Society Press, Los Alamitos, CA, USA (1999)

167. de Jong, G., Verdonck, B., Wuytack, S., Catthoor, F.: Background Memory Management for Dynamic Data Structure Intensive Processing Systems. In: Proc. of the 1995 IEEE/ACM Intl. Conf. on Computer-Aided Design (ICCAD'95), pp. 515–520. IEEE Computer Society Press, Washington, DC, USA (1995)
168. Kastrup, B., Bink, A., Hoogerbrugge, J.: ConCISe: A Compiler-Driven CPLD-based Instruction Set Accelerator. In: Proc. of the 7th IEEE Symp. on Field-Programmable Custom Computing Machines (FCCM'99), pp. 92–101. IEEE Computer Society, Washington, DC, USA (1999)
169. Kaul, M., Vemuri, R.: Optimal Temporal Partitioning and Synthesis for Reconfigurable Architectures. In: Proc. of the Conf. on Design, Automation and Test in Europe (DATE'98), pp. 389–396. IEEE Press, Piscataway, NJ, USA (1998)
170. Kaul, M., Vemuri, R.: Temporal Partitioning Combined with Design Space Exploration for Latency Minimization of Run-Time Reconfigured Designs. In: Proc. of the Conf. on Design, Automation and Test in Europe (DATE'98), pp. 202–209. IEEE Press, Piscataway, NJ, USA (1998)
171. Kaul, M., Vemuri, R., Govindarajan, S., Ouaiss, I.: An Automated Temporal Partitioning and Loop Fission Approach for FPGA based Reconfigurable Synthesis of DSP Applications. In: Proc. of the 36th IEEE/ACM Design Automation Conference (DAC'99), pp. 616–622. ACM Press, New York, NY, USA (1999)
172. Kerkiz, N.: Development and Experimental Evaluation of Partitioning Algorithms for Adaptive Computing Systems. Ph.D. thesis, University of Tennesse, Knoxville, Tennessee, USA (2000)
173. Kernighan, B., Lin, S.: An Efficient Heuristic Procedure for Partitioning Graphs. Bell Sys. Tech. J. **49**, 291–308 (1970)
174. Kiczales, G., Lamping, J., Menhdhekar, A., Maeda, C., Lopes, C., Loingtier, J.M., Irwin, J.: Aspect-Oriented Programming. In: M. Akşit, S. Matsuoka (eds.) Proc. of the European Conference on Object-Oriented Programming (ECOOP'97), *Lecture Notes in Computer Science (LNCS)*, vol. 1241, pp. 220–242. Springer-Verlag, Berlin, Heidelberg, and New York (1997)
175. Kilts, S.: Advanced FPGA Design: Architecture, Implementation, and Optimization. Wiley-IEEE Press (2007)
176. Kirkpatrick, S., Gellat, C., Jr., M.V.: Optimization by Simulated Annealing. Science **220**(4598), 671–680 (1983)
177. Kobayashi, S., Kozuka, I., Tang, W., Landmann, D.: A Software/Hardware Codesigned Hands Free System on a Resizable Block-floating-point DSP. In: Proc. of the IEEE Intl. Conf. on Acoustics, Speech, and Signal Processing (ICASSP'04), Montreal, Canada, May, pp. 149–152 (2004)
178. Koren, I., Mendelsom, B., Peled, I., Silberman, G.M.: A Data-Driven VLSI Array for Arbitrary Algorithms. Computer **21**(10), 30–43 (1988)
179. Krupnova, H., Saucier, G.: A Data Reuse Based Compiler Optimization for FPGAs. In: Proc. of the 9th Intl. Conf. on Field Programmable Logic and Applications (FPL'99), *Lecture Notes on Computer Science (LNCS)*, vol. 1673, pp. 101–110. Springer-Verlag (1999)
180. Kulkarni, D., Najjar, W., Rinker, R., Kurdahi, F.: Compile-time Area Estimation for LUT-based FPGAs. ACM Trans. Des. Autom. Electron. Syst. **11**(1), 104–122 (2006)
181. Kung, S., Lo, S., Jean, S., Hwang, J.: Wavefront Array Processors-Concept to Implementation. Computer **20**(7), 18–33 (1987)
182. Kuzmanov, G., Gaydadjiev, G., Vassiliadis, S.: The MOLEN Media Processor: Design and Evaluation. In: Proc. of the Intl. Workshop on Application Specific Processors (WASP'05), New York, USA, September 22, pp. 26–33 (2005)
183. Lakshmikanthan, P., Govindarajan, S., Srinivasan, V., Vemuri, R.: Behavioral Partitioning with Synthesis for Multi-FPGA Architectures under Interconnect, Area, and Latency Constraints. In: Proc. of the 7th Reconfigurable Architectures Workshop (RAW'00), *Lecture Notes on Computer Science (LNCS)*, vol. 1800, pp. 924–931. Springer-Verlag (2000)
184. Lakshminarayana, G., Khouri, K., Jha, N.: Wavesched: A Novel Scheduling Technique for Control-Flow Intensive Designs. IEEE Trans. Computer-Aided Design Integrated Circuits Syst. **18**(5), 505–523 (1999)

185. Lam, M.: Software Pipelining: An Effective Scheduling Technique for VLIW Machines. In: Proc. of the 1988 ACM Conf. on Programming Language Design and Implementation (PLDI'88), pp. 318–328. ACM Press, New York, NY, USA (1988)
186. Lam, M., Wolf, M.: A Data Locality Optimizing Algorithm. In: Proc. of the ACM Conf. on Programming Language Design and Implementation (PLDI'91), pp. 30–44. ACM Press, New York, NY, USA (1991)
187. Lau, D., Pritchard, O., Molson, P.: Automated Generation of Hardware Accelerators with Direct Memory Access from ANSI/ISO Standard C Functions. In: Proc. of the 14th IEEE Symp. on Field-Programmable Custom Computing Machines (FCCM'06), pp. 45–56. IEEE Computer Society, Washington, DC, USA (2006)
188. Lee, H., Sobelman, G.: FPGA-Based FIR Filters Using Digit-Serial Arithmetic. In: Proc. of IEEE Intl. ASIC Conference (ASIC'97), Portland, OR, USA, Sept. 7–10, pp. 225–228 (1997)
189. Lee, W., Barua, R., Frank, M., Srikrishna, D., Babb, J., Sarkar, V., Amarasinghe, S.: Space-Time Scheduling of Instruction-Level Parallelism on a RAW Machine. In: Proc. of the 8th Intl. Conf. on Architectural Support for Programming Languages and Operating Systems (ASPLOS-VIII), pp. 46–57. ACM Press, New York, NY, USA (1998)
190. Leong, M., Yeung, M., Yeung, C., Fu, C., Heng, P., Leong, P.: Automatic Floating to Fixed Point Translation and Its Application to Post-Rendering 3D Warping. In: Proc. of the 7th IEEE Symp. on Field-Programmable Custom Computing Machines (FCCM'99), pp. 240–248. IEEE Computer Society Press, Los Alamitos, CA, USA (1999)
191. Lewis, D., van Ierssel, M., Rose, J., Chow, P.: The Transmogrifier-2: a 1 million gate rapid-prototyping system. IEEE Trans. Very Large Scale Integr. Syst. **6**(2), 188–198 (1998)
192. Li, Y., Callahan, T., Darnell, E., Harr, R., Kurkure, U., Stockwood, J.: Hardware-Software Co-Design of Embedded Reconfigurable Architectures. In: Proc. of the 37th ACM/IEEE Design Automation Conference (DAC'00), pp. 507–512. ACM Press, New York, NY, USA (2000)
193. Lindholm, T., Yellin, F.: The Java Virtual Machine Specification. Prentice-Hall, Inc. (1996)
194. Ling, X., Amano, H.: WASMII: A Data Driven Computer on a Virtual Hardware. In: Proc. of the IEEE Workshop on FPGAs for Custom Computing Machines (FCCM'93), pp. 33–42. IEEE Computer Society Press, Los Alamitos, CA, USA (1993)
195. Ling, X., Amano, H.: WASMII: An MPLD with Data-driven Control on a Virtual Hardware. J. Supercomputing **9**(3), 253–276 (1995)
196. Liu, H., Wong, D.: Circuit Partitioning for Dynamically Reconfigurable FPGAs. In: Proc. of the 7th ACM Intl. Symp. on Field Programmable Gate Arrays (FPGA'99), pp. 187–194. ACM Press, New York, NY, USA (1999)
197. Luk, W., Wu, T.: Towards a Declarative Framework for Hardware-Software Codesign. In: Proc. of the 3rd Intl. Workshop on Hardware/software Co-design (CODES'94), pp. 181–188. IEEE Computer Society Press, Los Alamitos, CA, USA (1994)
198. Lynch, N., Merritt, M., Weihl, W., Fekete, A.: Atomic Transactions: In Concurrent and Distributed Systems. Morgan Kaufmann Pub., Inc., San Francisco, CA, USA (1993)
199. Magenheimer, D., Peters, L., Pettis, K., Zuras, D.: Integer Multiplication and Division on the HP Precision Architecture. IEEE Trans. Comput. **37**(8), 980–990 (1988)
200. Mahlke, S., Lin, D., Chen, W., Hank, R., Bringmann, R.: Effective Compiler Support for Predicated Execution Using the Hyperblock. In: Proc. of the 25th IEEE/ACM Intl. Symp. on Microarchitecture (MICRO), Portland, Oregon, USA, pp. 45–54, IEEE Computer Society Press, Los Alamitos, CA, USA (1992)
201. Markovskiy, Y., Caspi, E., Huang, R., Yeh, J., Chu, M., Wawrzynek, J., DeHon, A.: Analysis of Quasi-Static Scheduling Techniques in a Virtualized Reconfigurable Machine. In: Proc. of the 10th ACM Intl. Symp. on Field-Programmable Gate arrays (FPGA'02), pp. 196–205. ACM Press, New York, NY, USA (2002)
202. Maruyama, T., Hoshino, T.: A C to HDL Compiler for Pipeline Processing on FPGAs. In: Proc. of the 8th IEEE Symp. on FPGA for Custom Computing Machines (FCCM'00), pp. 101–110. IEEE Computer Society Press, Los Alamitos, CA, USA (2000)

203. MathStar, Inc.: URL http://www.mathstar.com
204. McCanny, J., McWhirter, J., Swartzlander, E.J., (eds.): Systolic Array Processors. Prentice-Hall, Inc., Upper Saddle River, NJ, USA (1989)
205. McKinley, K.S., Carr, S., Tseng, C.W.: Improving Data Locality with Loop Transformations. ACM Trans. Prog. Lang. Syst. **4**(18), 424–453 (1996)
206. Mei, B., Lambrechts, A., Verkest, D., Mignolet, J.Y., Lauwereins, R.: Architecture Exploration for a Reconfigurable Architecture Template. IEEE Design Test Comput. **22**(2), 90–101 (2005)
207. Mei, B., Vernalde, S., Verkest, D., Man, H.D., Lauwerein, R.: DRESC: A Retargetable Compiler for Coarse-Grained Reconfigurable Architectures. In: Proc. of the IEEE Intl. Conf. Field-Programmable Technology (FPT'02), pp. 166–173. IEEE Computer Society Press (2002)
208. Mei, B., Vernalde, S., Verkest, D., Man, H.D., Lauwereins, R.: ADRES: An Architecture with Tightly Coupled VLIW Processor and Coarse-Grained Reconfigurable Matrix. In: Proc. of the 13th Intl. Conf. on Field Programmable Logic and Application (FPL'03), *Lecture Notes on Computer Science (LNCS)*, vol. 2778, pp. 61–70. Springer-Verlag (2003)
209. Mencer, O., Morf, M., Flynn, M.: PAM-Blox: High Performance FPGA Design for Adaptive Computing. In: Proc. of the 6th IEEE Symp. on FPGAs for Custom Computing Machines (FCCM'98), pp. 167–174. IEEE Computer Society, Washington, DC, USA (1998)
210. Micheli, G.D.: Synthesis and Optimization of Digital Circuits. McGraw-Hill Pub. (1994)
211. Micheli, G.D., Benini, L.: Networks on Chips. Elsevier Science & Technology (2006)
212. Micheli, G.D., Ernst, R., Wolf, W. (eds.): Readings in Hardware/Software Co-Design. Kluwer Academic Pub., Norwell, MA, USA (2002)
213. Micheli, G.D., Gupta, R.: Hardware/Software Co-Design. Proc. IEEE **85**(3), 349–365 (1997)
214. Mick, J., Brick, J.: Bit-Slice Microprocessor Design. McGraw-Hill, Inc., New York, NY, USA (1980)
215. Miller, R., Cocker, J.: Configurable Computers: A New Class of General Purpose Machines. In: Proc. of the Intl. Symp. on Theoretical Programming, *Lecture Notes on Computer Science (LNCS)*, vol. 5, pp. 285–298. Springer-Verlag (1972)
216. Mirsky, E., DeHon, A.: MATRIX: A Reconfigurable Computing Device with Reconfigurable Instruction Deployable Resources. In: Proc. of the 4th IEEE Symp. on FPGAs for Custom Computing Machines (FCCM'96), pp. 51–72. IEEE Computer Society Press, Los Alamitos, CA, USA (1996)
217. Mitrionics, Inc.: URL http://www.mitrionics.com
218. Miyamori, T., Olukotun, K.: A Quantitative Analysis of Reconfigurable Coprocessors for Multimedia Applications. In: Proc. of the 6th IEEE Symp. on FPGAs for Custom Computing Machines (FCCM'98), pp. 2–11. IEEE Computer Society Press, Los Alamitos, CA,USA (1998)
219. Mo, F., Tabbara, A., Brayton, R.: A Force-Directed Macro-Cell Placer. In: Proc. of the 2000 IEEE/ACM Intl. Conf. on Computer-Aided Design (ICCAD'00), pp. 177–181. IEEE Computer Society Press, Los Alamitos, CA, USA (2000)
220. Moll, L., Vuillemin, J., Boucard, P.: High-Energy Physics on DECPeRLe-1 Programmable Active Memory. In: Proc. of the 3rd ACM Intl. Symp. on Field-Programmable Gate Arrays (FPGA'95), pp. 47–52. ACM Press, New York, NY, USA (1995)
221. Moore, G.: Cramming More Components onto Integrated Circuits. Electronics **38**(8) (1965)
222. Muchnick, S.: Advanced Compiler Design and Implementation. Morgan Kaufmann Pub., Inc., San Francisco, CA, USA (1997)
223. Nallatech, Inc.: URL http://www.nallatech.com
224. Nayak, A., Haldar, M., Choudhary, A., Banerjee, P.: Parallelization of Matlab Applications for a Multi-FPGA System. In: Proc. of the 9th IEEE Symp. on Field-Programmable Custom Computing Machines (FCCM'01), pp. 1–9. IEEE Computer Society Press, Los Alamitos, CA, USA (2001)
225. Nayak, A., Haldar, M., Choudhary, A., Banerjee, P.: Precision and Error Analysis of Matlab Applications During Automated Hardware Synthesis for FPGAs. In: Proc. of the Conf. on Design, Automation and Test in Europe (DATE'01), pp. 722–728. IEEE Press, Piscataway, NJ, USA (2001)

226. Nisbet, S., Guccione, S.: The XC6200DS Development System. In: Proc. of the 7th Intl. Workshop on Field-Programmable Logic and Applications (FPL'97), London, UK, September 1–3, 1997, *Lecture Notes on Computer Science (LNCS)*, vol. 1304, pp. 61–68. Springer-Verlag, Heidelberg, Germany (1997)
227. Ogawa, O., Takagi, K., Itoh, Y., Kimura, S., Watanabe, K.: Hardware Synthesis from C Programs with Estimation of Bit Length of Variables. IEICE Trans. Fundam. Electron. Commun. Comput. Sci. **E82-A**(11), 2338–2346 (1999)
228. Ogras, U., Marculescu, R., Lee, H., Choudhary, P., Marculescu, D., Kaufman, M., Nelson, P.: Challenges and Promising Results in NoC Prototyping Using FPGAs. IEEE Micro **27**(5), 86–95 (2007)
229. Ong, S.W., Kerkiz, N., Srijanto, B., Tan, C., Langston, M., Newport, D., Bouldin, D.: Automatic Mapping of Multiple Applications to Multiple Adaptive Computing Systems. In: Proc. of the 9th IEEE Intl. Symp. on Field-Programmable Custom Computing Machines (FCCM'01), pp. 10–20. IEEE Computer Society Press, Los Alamitos, CA, USA (2001)
230. Ouaiss, I., Govindarajan, S., Srinivasan, V., Kaul, M., Vemuri, R.: An Integrated Partitioning and Synthesis System for Dynamically Reconfigurable Multi-FPGA Architectures. In: Proc. of the Reconfigurable Architectures Workshop (RAW'98), Springer, 1998, vol. 1388, Berlin/Heidelberg, pp. 31–36 (1998)
231. Ouaiss, I., Govindarajan, S., Srinivasan, V., Kaul, M., Vemuri, R.: A Unified Specification Model of Concurrency and Coordination for Synthesis from VHDL. In: Proc. of the Intl. Conf. on Information Systems Analysis and Synthesis (ISAS'98), Orlando, Florida, USA, pp. 771–778 (1998)
232. Ouaiss, I. Vemuri, R.: Efficient Resource Arbitration in Reconfigurable Computing Environments. In: Proc. of the Conf. on Design, Automation and Test in Europe (DATE'00), pp. 560–566. IEEE Press, Piscataway, NJ, USA (2000)
233. Ouaiss, I., Vemuri, R.: Hierarchical Memory Mapping During Synthesis in FPGA-Based Reconfigurable Computers. In: Proc. of the Conf. on Design, Automation and Test in Europe (DATE'01), pp. 650–657. IEEE Press, Piscataway, NJ, USA (2001)
234. PACT Technologies AG, Munich, Germany: XPP: The eXtreme Processor Platform. URL http://www.pactxpp.com
235. Page, I.: Constructing Hardware-Software Systems from a Single Description. J. VLSI Signal Processing **12**(1), 87–107 (1996)
236. Page, I., Luk, W.: Compiling Occam into Field-Programmable Gate Arrays. In: FPGAs, Oxford Workshop on Field Programmable Logic and Applications, pp. 271–283. Abingdon EE&CS Books, 15 Harcourt Way, Abingdon OX14 1NV, UK (1991)
237. Panainte, E., Bertels, K., Vassiliadis, S.: The MOLEN Compiler for Reconfigurable Processors. ACM Trans. Embedded Comput. Syst. (TECS) **6** (2007)
238. Pandey, A., Vemuri, R.: Combined Temporal Partitioning and Scheduling for Reconfigurable Architectures. In: Proc. SPIE Photonics East Conference, Reconfigurable Technology: FPGAs for Computing and Applications, pp. 93–103 (1999)
239. Parhi, K.: A Systematic Approach for Design of Digit-Serial Signal Processing Architectures. IEEE Trans. Circuits Syst. **38**(4), 358–375 (1991)
240. Park, H., Fan, K., Kudlur, M., Mahlke, S.: Modulo Graph Embedding: Mapping Applications onto Coarse-Grained Reconfigurable Architectures. In: Proc. of the 2006 Intl. Conf. on Compilers, Architecture, and Synthesis for Embedded Systems (CASES'06), pp. 136–146. ACM Press, New York, NY, USA (2006)
241. Park, J., Diniz, P.: Synthesis of Memory Access Controller for Streamed Data Applications for FPGA-based Computing Engines. In: Proc. of the 14th Intl. Symp. on Systems synthesis (ISSS'01), pp. 221–226. ACM Press, New York, NY, USA (2001)
242. Park, J., Diniz, P., Shayee, K.: Performance and Area Modeling of Complete FPGA Designs in the Presence of Loop Transformations. IEEE Trans. Comput. **53**(11), 1420–1435 (2004)
243. Pellerin, D., Thibault, S.: Practical FPGA Programming in C. Prentice-Hall, Inc. (2005)
244. Peterson, J., O'Connor, R., Athanas, P.: Scheduling and Partitioning ANSI-C Programs onto Multi-FPGA CCM Architectures. In: Proc. of the 4th IEEE Symp. on FPGA for Custom

Computing Machines (FCCM'96), pp. 178–179. IEEE Computer Society Press, Los Alamitos, CA, USA (1996)
245. Pinter, S., Pinter, R.: Program Optimization and Parallelization Using Idioms. In: Proc. of the 18th ACM Symp. on Principles of Programming Languages (POPL'91), pp. 79–92. ACM Press, New York, NY, USA (1991)
246. Pozzi, L., Atasu, K., Ienne, P.: Exact and Approximate Algorithms for the Extension of Embedded Processor Instruction Sets. IEEE Trans. Computer-Aided Design Integrated Circuits Syst. **25**(7), 1209–1229 (2006)
247. Praun, C., Ceze, L., Cascaval, C.: Implict Parallelism with Ordered Transaction. In: Proc. of the 2007 ACM Symp. on Principles and Practice of Parallel Programming (PPoPP'07). ACM Press, New York, NY, USA (2007)
248. Purna, K., Bhatia, D.: Temporal Partitioning and Scheduling Data Flow Graphs for Reconfigurable Computers. IEEE Trans. Comput. **48**(6), 579–591 (1999)
249. von Radetski, M.: Synthesis of Digital Circuits from Object-Oriented Specifications. Ph.D. thesis, Oldenburg University, Oldenburg, Germany (2000)
250. Raimbault, F., Lavenier, D., Rubini, S., Pottier, B.: Fine Grain Parallelism on a MIMD Machine Using FPGAs. In: IEEE Workshop on FPGAs for Custom Computing Machines, pp. 2–8. IEEE Computer Society Press, Los Alamitos, CA, USA (1993)
251. Rajan, J., Thomas, D.: Synthesis by Delayed Binding of Decisions. In: Proc. of the 22nd ACM/IEEE Design Automation Conference (DAC'85), pp. 367–373. ACM Press, New York, NY, USA (1985)
252. Ralev, K., Bauer, P.: Realization of Block Floating Point Digital Filters and Application to Block Implementations. IEEE Trans. Signal Processing **47**(4), 1076–1086 (1999)
253. Ramachandran, L., Narayan, S., Vahid, F., Gajski, D.: Synthesis of Functions and Procedures in Behavioral VHDL. In: Proc. of the 1993 European Design Automation Conference (EURO-DAC'93), pp. 560–565. IEEE Computer Society Press, Los Alamitos, CA, USA (1993)
254. Ramanujam, J., Sadayappan, P.: Compile-Time Techniques for Data Distribution in Distributed Memory Machines. IEEE Trans. Parallel Distrib. Syst. **2**(4), 472–482 (1991)
255. Rau, B.: Iterative Modulo Scheduling: An Algorithm for Software Pipelining Loops. In: Proc. of the 27th Intl. Symp. on Microarchitecture (MICRO), pp. 63–74. ACM Press, New York, NY, USA (1994)
256. Rau, B.R., Fisher, J.A.: Instruction-Level Parallel Processing: History, Overview, and Perspective. J. Supercomputing **7**(1–2), 9–50 (1993)
257. Razdan, R.: PRISC: Programmable Reduced Instruction Set Computers. Ph.D. thesis, Harvard University, Cambridge, MA, USA (1994)
258. Razdan, R., Smith, M.: A High-Performance Microarchitecture with Hardware-Programmable Functional Units. In: Proc. of the 27th IEEE/ACM Intl. Symp. on Microarchitecture (MICRO), pp. 172–180. ACM Press, New York, NY, USA (1994)
259. Reddi, S., Feustel, E.: A Restructurable Computer System. IEEE Trans. Comput. **27**(1), 1–20 (1978)
260. Rinker, R., Carter, M., Patel, A., Chawathe, M., Ross, C., Hammes, J., Najjar, W., Böhm, W.: An Automated Process for Compiling Dataflow Graphs into Hardware. IEEE Trans. Very Large Scale Integration (VLSI) Syst. **9**(1), 130–139 (2001)
261. Rivera, G., Tseng, C.W.: Data Transformations for Eliminating Conflict Misses. In: Proc. of the ACM Conf. on Programming Language Design and Implementation (PLDI'98), pp. 38–49. ACM Press, New York, NY, USA (1998)
262. Robinett, W., Snider, G., Kuekes, P., Williams, R.: Computing with a Trillion Crummy Components. Commun. of the ACM **50**(9), 35–39 (2007)
263. Rodrigues, R., Cardoso, J., Diniz, P.: A Data-Driven Approach for Pipelining Sequences of Data-Dependent Loops. In: Proc. of the 15th IEEE Symp. on FPGAs for Custom Computing Machines (FCCM'07), pp. 219–228. IEEE Computer Society Press, Los Alamitos, CA, USA (2007)

264. Rupp, C., Landguth, M., Garverick, T., Gomersall, E., Holt, H., Arnold, J., Gokhale, M.: The NAPA Adaptive Processing Architecture. In: Proc. of the 6th IEEE Symp. on FPGAs for Custom Computing Machines (FCCM'98), p. 28. IEEE Computer Society Press, Los Alamitos, CA, USA (1998)
265. Rusu, S., Sachdev, M., Svensson, C., Nauta, B.: Trends and Challenges in VLSI Technology Scaling Towards 100 nm. Tutorial, Proceedings of the ASPDAC 2002/VLSI Design 2002, Bangalore, India, Jan. 7–11, pp. 16–17 (2002)
266. Sait, S., Youssef, H.: VLSI Physical Design Automation. McGraw-Hill, Inc., New York, NY, USA (1994)
267. Salefski, B., Caglar, L.: Re-configurable Computing in Wireless. In: Proc. of the 38th ACM/IEEE Design Automation Conference (DAC'01), pp. 178–183. ACM Press, New York, NY, USA (2001)
268. Sanchis, L.A.: Multiple-Way Network Partitioning. IEEE Trans. Comput. **38**(1), 62–81 (1989)
269. Sankar, Y., Rose, J.: Trading Quality for Compile Time: Ultra-Fast Placement for FPGAs. In: Proc. of the 7th ACM Intl. Symp. on Field Programmable Gate Arrays (FPGA'99), pp. 157–166. ACM Press, New York, NY, USA (1999)
270. Sankaralingam, K., Nagarajan, R., McDonald, R., Desikan, R., Drolia, S., Govindan, M., Gratz, P., Gulati, D., Hanson, H., Kim, C., Liu, H., Ranganathan, N., Sethumadhavan, S., Sharif, S., Shivakumar, P., Keckler, S., Burger, D.: Distributed Microarchitectural Protocols in the TRIPS Prototype Processor. In: Proc. of the 39th IEEE/ACM Intl. Symp. on Microarchitecture (MICRO), pp. 480–491. IEEE Computer Society, Washington, DC, USA (2006)
271. dos Santos, L., Heijligers, M., van Eijk, C., van Eijndhoven, J., Jess, J.: A Code-Motion Pruning Technique for Global Scheduling. ACM Trans. Design Automation Electronic Syst. **5**(1), 1–38 (2000)
272. Schlansker, M., Rau, B.: EPIC: Explicitly Parallel Instruction Computing. Computer **33**(2), 37–45 (2000)
273. Schmit, H., Arnstein, L., Thomas, D., Lagnese, E.: Behavioral Synthesis for FPGA-based Computing. In: Proc. of the 2nd IEEE Workshop on FPGA for Custom Computing Machines (FCCM'94), pp. 125–132. IEEE Computer Society Press, Los Alamitos, CA, USA (1994)
274. Schmit, H., Levine, B., Ylvisaker, B.: Queue Machines: Hardware Compilation in Hardware. In: Proc. of the 10th IEEE Symp. on FPGA for Custom Computing Machines (FCCM'02), pp. 77–86. IEEE Computer Society Press (2002)
275. Schmit, H., Thomas, D.: Address Generation for Memories Containing Multiple Arrays. IEEE Trans. Computer-Aided Design Integrated Circuits Syst. **17**(5), 377–385 (1998)
276. Séméria, L., Sato, K., Micheli, G.D.: Synthesis of Hardware Models in C with Pointers and Complex Data Structures. IEEE Trans. Very Large Scale Integration (VLSI) Syst. **9**, 743–756 (2001)
277. Semiconductor Industry Association: International Technology Roadmap for Semiconductors (2001). URL http://public.itrsitrs.net/Files/2001ITRS/.net/Files/2001ITRS/ExecSumExecSum.pdf
278. Sharp, R. , Mycroft, A.: A Higher-Level Language for Hardware Synthesis. In: Proc. of the 11th IFIP WG 10.5 Advanced Research Working Conference on Correct Hardware Design and Verification Methods (CHARME'01), pp. 228–243. Springer-Verlag, London, UK (2001)
279. Shirazi, N., Walters, A., Athanas, P.: Quantitative Analysis of Floating Point Arithmetic on FPGA-based Custom Computing Machines. In: Proc. of the 3rd IEEE Workshop on FPGA's for Custom Computing Machines (FCCM'95), p. 155. IEEE Computer Society Press, Los Alamitos, CA, USA (1995)
280. Sikha, E., Simpson, R.: The PowerPC® Architecture: A Specification for a New Family of RISC Processors. Morgan Kaufmann Pub., Inc., San Francisco, CA, USA (1994)
281. Singh, H.: Reconfigurable Architectures for Multimedia and Data-Parallel Application Domains. Ph.D. thesis, University of California, Irvine, Irvine, Calif., USA (2000)

282. Singh, H., Lee, M., Lu, G., Kurdahi, F., Bagherzadeh, N., Filho, E.: MorphoSys: An Integrated Reconfigurable System for Data-Parallel and Computation-Intensive Applications. IEEE Trans. Comput. **49**(5), 465–481 (2000)
283. Smith, B.: A Pipelined, Shared Resource MIMD Computer. In: Proc. of the 1978 Intl. Conf. on Parallel Processing (ICPP'78), pp. 6–8. IEEE Computer Society Press, Los Alamitos, CA, USA (1978)
284. Smith, M.: Extending SUIF for Machine-dependent Optimizations. In: Proc. First SUIF Compiler Workshop, Stanford University, Stanford, CA, USA (1996)
285. Snider, G.: Performance-constrained Pipelining of Software Loops onto Reconfigurable Hardware. In: Proc. of the 10th ACM Intl. Symp. on Field-Programmable Gate Arrays (FPGA'02), pp. 177–186. ACM Press, New York, NY, USA (2002)
286. Snider, G., Williams, R.: Nano/CMOS Architectures Using a Field-Programmable Nanowire Interconnect. Nanotechnology **18**(3), 035204 (11pp) (2007)
287. Snider, G. Shackleford, B., Carter, R.: Attacking the Semantic Gap Between Application Programming Languages and Configurable Hardware. In: Proc. of the 9th ACM Intl. Symp. on Field-Programmable Gate Arrays (FPGA'01), pp. 115–124. ACM Press, New York, NY, USA (2001)
288. So, B., Diniz, P., Hall, M.: Using Estimates from Behavioral Synthesis Tools in Compiler-Directed Design Space Exploration. In: Proc. of the 40th ACM/IEEE Design Automation Conference (DAC'03). ACM Press, New York, N.Y, USA (2003)
289. So, B., Hall, M.: Increasing the Applicability of Scalar Replacement. In: Proc. of the Intl. Conf. on Compiler Construction, *Lecture Notes on Computer Science (LNCS)*, vol. 2985, pp. 185–201. Springer, Berlin/Heidelberg (2004)
290. So, B., Hall, M., Diniz, P.: A Compiler Approach to Fast Hardware Design Space Exploration in FPGA-based Systems. In: Proc. of the ACM Conf. on Programming Language Design and Implementation (PLDI'02), pp. 165–176. ACM Press, New York, NY, USA (2002)
291. So, B., Hall, M., Ziegler, H.: Custom Data Layout for Memory Parallelism. In: Proc. of the Intl. Symp. on Code Generation and Optimization (CGO'04), pp. 291–302. IEEE Computer Society Press, Los Alamitos, CA, USA (2004)
292. SRC Computers, Inc.: URL http://www.srccomp.com
293. Starbridge Systems, Inc.: URL http://www.starbridgesystems.com
294. Steele, R.: SRAM Based Cell for Programmable Logic Devices. US Patent 5,144,582 (1992)
295. Stefanovic, D., Matonosi, M.: On Availability of Bit-Narrow Operations in General-Purpose Applications. In: Proc. of the 10th Intl. Workshop on Field-Programmable Logic and Applications (FPL'00), *Lecture Notes on Computer Science (LNCS)*, vol. 1896, pp. 412–421. Springer-Verlag, London, UK (2000)
296. Stephenson, M., Babb, J., Amarasinghe, S.: Bidwidth Analysis with Application to Silicon Compilation. In: Proc. of the 2000 ACM Conf. on Programming Language Design and Implementation (PLDI'00), pp. 108–120. ACM Press, New York, NY, USA (2000)
297. Stretch, Inc.: URL http://www.stretchinc.com
298. Styles, H., Thomas, D., Luk, W.: Pipelining Designs with Loop-Carried Dependencies. In: Proc. of the 2004 IEEE Intl. Conf. on Field-Programmable Technology (FPT'04), pp. 255–262. IEEE Computer Society Press, Los Alamitos, CA, USA (2004)
299. Sutter, B., Mei, B., Bartic, A., Aa, T.V., Berekovic, M., Mignolet, J.Y., Croes, K., Coene, P., Cupac, M., Couvreur, A., Folens, A., Dupont, S., Thielen, B., Kanstein, A., Kim, H.S., Kim, S.: Hardware and a Tool Chain for ADRES. In: Proc. of the Intl. Workshop on Applied Reconfigurable Computing (ARC'06), *Lecture Notes on Computer Science (LNCS)*, vol. 3985, pp. 425–430. Springer, Berlin/Heidelberg (2006)
300. Synopsys, Inc.: CoCentric™ Fixed-Point Designer. URL http://www.synopsys.com/ %20products/cocentric_fixedpoint/ cocentric_fixedpoint_ds.html
301. Synplicity, Inc.: URL http://www.synplicity.com
302. Takayama, A., Shibata, Y., Iwai, K., Amano, H.: Dataflow Partitioning and Scheduling Algorithms for WASMII, a Virtual Hardware. In: Proc. of the 10th Intl. Conf. on Field Programmable Logic and Applications (FPL'01), *Lecture Notes on Computer Science (LNCS)*, vol. 2147, pp. 685–694. Springer, Heidelberg/New York (2000)

303. Taylor, M., Kim, J., Miller, J., Wentzlaff, D., Ghodrat, F., Greenwald, B., Hoffman, H., Johnson, P., Lee, J.W., Lee, W., Ma, A., Saraf, A., Seneski, M., Shnidman, N., Strumpen, V., Frank, M., Amarasinghe, S., Agarwal, A.: The RAW Microprocessor: A Computational Fabric for Software Circuits and General-Purpose Programs. IEEE Micro **22**(2), 25–35 (2002)
304. Teifel, J., Manohar, R.: Highly Pipelined Asynchronous FPGAs. In: Proc. of the 12th ACM Intl. Symp. on Field Programmable Gate Arrays (FPGA'04), pp. 133–142. ACM Press, New York, NY, USA (2004)
305. Tensilica, Inc.: URL http://www.tensilica.com
306. Tessier, R., Burleson, W.: Reconfigurable Computing and Digital Signal Processing: A Survey. J. VLSI Signal Processing pp. 7–27 (2001)
307. The MathWorks, Inc.: URL http://www.mathworks.com
308. Todman, T., Constantinides, G., Wilton, S., Mencer, O., Luk, W., Cheung, P.: Reconfigurable Computing: Architectures and Design Methods. IEE Proc. Comput. Digital Techniques **152**(2), 193–207 (2005)
309. Trimberger, S.: Scheduling Designs into a Time-Multiplexed FPGA. In: Proc. of the 6th ACM Intl. Symp. on Field Programmable Gate Arrays (FPGA'98), pp. 153–160. ACM Press, New York, NY, USA (1998)
310. Tripp, J., Jackson, P., Hutchings, B.: Sea Cucumber: A Synthesizing Compiler for FPGAs. In: Proc. of the Intl. Conf. on Field Programmable Logic (FPL'02), *Lecture Notes in Computer Science (LNCS)*, vol. 2438, pp. 51–72. Springer, Heidelberg/New York (2002)
311. Tripp, J., Peterson, K., Ahrens, C., Poznanovic, J., Gokhale, M.: Trident: An FPGA Compiler Framework for Floating-Point Algorithms. In: Proc. of the Intl. Conf. on Field Programmable Logic and Applications (FPL'05), vol. 3203, pp. 317–322. IEEE (2005)
312. Triscend, Corp.: Triscend A7 CSoC Family. URL http://www.triscend.com
313. Vahid, F.: Procedure Exlining: a Transformation for Improved System and Behavioral Synthesis. In: Proc. of the 8th Intl. Symp. on System Synthesis (ISSS'95), pp. 84–89. ACM Press, New York, NY, USA (1995)
314. Vahid, F.: Functional Partitioning Improvements over Structural Partitioning for Packaging Constraints and Synthesis: Tool Performance. ACM Trans. Design Automation Electronic Syst. **3**(3), 181–208 (1998)
315. Vasilko, M., Ait-Boudaoud, D.: Architectural synthesis techniques for dynamically reconfigurable logic, Proc. of the 6th Intl. Workshop on Field-Programmable Logic (FPL'96), *Lecture Notes in Computer Science (LNCS)*, vol. 1142, pp. 290–296, Springer-Verlag, London, UK (1996)
316. Vassiliadis, S., Wong, S., Cotofana, S.D.: The MOLEN $\rho\mu$ Processor. In: Proc. of the 11th International Conf. on Field-Programmable Logic and Applications (FPL'01), *Lecture Notes in Computer Science (LNCS)*, vol. 2147, pp. 275–285. Springer, Heidelberg/New York (2001)
317. Vassiliadis, S., Wong, S., Gaydadjiev, G., Bertels, K., Kuzmanov, G., Panainte, E.: The MOLEN Polymorphic Processor. IEEE Trans. Comput. **53**(11), 1363–1375 (2004)
318. Venkataramani, G., Najjar, W., Kurdahi, F., Bagherzadeh, N., Böhm, W., Hammes, J.: Automatic Compilation to a Coarse-Grained Reconfigurable System-On-Chip. Trans. Embedded Computing Syst. **2**(4), 560–589 (2003)
319. Waingold, E., Taylor, M., Srikrishna, D., Sarkar, V., Lee, W., Lee, V., Kim, J., Frank, M., Finch, P., Barua, R., Babb, J., Amarasinghe, S., Agarwal, A.: Baring It All to Software: RAW Machines. Computer **30**(9), 86–93 (1997)
320. Walker, R.A., Thomas, D.E.: A Model of Design Representation and Synthesis. In: Proc. of the 22nd ACM/IEEE Design Automation Conference (DAC'85), pp. 453–459. ACM Press, New York, NY, USA (1985)
321. Weinhardt, M.: Portable Pipeline Synthesis for FCCMs. In: Proc. of the 6th Intl. Workshop on Field-Programmable Logic, Smart Applications, New Paradigms and Compilers (FPL'96), vol. 1142, pp. 1–13. Springer-Verlag, London, UK (1996)
322. Weinhardt, M., Luk, W.: Memory Access Optimisation for Reconfigurable Systems. IEE Proc. Computers Digital Techniques **148**(3) (2001)
323. Weinhardt, M., Luk, W.: Pipeline Vectorization. IEEE Trans. Computer-Aided Design Integrated Circuits Syst. **20**(2), 234–233 (2001)

324. Willems, M., Bürsgens, V., Keding, H., Grötker, T., Meyr, H.: System Level Fixed-Point Design Based on an Interpolative Approach. In: Proc. of the 34th ACM/IEEE Design Automation Conference (DAC'97), pp. 293–298. ACM Press, New York, NY, USA (1997)
325. Wilson, R., French, R., Wilson, C., Amarasinghe, S., Anderson, J., Tjiang, S., Liao, S.W., Tseng, C.W., Hall, M., Lam, M., Hennessy, J.: SUIF: an Infrastructure for Research on Parallelizing and Optimizing Compilers. SIGPLAN Not. **29**(12), 31–37 (1994). URL http://suif.stanford.edu
326. Wirth, N.: Hardware Compilation: Translating Programs into Circuits. IEEE Computer **31**(6), 25–31 (1998)
327. Wirthlin, M., Hutchings, B.: A Dynamic Instruction Set Computer. In: Proc. of the 3rd IEEE Workshop on FPGAs for Custom Computing Machines (FCCM'95), pp. 99–107. IEEE Computer Society Press, Los Alamitos, CA, USA (1995)
328. Wirthlin, M.J., Hutchings, B., Worth, C.: Synthesizing RTL Hardware from Java Byte Codes. In: Proc. of the 11th Intl. Conf. on Field-Programmable Logic and Applications (FPL'01), pp. 123–132. Springer-Verlag, London, UK (2001)
329. Wittig, R., Chow, P.: OneChip: An FPGA Processor with Reconfigurable Logic. In: Proc. of the 4th IEEE Symp. on FPGAs for Custom Computing Machines, pp. 126–135. IEEE Computer Society Press, Los Alamitos, CA, USA (1996)
330. Wo, D., Forward, K.: Compiling to the Gate Level for a Reconfigurable Coprocessor. In: Proc. of the 2nd IEEE Workshop on FPGA for Custom Computing Machines (FCCM'94), pp. 147–154. IEEE Computer Society Press, Los Alamitos, CA, USA (1994)
331. Wolfe, A., Shen, P.: Flexible Processors: A Promising Application-Specific Processor Design Approach. In: Proc. of the 21st Workshop on Microprogramming and Microarchitecture (MICRO), pp. 30–39. IEEE Computer Society Press, Los Alamitos, CA, USA (1988)
332. Wolfe, M.: High Performance Compilers for Parallel Computing. Addison-Wesley Longman Publishing Co., Inc., Boston, MA, USA (1996)
333. Wolinski, C., Gokhale, M., McCabe, K.: A Polymorphous Computing Fabric. IEEE Micro **22**(5), 56–68 (2002)
334. Wong, D., Leong, H., Liu, C.: Simulated Annealing for VLSI Design. Kluwer Academic Pub., Norwell, MA, USA (1988)
335. Wrighton, M., DeHon, A.: Hardware-assisted Simulated Annealing with Application for Fast FPGA Placement. In: Proc. of the 11th ACM Intl. Symp. on Field Programmable Gate Arrays (FPGA'03), pp. 33–42. ACM Press, New York, NY, USA (2003)
336. Wu, P., Michael, M., Praun, C., Nakaike, T., Bordawekar, R., Cain, H., Cascaval, C., Chatterjee, S., Chiras, S., Hou, R., Mergen, M., Shen, X., Spear, M., Wang, H., Wang, K.: Compiler and Runtime Techniques for Software Transactional Memory Optimization. Concurrency and Computation: Practice and Experience (Special Issue devoted to the 13th Intl. Workshop on Compilers for Parallel Computing (CPC'07)) **20**(1) (2008)
337. Wuytack, S., Catthoor, F., de Jong, G., Man, H.D.: Minimizing the Required Memory Bandwidth in VLSI System Realizations. IEEE Trans. VLSI Syst. **7**(4), 433–441 (1999)
338. Xilinx, Corp.: URL http://www.xilinx.com
339. Xilinx, Corp.: Forge compiler. URL http://www.lavalogic.com
340. Xilinx Corp.: Virtex-II Pro™ and Virtex-II Pro X™ Platform FPGAs: Complete Data Sheet (2007). URL http://www.xilinx.com
341. Xilinx, Inc.: XC6200 Field Programmable Gate Arrays (1997)
342. Xilinx, Inc.: Virtex-5™ 1.5V, Field-Programmable Gate Arrays (v1.7) – Advance Product Specification (2001). URL http://www.xilinx.com
343. Xilinx, Inc.: Virtex-II™ 1.5v, Field-Programmable Gate Arrays (v1.7) – Advance Product Specification (2001). URL http://www.xilinx.com
344. Xilinx, Inc.: PowerPC® 405 Processor Block Reference Guide (2005). URL http://www.xilinx.com
345. Xilinx, Inc.: MicroBlaze® Processor Reference Guide (2007). URL http://www.xilinx.com

346. Yankova, Y., Kuzmanov, G., Bertels, K., Gaydadjiev, G., Lu, Y., Vassiliadis, S.: DWARV: Delft Workbench Automated Reconfigurable VHDL Generator. In: Proc. of the 17th Intl. Conf. on Field Programmable Logic and Applications (FPL'07), pp. 697–701. Amsterdam, The Netherlands, August 27–29 (2007)
347. Ye, Z., Shenoy, N., Baneijee, P.: A C Compiler for a Processor with a Reconfigurable Functional Unit. In: Proc. of the 8th Intl. Symp. on Field Programmable Gate Arrays (FPGA'00), pp. 95–100. ACM Press, New York, NY, USA (2000)
348. Ye, Z.A., Moshovos, A., Hauck, S., Banerjee, P.: Chimaera: A High-Performance Architecture with a Tightly-Coupled Reconfigurable Functional Unit. In: Proc. of the 27th Annual Intl. Symp. on Computer Architecture (ISCA'00), pp. 225–235. ACM Press, New York, NY, USA (2000)
349. Young, M., Argiro, D., Kubica, S.: Cantata®: Visual Programming Environment for the Khoros System. Comput. Graphics **29**(2), 22–26 (1995)
350. Zhang, X., Ng, K.: A Review of High-Level Synthesis for Dynamically Reconfigurable FPGAs. Microprocessors Microsystems **24**(1), 199–211 (2000)
351. Ziegler, H., Hall, M., Diniz, P.: Compiler-Generated Communication for Pipelined FPGA Applications. In: Proc. of the 40th ACM/IEEE Design Automation Conference (DAC'03), pp. 610–615. ACM Press, New York, NY, USA (2003)
352. Ziegler, H., Malusare, P., Diniz, P.: Array Replication to Increase Parallelism in Applications Mapped to Configurable Architectures. In: Proc. of the 18th Intl. Workshop on Languages and Compilers for Parallel Computing (LCPC'05), *Lecture Notes on Computer Science (LNCS)*, vol. 4339, pp. 63–72. Springer, Heidelberg/New York (2005)
353. Ziegler, H., So, B., Hall, M., Diniz, P.: Coarse-Grain Pipelining on Multiple FPGA Architectures. In: Proc. of the 10th IEEE Symp. on FPGA for Custom Computing Machines (FCCM'02), pp. 77–86. IEEE Computer Society Press, Los Alamitos, CA, USA (2002)

List of Acronyms

ADRES	Architecture for dynamically reconfigurable embedded systems
ALAP	As late as possible
ALU	Arithmetic-logic unit
AOP	Aspect oriented programming
API	Application programming interface
ASAP	As soon as possible
ASIC	Application-specific integrated circuit
ASIP	Application-specific instruction processor
AST	Abstract syntax tree
CCM	Custom computing machine
CDFG	Control/data flow graph
CDG	Control dependence graph
CFG	Control-flow graph
CISC	Complex instruction-set computer
CLB	Configurable logic block
CPLD	Complex programmable logic Devices
CPU	Central processing unit
CSD	Common signed digit
CSP	Communicating sequential processes
DAG	Directed acyclic graph
DDG	Data dependence graph
DFG	Data flow graph
DIL	Dataflow intermediate language
DISC	Dynamic instruction set computer
DRESC	Dynamically reconfigurable embedded system compiler
DRLE	Dynamically reconfigurable logic engine
DSE	Design space exploration
DSL	Domain specific language
DSP	Digital signal processor
EDIF	Electronic design interchange format
EPIC	Explicitly parallel instruction computing

FCCM	Field-custom computing machine
FDCT	Fast discrete cosine transform
FFT	Fast Fourier transform
FIFO	First in first out
FPAA	Field-programmable ALU arrays
FPGA	Field-programmable gate arrays
FSM	Finite-state machine
FSMD	Finite-state machine with data-path
FU	Functional unit
GPP	General purpose processor
HDL	Hardware description language
HLS	High-level synthesis
HPDG	Hierarchical program dependence graph
HTG	Hierarchical task graphs
IEEE	Institute of electrical and electronic engineers
ILP	Instruction level parallelism
IP	Intellectual property
IR	Intermediate representation
ISA	Instruction set architecture
I/O	Input/output
JIT	Just in time
JVM	Java virtual machine
LSB	Least significant bit/byte
LARA	LAnguage for Reconfigurable Architectures
LUT	Look-up table
MARGE	Malleable architecture generator
MSB	Most significant bit/byte
P&R	Placement and routing
PE	Processing element
PLD	Programmable logic device
PRISC	Programmable reduced instruction set computers
RAM	Random-access memory
ROM	Read-only memory
rDPA	re-configurable data-path architecture
REMARC	Reconfigurable multimedia array coprocessor
RFU	Reconfigurable functional unit
RISC	Reduced instruction-set computer
RPU	Reconfigurable processing unit
RTL	Register transfer level
SIMD	Single instruction multiple data
SRAM	Static random-access memory
SSA	Static single assignment
STG	State transition graph

TDF	Task description format
VHDL	VHSIC (very high speed integrated circuit) hardware description language
VLIW	Very-long instruction width
VLSI	Very large scale integration

Index

A

Abstract-machines compiler, 161–162
Abstract-Syntax-Tree, 52
ADRES. *See* Architecture for Dynamically Reconfigurable Embedded Systems
ALU. *See* Arithmetic Logic Unit
Application Programming Interfaces (APIs), 38, 61
Application-specific instruction-set processors, 182
Application-Specific Integrated Circuit, 2
Architecture for Dynamically Reconfigurable Embedded Systems, 16, 17
Arithmetic Logic Unit, 8
Array mapping approaches, 148
ASIC. *See* Application-Specific Integrated Circuit
ASIPs. *See* Application-specific instruction-set processors
Aspect-Oriented programming technique, 187, 188
AST. *See* Abstract-Syntax-Tree
Augmenting imperative languages, 178

B

Backward propagation, 70
Bit reversing, 74–75
Bit-level operation specialization, 78–79
Bit-level transformations
  bit-level optimizations
    bit-value results, 74
    definition, 72
    of compiler, 73
  bit-width narrowing
    bit-width propagation, 70–71
    in loop control variables, 68
    static, 71–72
  by nonstandard floating-point formats, 77
  floating-point to fixed-point conversion, 76–77
Bit-width analysis
  based on
    dynamic run-time techniques, 70
    run-time profiling, 69
  by DeepC silicon compiler, 158
  of variables, 68–69
  static, 70
BitValue analysis, 70
Block floating-point formats. *See* Nonstandard floating-point formats

C

C programming language
  COBRA-ABS tool, 158
  SPC compiler for, 157
Cameron compiler, 160
Canonical Signed Digit representation, 79–80
CCA. *See* Configurable Compute Accelerator
CDG. *See* Control-dependence graph
CLBs. *See* Configurable-Logic-Blocks
Coarse-grained pipelining
  concurrency, 144
  fine-grained synchronization scheme, 144–145
Coarse-grained reconfigurable architectures, 14–16
  applicability of compilation techniques to, 106

Coarse-grained reconfigurable architectures (*Continued*)
bit reversal, 74–75
compiler
CoDe-X compiler, 165–166
data-flow intermediate language (DIL) compiler, 164
DRESC compiler (*see* Dynamically reconfigurable embedded system compiler)
RaPiD-C compiler (*see* RaPiD-C compiler)
XPP-VC compiler (*see* XPP-VC compiler)
FU sharing, 131
loop tiling, 91, 92
module generation techniques, 152
scaling operations, 77
Code motion
code hoisting and sinking, 84–85
in context of loops, 85–86
loop invariant, 86
Code transformations. *See* Bit-level transformations; Data-oriented transformations; Function-oriented transformations; Instruction-level transformations; Loop-level transformations
Communicating sequential processes, 61, 159, 161
Compiler. *See also* FPGA-based systems
bit-level optimizations, 73–74
for reconfigurable architectures
coarse-grained pipelining of, 144
function inlining and outlining
concurrency and resource sharing, balance between, 103–104
inner loop pipelining, 142
multiple data-path elements, 156, 165
scheduling algorithms, 151
software pipelining implementation, 143
temporal partitioning using loop distribution, 122–123
Compiler intermediate representation for reconfigurable computing (CIRRF), 163
Compiler techniques
for bit-width and type inference analyses, 69
for mapping of array data to memories
array mapping approaches, 148
memory bank disambiguation, 146–147
Configurable Compute Accelerator, 133, 134
Configurable-Logic-Blocks, 12, 65
Control Units, 9
Control-dependence graph, 63
CSD representation. *See* Canonical Signed Digit representation
CSP. *See* Communicating sequential processes
CUs. *See* Control Units
Custom computing machines, 2

D

Data strip-mining, 101
Data-dependence graph, 63
Data-Flow Graphs, 52
and DFG Builder, 164
and DIL compiler, 164–165
and SSA representation, 129
bit-width propagation, 71
for partitioning, 118
for THR, 83
hardware implementation for pipelined execution, 140–141
ILP, 110
without code hoisting, 85
Data-layout transformation, 100–101
Data-oriented transformations
and mapping, 55–58
data distribution, 95
data replication, 96
data reuse, 96–97
data-layout, reorganization of, 100–101
data-permutation, 101
scalar expansion, 99–100
scalar replacement
in RAM, 99
in registers, 97–99
Data-path synthesis tool, 166
DDG. *See* Data-dependence graph
Delft Workbench Automated Reconfigurable VHDL (DWARV) compiler, 163–164
Design Environment for Adaptive Computing Technology compiler, 159
Design-space exploration, 65
techniques for solving, 122, 183–184
DFGs. *See* Data-Flow Graphs
Digital signal processing, 12
DISC. *See* Dynamic Instruction Set Computer
Distributive transformation, 80–81
Domain-specific languages, 178–179, 181
DPSS. *See* Data-path synthesis tool
DSE. *See* Design-space exploration
DSP. *See* Digital signal processing
Dynamic Instruction Set Computer, 11
Dynamic run-time approach, 70
Dynamically reconfigurable embedded system compiler (DRESC), 166–167

E

Electronic design interchange format (EDIF), 161

F

Fast Fourier transform, 2
Fast prototyping and emulation systems, 2
FCCM. *See* Field-Programmable Custom Computing Machines
FFT. *See* Fast Fourier transform
Field-Programmable ALU Arrays, 11
Field-Programmable Custom Computing Machines, 8
Field-Programmable Logic and Applications, 8
Field-programmable-gate-arrays, 1, 8, 155. *See also* FPGA-based systems
Fine-grained reconfigurable architectures, 12–13
 applicability of compilation techniques to, 106
 FU sharing, 131
 loop tiling for, 91, 92
 module generation techniques, 151–152
 shift operation, 77
Fine-grained synchronization scheme, 144–145
Finite-state machine, 9, 156
 for control unit, 43–44
Fixed-point and floating-point data representation, 75
Floating-point to fixed-point conversion, 76
Fortran language, DEFACTO compiler for, 159
FPAAs. *See* Field-Programmable ALU Arrays
FPGA-based systems
 compilers for (*see also* MATCH Compiler)
  A C to fine-grained pipelining compiler, 158
  abstract-machines compiler (*see* Abstract-machines compiler)
  Cameron compiler (*see* Cameron compiler)
  CHAMPION software design environment, 162
  COBRA-ABS tool, 158–159
  DeepC silicon compiler, 158
  DEFACTO compiler (*see* Design Environment for Adaptive Computing Technology compiler)
  DWARV compiler (*see* Delft Workbench Automated Reconfigurable VHDL)
  Galadriel compiler, 161
  MATCH compiler (*see* MATCH Compiler)
  Nenya compiler, 161
  ROCCC compiler (*see* Riverside optimizing compiler for configurable computing compiler)
  Sea cucumber (SC) compiler (*see* Sea Cucumber (SC) compiler)
  SPARCS tool (*see* Synthesis and partitioning for adaptive reconfigurable computing systems tool)
  SPC compiler (*see* SUIF Pipeline Compiler (SPC))
  Streams-C compiler (*see* Streams-C compiler)
FPGAs. *See* Field-programmable-gate-arrays
FPL. *See* Field-Programmable Logic and Applications
FSM. *See* Finite-state machine
FU merging technique. *See* RaPiD-C compiler
Function-oriented transformations
 function inlining, 101
  and noninlined hardware implementation, 102–103
 function outlining, 101
  applications of, 103
 recursive functions, 105
Functional unit (FU), 1, 8
 ALU operation of, 24
 data-path, 1
 mapping of operations to, 129–130
 merging of, 165
 sharing, 131–133
 with 2-input LUT, 12

G

Galadriel compiler, for Java bytecodes translation, 161
Garp architecture, 18
General purpose processor (GPP), 1, 21, 33, 156, 182
 CoDe-X compiler, 165

H

Handel-C compiler, 156
Hardware compilation
 and high-level synthesis, 39–40

Hardware compilation (*Continued*)
customized, 41–45
for coarse-grained reconfigurable architectures, 48–49
generic, 40–41
placement and routing, 49–50
Register-Transfer-Level/logic synthesis, 45–47
coarse-grained reconfigurable architecture, 156–157
Hardware execution techniques, 110
instruction-level parallelism
loop unrolling and, 111–112
nonhomogeneous execution units, 110–111
multitasking, 116
and access to shared resources, 117–118
coarse-grained, 117
partitioning, 118
predication and if-conversion, 114–116
hardware implementations for, 117
speculative execution
concurrent evaluation, 112–113
memory access, 113
Hardware retiming, 137
Height reduction, 80. *See also* Tree-height reduction
Hierarchical Task Graph, 63
High-level programming constructs, mapping of
data selection constructs, 130–131
FU resource sharing, 131–132
operations to FUs, 129–130
reconfigurable function units, 132–134
scalar variables to registers, 127
SSA representation approach, 129
syntax-oriented hardware compilation, 128
High-level synthesis, 4, 39–40
customized, 41–45
for coarse-grained reconfigurable architectures, 48–49
generic, 40–41
placement and routing, 49–50
register-transfer-level/logic synthesis, 45–47
scheduling and temporal partitioning, 121
tools, 156
High-performance computing, 2
History-based and Learning based techniques, 187
HLS. *See* High-level synthesis
HTG. *See* Hierarchical Task Graph
Hybrid reconfigurable architectures, 16–18
compilers for
Chimaera-C compiler, 167
Garp and Nimble C compiler, 168
NAPA-C compiler (*see* NAPA-C compiler)

I

Impulse-C, for targeting FPGA, 156
Input/Output Buffers, 9
Instruction-level parallelism (ILP)
abstract-machines compiler, 161
loop unrolling and, 111–112
nonhomogeneous execution units, 110–111
Instruction-level transformations
algebraic transformations, 77–78
code motion (*see* Code motion)
height reduction (*see* Height reduction)
operator strength reduction (*see* Operator strength reduction)
Instruction-set architectures, 33, 179
Integer linear programming approach
inference of on-chip memories, for, 148
temporal partitioning, for, 121
Interconnection resources, 9, 30
Intermediate representation, 58, 181–182
IOBs. *See* Input/Output Buffers
IR. *See* Intermediate representation
IRs. *See* Interconnection resources
ISA. *See* Instruction-set architectures

J

Java thread model, 161
Just-In-Time (JIT), 186

L

Language for Reconfigurable Architectures (LARA), 187–188
Latency-hiding techniques, 145–146
Look-up table, 12
Loop dissevering, 122–123
Loop invariant code motion, 85–86
Loop pipelining
for hardware, 139
in reconfigurable architectures, 184–185
innermost loops
nonpipelined hardware implementation for, 142–143
pipeline vectorization, based on, 140
software pipelining, based on, 141–142
schemes, comparison of, 143

Loop strip-mining, 94
definition of, 90
hardware implementation, 92–93
source code, to, 91–92
Loop-level transformations
loop merging and loop distribution, 94
scalar expansion and, 99–100
loop tiling, 94
loop strip-mining (*see* Loop strip-mining)
matrix multiplication, 90, 92
nested loops, 90
loop unrolling
data availability requirements, 88
hardware implementations, 91
instruction-level parallelism, 87, 89–90, 111–112
LUT. *See* Look-up table

M

Malleable architecture generator (MARGE) tool, 159–160. *See also* Streams-C compiler
Mapped occam program, 156
Mask operation, 70
MATCH compiler, 160
MATLAB, in reconfigurable computing, 3, 62
Memory accesses
array mapping approaches for, 148
memory bank disambiguation, 146–147
techniques improving, 148
data packing/unpacking, 149–150
pipelining, 148
Memory Elements, 9
Memory mapping optimizations, 185
MEMs. *See* Memory Elements
MIMO (Multiple-Input, Multiple-Output) region, 134
MISO (Multiple-Input, Single-Output) region, 134
Module generation techniques, 151–152
Modulo graph embedding and modulo scheduling technique, 50
Molen polymorphic processor system, 23–24
MorphoSys architecture, 18
Multiple computing engines, mapping of, 182
Multiplexer merging technique. *See* RaPiD-C compiler
Multitasking, 116
and access to shared resources, 117–118
coarse-grained, 117

N

NAPA-C compiler
C program mapping, 168
malleable architecture generator (MARGE) use by, 169
stream-C language, 168
Nenya compiler, 161
Network-on-a-Chip (NoC), 10
Nonstandard floating-point formats, 77

O

Operator strength reduction (OSR)
bit manipulation operations, 78
on integer multiplications by constants, 79–80

P

P&R. *See* Place and routing
Packing and unpacking of data items
5-bit array elements, 149–150
and memory access, 149
Partitioning, 118
spatial (*see* Spatial partitioning)
temporal (*see* Temporal partitioning)
Peripheral Controller Interface (PCI), 22
PEs. *See* Processing elements
Pipeline vectorization, 140, 157
Pipelined execution. *See* Pipelining
Pipelining, 134
coarse-grained (*see* Coarse-grained pipelining)
configuration, 145–146
data-path, 136–137
hardware retiming, 137
latency models for multiplier, 135–136
of memory accesses, 138–139, 149
PipeRench reconfigurable architecture, 15, 16
Place and routing, 9, 19, 49–50
PLDs, 155
Prefetching techniques, 145
Processing elements, 33

R

Range propagation analysis, 71
Rapid prototyping, 156
RaPiD reconfigurable architecture, 15

RaPiD-C compiler
during compilation, 165
space-loop notion, 165
RAW Machine architecture, 18
rDPA. *See* Reconfigurable Data-Path Array architecture
Reconfigurable architectures, 1, 4–5
and nanotechnology, 189
back-end support
allocation, scheduling, and binding, 150–151
mapping, placement, and routing, 153
module generation, 151–152
challenges of, 191–192
characteristics features of, 8–10
coarse-grained (*see* Coarse-grained reconfigurable architectures)
compilation process
research for, 181–187
solving challenges of, 187–188
computational and execution models, 29–31
computing domains of, 2–3
development of
high-level programming tool, 178–179
performance portability, approaches for solving, 180
program portability and legacy code migration, 179–180
dynamic reconfiguration of, 24–28
fine-grained (*see* Fine-grained reconfigurable architectures)
granularity, 10–11
and mapping, 19–20
coarse-grained reconfigurable architectures, 14–16
fined-grained reconfigurable architectures, 12–13
hybrid reconfigurable architectures, 16–18
hardware compilation and high-level synthesis, 39–40
customized high-level synthesis, 41–45
generic high-level synthesis, 40–41
high-level compilation for coarse-grained reconfigurable architectures, 48–49
placement and routing, 49–50
Register-Transfer-Level/logic synthesis, 45–47
hardware execution techniques (*see* Hardware execution techniques)
input and output data bandwidth, 31
interconnection topologies, 20–21
limitations of, 3–4
origin of, 7–8
pipelined execution enabled by (*see* Pipelining)
system-level integration, 21–24
Reconfigurable Data-Path Array architecture, 14
Reconfigurable functional units, 22, 132
mapping computation to, 133–134
Reconfigurable processing unit, 4, 8, 33
computation operations, 153
focus on low-level optimization, 156
Reconfigurable processor, 23
Reconfigurable systems
generic compilation and synthesis flow of
back end phase, 37–38
computation translation to hardware, 58–59
computation-oriented mapping and scheduling, 53–55
data-flow representation, 52–53
data-oriented mapping and transformations, 55–58
front end phase, 34–35
high-level source code, 51–52
middle end phase, 35–37
reconfigurable computing issues and, 59–65
Recursive functions, 105
Register-Transfer-Level, 45
Relatively Placed Macros, 19
Remote-procedure-call, 23
Resource Virtualization techniques, 187
Resource virtualization, in reconfigurable architectures, 186
RFU. *See* Reconfigurable functional unit
Riverside optimizing compiler for configurable computing compiler, 163
RP. *See* Reconfigurable processor
RPC. *See* Remote-procedure-call
RPMs. *See* Relatively Placed Macros
RPU. *See* Reconfigurable processing unit
RTL. *See* Register-Transfer-Level
RTL/logic synthesis, 45–47
Run-time profiling, 69

S

SA-C language, 62, 160
Scalar expansion, 99–100
SCORE. *See* Stream Computations Organized for Reconfigurable Execution
Sea cucumber (SC) compiler, 161
Single-instruction-multiple-data (SIMD), 64
Single-Program-Multiple-Data, 64

SoC. *See* System-on-a-Chip
Software pipelining
compiler implementations of, 143
inner loop pipelining based on, 140–141
Spatial partitioning
applications of, 124–127
minimization of communication between partitions, 124
Spatial partitioning, for compilation, 156
Speculative execution
concurrent evaluation, 112–113
memory access, 113
SPMD. *See* Single-Program-Multiple-Data
SSA intermediate representation
for constructs mapping, 129
Stream Computations Organized for Reconfigurable Execution, 18
Streams-C compiler, 159–160
Submicron and nanoscale computing systems, 2–3
SUIF pipeline compiler (SPC), 157
use by DEFACTO, 159
Synthesis and partitioning for adaptive reconfigurable computing systems tool, 163
System-on-a-Chip, 22
Systolic array, 157

T

Task Description Format, 18
Task-and loop-level scheduling schemes, 53–54
TDF. *See* Task Description Format
Temporal partitioning
advantages of, 119
algorithmic approach, 121–122
applications of, 120, 125–127
in high-level compilation, 121
design-space exploration techniques, 122
spatial and, 118–119
using loop distribution, 122–123
with different communications costs, 119–120
Temporal partitions
loop splitting across, 123
minimizing number of, 122
THR. *See* Tree-height reduction
Transactional-based languages, 178
Tree-height minimization. *See* Tree-height reduction
Tree-height reduction
distributive property, 80–81
reduction in execution latency, 82
schedule length, 83
selection points in control-flow intensive constructs, 83–84

U

Unified Specification Model (USM), 63

V

Value range analysis. *See* Range propagation analysis
Very Long Instruction Word (VLIW), 9

X

XPP-VC compiler, 166
Xputer architecture, 14

Printed in the United States of America